Life-Threatening Disorders

Life-Threatening Disorders

Springhouse Corporation
Springhouse, Pennsylvania

Staff

Executive Director, Editorial
Stanley Loeb

Senior Publisher
Matthew Cahill

Clinical Manager
Cindy Tryniszewski, RN, MSN

Art Director
John Hubbard

Senior Editor
June Norris

Clinical Project Editor
Marlene Ciranowicz, RN, MSN

Drug Information Editor
George J. Blake, RPh, MS

Editors
Jane V. Cray, Edith McMahon, Marylou Ambrose, Gale
Sloan, Jean Wallace

Copy Editors
Cynthia C. Breuninger (supervisor), Priscilla DeWitt, Jennifer
George Mintzer, Nancy Papsin, Doris Weinstock

Designers
Stephanie Peters (associate art director), Matie Patterson
(senior designer)

Illustrators
Jackie Facciolo, Rhonda Forbes, Jean Gardner, Tom
Herbert, Robert Jackson, Robert Neumann, Judy Newhouse,
Mary Stangl, Larry Ward

Typography
Diane Paluba (manager), Elizabeth Bergman, Joyce Rossi
Biletz, Phyllis Marron, Robin Mayer, Valerie Rosenberger

Manufacturing
Deborah Meiris (director), Anna Brindisi, Kate Davis,
T. A. Landis

Production Coordinator
Patricia W. McCloskey

Editorial Assistants
Maree DeRosa, Beverly Lane, Mary Madden

Indexer
Robin Hipple

R A member of the Reed Elsevier plc group

Library of Congress Cataloging-in-Publication Data

Life-threatening disorders.
   p. cm.
   Includes bibliographical references and index.
   1. Intensive care nursing. I. Springhouse Corporation.
   [DNLM: 1. Critical Care—handbooks. 2. Catastrophic
   Illness—nursing—handbooks. QS 504 K913e 1994]
RT120.I5L54 1994
610.73'61—dc20
DNLM/DLC   93-44371
ISBN 0-87434-542-1   CIP

Contents

Consultants

Sandra J. Bixler, RN, MSN, CCRN
Clinical Nurse Specialist
Berks Cardiologists, Ltd.
Reading, Pa.

Kathleen M. Donahue, RN,C, MSN
Maternal/Child Health Staff Development Educator
North Penn Hospital, Lansdale, Pa.

Paulette Dorney, RN, MSN, CCRN
Critical Care Staff Development Instructor
North Penn Hospital, Lansdale, Pa.

Michelle C. Quigel, RN, BSN, CETN
Enterostomal Therapy Nurse
Holy Redeemer Hospital and Medical Center
Meadowbrook, Pa.

Gerarda Savinski-Bozinko, RN, BSN, CCRN
Clinical Educator
Crozer-Chester Medical Center, Upland, Pa.

Gwendolyn A. Smith, RN, MBA, MSN, CCRN
Clinical Coordinator, Burn Treatment Center
Crozer-Chester Medical Center, Upland, Pa.

Jo Ann Zack, RN, MSN, CDE
Diabetes Clinical Nurse Specialist
Albert Einstein Medical Center, Philadelphia

Foreword

Your ability to act quickly could mean the difference between life and death for a patient in crisis. No matter what your work setting, life-threatening disorders—such as anaphylaxis, septic shock, acute respiratory failure, myocardial infarction, and diabetic ketoacidosis—can occur suddenly. And your patient's condition can deteriorate rapidly. However, your astute assessment skills and timely interventions can help slow the disorder's progression or reduce its severity.

To be fully effective, you must be able to detect both subtle and gross changes in your patient's condition, provide emotional support, interpret the results of diagnostic testing, give emergency drugs, and perform other rapid interventions. After the crisis is over, your supportive nursing care— such as early recognition and treatment of complications—is crucial to ensuring your patient's optimal recovery. To help you provide the most efficient and effective nursing care in these life-threatening situations you need an up-to-date, comprehensive reference.

Life-Threatening Disorders meets these requirements. It provides all the information you'll need to care for any patient with an acute and possibly fatal disorder. Organized by body system, with additional chapters on trauma and infection, this book covers nearly 90 life-threatening disorders.

Each entry begins with an introduction, a discussion of causes (which may include risk factors and pathophysiology), and a list of potential complications. Assessment information from the patient history and physical examination and a list of typically ordered diagnostic tests follow. The treatment section summarizes medical and surgical interventions. Next, the section on key nursing diagnoses and patient outcomes helps you focus your assessment and plan interventions. Finally, nursing interventions (including monitoring and patient teaching) conclude the entry.

Noteworthy features are highlighted by a special graphic symbol. The first example, a *Priority Checklist* of assessment steps and nursing actions, introduces each chapter. The checklist that precedes the cardiovascular chapter advises you to check the patient's history for signs and symptoms—such as chest pain, palpitations, shortness of breath, edema, or fatigue—then lists interventions, such as inserting an I.V. line, obtaining a 12-lead electrocardiogram, and preparing the patient for hemodynamic monitoring. This at-a-glance format is invaluable, especially when quick action is required.

Another feature, *Dosage Finder,* briefly lists indications and dosage recommendations for crisis drugs; *Nursing Alert* highlights important cautions, warnings, or advice. In selected disorders, a *Priority Flowchart* quickly guides you through the decision-making process for priority assessment steps, nursing diagnoses, interventions, and evaluation. And finally, the appendices provide an in-depth reference on code management, cardiopulmonary resuscitation, and manual ventilation.

This up-to-date guide to priority nursing care in life-threatening situations is an indispensable reference. *Life-Threatening Disorders* can help you gain confidence as you skillfully assess your acutely ill patient, plan his care, quickly intervene, and provide essential teaching. Not only will this book help you provide your patients with better care in today's fast-paced and continually changing health care environment, but by doing so it will also help you grow professionally and derive more satisfaction from your practice.

Edwina A. McConnell, RN, PhD
Independent Nurse Consultant
Madison, Wis.

1

Trauma

Broadly defined, trauma is bodily injury produced by violence or any thermal, chemical, or other extrinsic agent. It can range from a minor injury, such as a small abrasion, to a life-threatening injury, such as a high-voltage electric shock. Trauma is the third leading cause of death in North America, out-ranked only by cardiovascular disease and cancer. In people under age 35, it's the leading cause of death.

Although death can't always be prevented when trauma is severe and emergency care is delayed, your skilled care can mean the difference between life and death for many patients. You'll need to know how to assess and maintain ABCs (airway, breathing, and circulation), protect the patient from further injury, assess level of consciousness and, if necessary, prepare him for transfer or surgery.

The information you'll find in this section will prepare you to care for patients with such life-threatening traumatic injuries as burns, heat syndrome, cold injuries, electric shock, and poisoning.

PRIORITY CHECKLIST

Initial trauma care

Check for:
- □ history of the traumatic event
- □ medical conditions that may complicate trauma or recovery
- □ drug history, especially of drugs that shouldn't be stopped abruptly
- □ ABCs (airway, breathing, circulation)
- □ abnormal vital signs (especially extremely high or low)
- □ irregular heartbeat
- □ severity of injury
- □ multiple injury sites
- □ other injuries sustained during or just after the trauma
- □ altered level of consciousness
- □ altered sensory or motor function or both
- □ signs and symptoms of hypovolemia
- □ changes in skin color and temperature
- □ edema
- □ associated findings for the specific type of trauma.

Intervene by:
- □ initiating cardiopulmonary resuscitation, if indicated
- □ notifying the doctor
- □ starting an I.V. line
- □ taking precautions to prevent further injury or infection.

Prepare for:
- □ oxygen therapy
- □ hemodynamic monitoring
- □ emergency drug administration
- □ noninvasive or invasive procedures specific to the type of trauma.

BURNS

In the United States, about 2 million people annually receive burn injuries. Of these, 300,000 are seriously burned, and more than 6,000 die of burn injuries, making burns this nation's third largest cause of accidental death.

CAUSES

Thermal burns, the most common type, frequently result from residential fires, motor vehicle accidents, playing with matches, improperly stored gasoline, space heater or electrical malfunctions, and arson. Other causes include improper handling of firecrackers, scalding accidents, and kitchen accidents (for example, resulting from a child climbing on top of a stove or grabbing a hot iron). Sometimes burns are traced to child or elder abuse.

Chemical burns result from the contact, ingestion, inhalation, or injection of acids, alkalies, or vesicants. Electrical burns commonly occur after contact with faulty electrical wiring or with high-voltage power lines, or when electric cords are chewed (by young children). Friction, or abrasion, burns happen when the skin is rubbed harshly against a coarse surface. Sunburn follows excessive exposure to sunlight.

COMPLICATIONS

Possible complications of burns include respiratory distress, hypovolemic shock, anemia, malnutrition, and infection.

ASSESSMENT

The patient's history usually reveals the cause of the burn. It also may disclose preexisting medical conditions – such as a cardiac or pulmonary problem, diabetes mellitus, peripheral vascular disease, chronic alcohol or drug abuse, or a psychiatric disorder – that could complicate burn treatment and recovery.

If the patient is under age 4 or over age 60, he'll have a higher incidence of complications and, consequently, a higher risk of death. Obtain history information as soon as possible because medications, confusion resulting from the injury, or the use of an endotracheal tube may prevent the patient from giving an accurate history later.

Your assessment provides a general idea of burn severity. First, determine the depth of tissue damage. A partial-thickness burn damages the epidermis and part of the dermis, whereas a full-thickness burn also affects the subcutaneous tissue. The more traditional method is to gauge burns by degree, although most burns are a combination of degrees and thicknesses.

The following guidelines allow you to determine a burn's severity:
• *First degree.* Erythema appears, and the patient will complain of pain. Damage is limited to the epidermis.
• *Second degree.* Blisters and mild to moderate edema develop, and the patient will report pain. Both the epidermis and the dermis are damaged.
• *Third degree.* You'll see white, brown, or black leathery tissue and thrombosed vessels, although no blisters appear. Both the epidermis and dermis are damaged.
• *Fourth degree.* Damage extends through deeply charred subcutaneous tissue to muscle and bone.

Next, assess the size of the burn. This usually is expressed as the percentage of the body surface area (BSA) covered by the burn. Determine this percentage with an assessment tool, such as the Rule of Nines or the Lund and Browder Chart. (See *Estimating the extent of a burn.*) You usually don't need to calculate the total BSA in a patient with a first-degree burn.

Then estimate the severity of the burn by correlating its depth and size, as follows:
• *Major.* This category includes third-degree burns on more than 10% of the patient's BSA; second-degree burns on more than 25% of an adult's BSA or more than 20% of a child's BSA; burns of the hands, face, feet, or genitalia; burns complicated by fractures or respiratory damage; electrical burns; and all burns in high-risk patients.
• *Moderate.* This category covers third-degree burns on 2% to 10% of a patient's BSA, or second-degree burns on 15% to 25% of an adult's BSA or 10% to 20% of a child's BSA.

Estimating the extent of a burn

You can quickly estimate the extent of an adult patient's burns by using the Rule of Nines, shown below at left. This method divides the body surface into percentages.

To use this method, mentally transfer your patient's burns to the body chart shown here. Then add up the corresponding percentages for each burned body section. The total—a rough estimate of the extent of your patient's burns—enters into the formula to determine his initial fluid replacement needs.

You can't use this method with an infant or a child because his body section percentages differ from those of an adult. (For instance, an infant's head accounts for 17% of his total body surface, compared with 7% for an adult.) Instead, use the Lund and Browder chart.

Rule of Nines

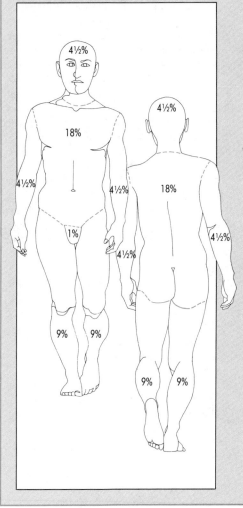

Lund and Browder chart

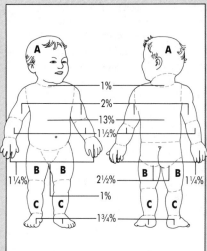

Relative percentages of areas affected by growth

	AT BIRTH	0 TO 1 YR	2 TO 4 YR	5 TO 9 YR	10 TO 15 YR	ADULT
A: Half of head						
	9½%	8½%	6½%	5½%	4½%	3½%
B: Half of thigh						
	2¾%	3¼%	4%	4¼%	4½%	4¾%
C: Half of leg						
	2½%	2½%	2¾%	3%	3¼%	3½%

• *Minor.* Third-degree burns that appear on less than 2% of a patient's BSA, or second-degree burns on less than 15% of an adult's BSA or 10% of a child's BSA make up this category.

Inspection reveals other characteristics of the burn as well, including location and extent. Keep in mind that burns on the face, hands, feet, and genitalia are most serious because of a possible loss of function or severe impact on body image. Also note the burn's configuration. If the patient has a circumferential burn, he runs the risk of edema totally occluding circulation in his extremity. If he has burns on his neck, he may suffer airway obstruction; burns on the chest can lead to restricted respiratory excursion.

Inspect the patient for other injuries that may complicate his recovery. In particular, look for signs of pulmonary damage from smoke inhalation – singed nasal hairs, mucosal burns, voice changes, coughing, wheezing, soot in the mouth or nose, and darkened sputum.

Palpation reveals edema and pulse rate, strength, and regularity. (If edema makes peripheral pulses difficult to find, palpate the femoral pulse or use a Doppler ultrasound device.)

Auscultation of the lungs may reveal respiratory distress, including stridor, wheezing, crackles, and rhonchi. Auscultation of the heart may detect an S_3 or S_4 gallop or murmur, an indication of myocardial injury or decompensation. The patient with severe burns may be hypotensive, indicating hypovolemia and, possibly, shock.

You can take this patient's blood pressure even if all his extremities are burned by placing a sterile $4'' \times 4''$ gauze pad or sterile towel on his extremity before applying the blood pressure cuff.

Abdominal auscultation may disclose absent bowel sounds if the patient has an ileus, which almost always accompanies a burn that covers more than 25% of the patient's total BSA.

DIAGNOSTIC TESTS

Routine blood studies for a patient with a burn injury include a complete blood count, a platelet count, clotting studies, liver function studies, and carboxyhemoglobin, electrolyte, blood urea nitrogen, glucose, and creatinine levels. A urinalysis may reveal myoglobinuria and hemoglobinuria. If the patient is age 35 or older, he'll also need an electrocardiogram. Chest X-ray films and arterial blood gas (ABG) levels allow the evaluation of alveolar function. Fiber-optic bronchoscopy shows the condition of the trachea and bronchi.

TREATMENT

For a patient with severe facial burns or suspected pulmonary injury, treatment to prevent hypoxia includes endotracheal intubation, administration of high concentrations of oxygen, and positive-pressure ventilation.

Treatment for moderate or severe burns includes administration of lactated Ringer's solution through a large-bore I.V. line inserted above the waist to expand vascular volume. Central I.V. lines and arterial lines are inserted as necessary. The patient needs enough I.V. fluids to maintain a urine output of 30 to 50 ml/hour. An indwelling urinary catheter permits accurate monitoring of urine output. I.V. morphine (2 to 4 mg) alleviates pain and anxiety. The patient also will need a nasogastric (NG) tube to prevent gastric distention and accompanying ileus from hypovolemic shock.

All burn patients need a booster of 0.5 ml of tetanus toxoid given I.M. Most burn centers don't recommend administering prophylactic antibiotics because overuse of antibiotics fosters the development of resistant bacteria.

Treatment of the burn wound itself includes:
• initial debridement by washing the surface of the wound area with mild soap
• sharp debridement of loose tissue and blisters (blister fluid contains vasospastic agents that potentiate tissue ischemia)
• covering the wound with an antibacterial agent, such as silver sulfadiazine, and an occlusive cotton gauze dressing
• escharotomy, if the patient is at risk for vascular, circulatory, or respiratory compromise.

KEY NURSING DIAGNOSES AND PATIENT OUTCOMES

Fluid volume deficit related to fluid evaporation through the burn and release of fluid into interstitial space caused by the burn. Based on this nursing diagnosis, you'll establish these patient outcomes. The patient will:
• regain and maintain normal fluid and blood volume
• produce a urine output of at least 30 ml/hour
• exhibit no signs and symptoms of hypovolemic shock.

High risk for infection related to massive breaks in skin integrity caused by the burn. Based on this nursing diagnosis, you'll establish these patient outcomes. The patient will:
• maintain a normal body temperature and white blood cell count and differential
• have burn areas that appear free of purulent drainage and foul odor
• remain free of all other signs of infection.

Impaired gas exchange related to smoke inhalation caused by fire exposure. Based on this nursing diagnosis, you'll establish these patient outcomes. The patient will:
• maintain adequate ventilation with or without mechanical support
• maintain normal ABG and oxygen saturation values
• report breathing comfort.

NURSING INTERVENTIONS

• Provide immediate, aggressive burn treatment to increase the patient's chance for survival. Later, provide supportive measures and use strict aseptic technique to minimize the risk of infection. Keep in mind that good nursing care can make the difference between life and death in a burn patient.
• Make sure the patient with major or moderate burns has adequate airway, breathing, and circulation. If needed, assist with endotracheal intubation. Administer 100% oxygen, as ordered, and adjust the flow to maintain adequate gas exchange. Also draw blood samples as ordered.
• Take steps to control bleeding, and remove any clothing that's still smoldering. If it's stuck to the patient's skin, saturate it first with 0.9%

Fluid replacement: The first 24 hours

Use one of these two formulas as a general guideline for the amount of fluid replacement to give your patient, according to hospital protocol. Vary the specific infusions depending on his response, especially his urine output.

Baxter formula
Administer 4 ml of lactated Ringer's solution per kilogram of body weight per percentage of body surface area (BSA) over 24 hours. Give one-half of the total over the first 8 hours after the burn and the remainder over the next 16 hours.

Brooke formula
With this formula, you'll administer various fluids:
• 0.5 ml of a colloid (plasma, plasmanate, or dextran) per kilogram of body weight per percentage of BSA
• 1.5 ml of lactated Ringer's solution per kilogram of body weight per percentage of BSA
• 2,000 ml of dextrose 5% in water for adults (less for children).
    Give one-half of the total over the first 8 hours after the burn and the remainder over the next 16 hours.

sodium chloride solution. Also remove rings and other constricting items.
• Cover the burns with a clean, dry, sterile bed sheet.
    NURSING ALERT. *Never* cover large burns with dressings soaked in 0.9% sodium chloride solution, which can drastically lower body temperature.
• Start I.V. therapy at once to prevent hypovolemic shock and maintain cardiac output. Use lactated Ringer's solution or a fluid replacement formula, as ordered. (See *Fluid replacement: The first 24 hours.*)
• Assist with the insertion of a central venous pressure line and additional arterial and I.V. lines (using venous cutdown, if necessary). Insert an indwelling urinary catheter as ordered.

• Continue fluid therapy, as ordered, to combat fluid evaporation through the burn and the release of fluid into interstitial spaces (possibly resulting in hypovolemic shock).
• Maintain the patient's core body temperature by covering him with a sterile blanket and exposing only small areas of his body at a time.
• Insert an NG tube, as ordered, to decompress the stomach and avoid aspiration of stomach contents.
• Provide a diet high in potassium, protein, vitamins, fats, nitrogen, and calories to try to maintain the patient's preburn weight. If necessary, feed him through a small NG tube until he can tolerate oral feedings. (If he had a paralytic ileus, wait until bowel sounds return.)
• If the patient will be transferred to a specialized burn care unit within 4 hours after the injury, don't treat the burn wound itself in the emergency department. Instead, prepare him for transport by wrapping him in a sterile sheet and a blanket for warmth and elevating the burned extremity to decrease edema. Then transport him immediately.
• If the patient has only minor burns, immerse the burned area in cool saline solution (55° F [12.8° C]) or apply cool compresses. Next, soak the wound in a mild antiseptic solution to clean it, and give ordered pain medication.
• Debride the devitalized tissue. Cover the wound with an antibacterial agent and a nonstick bulky dressing, and administer tetanus prophylaxis, as ordered.

For a patient with an electrical or a chemical burn:
• If the electric shock caused ventricular fibrillation and cardiac and respiratory arrest, begin cardiopulmonary resuscitation at once.
• If the patient has a chemical burn, irrigate the wound with copious amounts of water or 0.9% sodium chloride solution. Using a weak base (such as sodium bicarbonate) to neutralize hydrofluoric acid, hydrochloric acid, or sulfuric acid on skin or mucous membranes is controversial, particularly in the emergent phase, because the neutralizing agent can produce more heat and tissue damage.

• If the chemical entered the patient's eyes, flush them with large amounts of water or 0.9% sodium chloride solution for at least 30 minutes. In an alkali burn, irrigate until the pH of the conjunctival cul-de-sacs returns to 7.0. Have the patient close his eyes, and cover them with a dry, sterile dressing. Note the type of chemical that caused the burn and any noxious fumes. The patient will need an ophthalmologic examination.

Monitoring
• Immediately assess the patient's ABCs, (airway, breathing, circulation) and monitor them frequently.
• Check vital signs every 15 minutes until they're stable and then as often as indicated by the patient's condition.
• Monitor the patient's cardiopulmonary status closely. Note any abnormal heart or breath sounds, and observe for signs of respiratory distress.
• Evaluate the patient's hydration status and intake and output. Be alert for signs and symptoms of hypovolemic shock.
• Monitor for signs and symptoms of nutritional deficits. Weigh the patient daily at the same time.
• Monitor temperature, white blood cell count, and differential count. Assess the burn area regularly for signs of infection, and be alert for signs and symptoms of sepsis. Monitor closely for other complications.
• Evaluate pain and its severity. Also monitor the effectiveness of any administered analgesics.
• Keep in mind that tissue damage from an electrical burn is difficult to assess because internal destruction along the conduction pathway usually is greater than the surface burn indicates. An electrical burn that ignites the patient's clothes may cause thermal burns as well. Always get an estimate of the voltage that caused the injury.
• Monitor the patient's emotional response throughout the recovery period. Assess for depression and suicidal tendencies.

Patient teaching

• Explain all procedures to the patient before performing them. Speak calmly and clearly to help alleviate his anxiety. Encourage him to actively participate in his care as much as possible.

• Give the patient opportunities to voice his concerns, especially about altered body image. If appropriate, arrange for him to meet a patient with similar injuries. When possible, show the patient how his bodily functions are improving. If necessary, refer him for mental health counseling.

• If the patient has only a minor burn, stress the importance of keeping his dressing dry and clean, elevating the burned extremity for the first 24 hours, taking analgesics as ordered, and returning for a wound check in 2 days.

• For a patient with a moderate or major burn, discharge teaching involves the entire burn team. Teaching topics include wound management; signs and symptoms of complications; use of pressure dressings, exercises, and splints; and resocialization. Make sure the patient understands the treatment plan, including why it's necessary and how it will help his recovery.

• Explain to the patient that a home health nurse can assist with wound care. Provide the patient with the phone number of a doctor or nurse who can answer questions.

• Give the patient written discharge instructions for later reference.

HEAT SYNDROME

The body normally adjusts to excessive temperatures by complex cardiovascular and neurologic changes, which are coordinated by the hypothalamus. Heat loss offsets heat production to regulate temperature. Such regulation requires evaporation (sweating) or vasodilation, which cools the body's surface by radiation, conduction, and convection.

Sometimes both environmental and internal factors can increase heat production or decrease heat loss beyond the body's ability to compensate. When this happens, heat syndrome results. This syndrome falls into three categories: heat cramps, heat exhaustion, and heatstroke. Heat exhaustion and heatstroke are potentially life-threatening, with heatstroke being the more emergent of the two.

CAUSES

Heat syndrome may result from conditions that increase heat production, such as excessive exercise, infection, and drugs (for example, amphetamines). It also can stem from factors that impair heat dissipation. These include high temperatures or humidity, lack of acclimatization, excess clothing, cardiovascular disease, obesity, dehydration, sweat gland dysfunction, and drugs, such as phenothiazines and anticholinergics.

Heatstroke often is seen in elderly people during excessively hot summer days, particularly when they are inside with windows and doors closed and have no air conditioning. In high-crime areas especially, elderly people may not open windows and doors because of their fears of injury or theft.

COMPLICATIONS

Heat exhaustion may lead to respiratory alkalosis. Heatstroke, a medical emergency, can lead to hypovolemic or cardiogenic shock, arrhythmias, and renal failure caused by rhabdomyolysis, disseminated intravascular coagulation, and hepatic failure.

ASSESSMENT

Signs and symptoms vary with the type of heat syndrome. The history of a patient with heat cramps almost always reveals vigorous activity immediately preceding onset. The patient typically appears alert and complains of pain.

On assessment, the patient usually has normal vital signs, with body temperature normal or slightly elevated. Inspection reveals muscle twitching and spasm. Palpation reveals moist, cool skin and muscle tenderness. Involved muscle groups may feel hard and lumpy. The neurologic examination usually is normal, although the patient may appear agitated.

The history of a patient with heat exhaustion usually reveals prolonged activity in a very warm or hot environment, without adequate salt intake. The patient may complain of muscle cramps. More often, he reports nausea and vomiting, thirst, weakness, and oliguria. He also may complain of headache and fatigue.

Assessment reveals a rectal temperature over 100° F (37.8° C). On inspection, you may note pale skin. The patient's pulse feels thready and rapid on palpation, and his skin is cool and moist. Auscultation reveals decreased blood pressure. When heat exhaustion is mainly due to water depletion, the neurologic examination may reveal mental confusion, giddiness, syncope, impaired judgment, and anxiety paresthesia. Assessment also may reveal hyperventilation, which can lead to respiratory alkalosis. If you note that sweating ceases, the patient may be progressing from heat exhaustion to heatstroke.

The history of a patient with heatstroke may reveal the specific cause, such as exposure to high temperature and humidity without any wind. The patient may exhibit weakness, dizziness, nausea, vomiting, and blurred vision.

Your assessment shows a rectal temperature of at least 106° F (41.1° C). On inspection and palpation, the patient's skin is red, diaphoretic, and hot in early stages; gray, dry, and hot in later stages. He may have a rapid pulse rate. On auscultation, his blood pressure is slightly elevated in early stages and decreased in later stages. The neurologic examination of the conscious patient may reveal dilated pupils, emotional lability, confusion, and – as heatstroke progresses – delirium, seizures, collapse and, finally, unconsciousness. You also may note hyperpnea at any time, which leads to respiratory alkalosis and compensatory metabolic acidosis. In late stages, you may note slow, deep respirations, which progress to Cheyne-Stokes respirations.

DIAGNOSTIC TESTS

Serum electrolyte and arterial blood gas (ABG) levels may reveal respiratory alkalosis, hyponatremia, and hypokalemia in heat exhaustion and heatstroke. In heatstroke, blood studies reveal leukocytosis, elevated blood urea nitrogen levels, hemoconcentration, and decreased serum potassium, calcium, and phosphorus levels. Blood studies also may reveal thrombocytopenia, increased bleeding and clotting times, fibrinolysis, and consumption coagulopathy. Urinalysis results show concentrated urine, with elevated protein levels, tube casts, and myoglobinuria.

TREATMENT

For heat cramps, treatment consists of moving the patient to a cool environment, providing rest, and administering oral or I.V. fluid and electrolyte replacement (for example, Rehydralyte for adults and Pedialyte for children). Salt tablets aren't recommended because of their comparatively slow absorption.

Treatment for heat exhaustion involves moving the patient to a cool environment, providing rest, and administering oral fluid and electrolyte replacement. If I.V. replacement is necessary, laboratory test results determine the choice of I.V. solution – usually 0.9% sodium chloride or isotonic glucose solution.

Heatstroke therapy focuses on lowering the body temperature as rapidly as possible. The patient's clothing is removed, and cool water is applied to the skin, followed by fanning with cool air. Shivering is controlled with diazepam or chlorpromazine. Application of hypothermia blankets and ice packs to the groin and axillae also helps lower body temperature. Treatment continues until the body temperature drops to 102.2° F (39° C). Supportive measures include oxygen therapy, central venous pressure (CVP) and pulmonary artery wedge pressure (PAWP) monitoring and, if necessary, endotracheal intubation. The patient is closely observed for complications.

KEY NURSING DIAGNOSES AND EXPECTED OUTCOMES

Fluid volume deficit related to excessive sweating. Based on this nursing diagnosis, you'll establish these patient outcomes. The patient will:
• regain normal fluid and electrolyte balance
• produce adequate urine volume exhibited by a urine output of 30 ml/hour or more

• identify factors that caused fluid volume deficit and preventive measures to avoid a recurrence.

Hyperthermia related to increased heat production and severe dehydration. Based on this nursing diagnosis, you'll establish these patient outcomes. The patient will:

• regain and maintain a normal body temperature

• not experience seizures associated with hyperthermia

• identify risk factors that exacerbate heat production.

Impaired gas exchange related to ineffective breathing pattern. Based on this nursing diagnosis, you'll establish these patient outcomes. The patient will:

• regain and maintain a normal respiratory rate and pattern

• report breathing comfort

• have ABG values return to normal.

NURSING INTERVENTIONS

• Perform or assist with the cooling procedure as necessary. If ordered, place the patient on a cooling mattress. If the patient has heatstroke, remove his clothing and place him in the lateral recumbent position, or support him in the knee-chest position so that as much skin as possible is exposed to the air. Then spray his entire body with water as cool air is passed over the body. Use fans to provide the air movement needed to increase heat loss through convection and evaporation. Alternatively, cover the patient with a sheet dampened with water or isopropyl alcohol, and fan him with cool air.

• Assist with supportive measures as necessary. These may include assisting with insertion of an endotracheal tube and caring for it to maintain an adequate airway. Provide supplemental oxygen as ordered.

• Encourage adequate fluid intake as required. If necessary, ensure peripheral I.V. access as ordered.

• Administer medication as ordered to inhibit shivering.

• Referral to a social service agency may be necessary for an elderly patient who experiences heat syndrome because of a compromised home environment.

Monitoring

• Evaluate the patient's vital signs. If he's unstable, use a rectal probe to assess his body temperature.

• Frequently assess the patient for complications. Note his level of consciousness, cardiac rhythm, and cardiac output. If a central line is in place, monitor CVP and PAWP.

• Evaluate the patient's intake and urine output. Insert an indwelling urinary catheter as needed.

• Monitor the patient's respiratory rate and pattern. Auscultate breath sounds regularly.

• Monitor electrolyte and ABG values as ordered.

Patient teaching

• Advise the patient to avoid immediate reexposure to high temperatures. He may remain sensitive to heat for a while.

• Teach him the importance of maintaining an adequate fluid intake, wearing loose clothing, and limiting activity in hot weather.

• Advise athletes to monitor fluid losses, replace fluids, and use a gradual approach to physical conditioning.

• Encourage older patients to seek out air-conditioned areas, such as shopping malls and libraries, in hot weather.

COLD INJURIES

Caused by overexposure, cold injuries occur in two major forms: localized injuries (frostbite) and systemic injuries (hypothermia).

Frostbite may be superficial or deep. Superficial frostbite affects skin and subcutaneous tissue, especially of the face, ears, extremities, and other exposed body areas. Deep frostbite extends beyond the subcutaneous tissue and usually affects the hands and feet. Untreated or improperly treated, frostbite can lead to gangrene, requiring amputation.

Hypothermia — core body temperature below 95° F (35° C) — effects chemical changes in the body. Severe hypothermia can be fatal.

Risk factors for serious cold injuries

The risk for serious cold injury—especially hypothermia—increases with the following factors:
• youth or old age
• lack of insulating body fat
• wet or inadequate clothing
• drug abuse
• cardiac disease
• smoking
• fatigue
• malnutrition and depletion of caloric reserves
• excessive alcohol intake.

CAUSES

Frostbite results from prolonged exposure to dry temperatures far below freezing. The cold causes ice crystals to form in the tissues, expanding extracellular spaces. With compression of tissue cells, cell membranes rupture, interrupting enzymatic and metabolic activities. Increased capillary permeability accompanies the release of histamine, resulting in the aggregation of red blood cells and microvascular occlusion.

Hypothermia results from near drowning in cold water and prolonged exposure to cold temperatures. It also can occur in normal temperatures if the patient's homeostasis is altered by disease or debility. (For a list of common risk factors, see *Risk factors for serious cold injuries*.) Administration of large amounts of cold blood or blood products can cause hypothermia. In hypothermia, chemical changes slow the functions of most major organ systems, resulting in decreased renal blood flow and decreased glomerular filtration, for example.

COMPLICATIONS

Tissue and muscle damage caused by frostbite may lead to renal failure and rhabdomyolysis. Avascular necrosis and gangrene also may result from frostbite.

Common complications associated with hypothermia include severe infection, aspiration pneumonia, cardiac arrhythmias, hypoglycemia or hyperglycemia, metabolic acidosis, pancreatitis, and renal failure.

ASSESSMENT

The history of a patient with a cold injury reveals the cause, the temperature to which the patient was exposed, and the length of exposure. A patient with superficial frostbite may report burning, numbness, tingling, and itching, although he may not notice symptoms until he returns to a warm place. A patient with deep frostbite reports paresthesia and stiffness while the part is still frozen, and a burning pain when the part thaws.

On inspection, an area with superficial frostbite appears swollen, with a mottled, blue-gray skin color. An area affected by deep frostbite appears white or yellow until it's thawed; then it turns purplish blue. You also may note edema, skin blisters, and necrosis.

Palpation of superficial frostbite reveals the extent and severity of swelling. Palpation of deep frostbite may reveal skin immobility. In either type of frostbite, palpation also reveals the presence or absence of associated peripheral pulses.

Your assessment findings in a patient with hypothermia vary with the patient's body temperature. A patient with moderate hypothermia—a core body temperature of 82.4° to 89.6° F (28° to 32° C)—is unresponsive, with peripheral cyanosis and muscle rigidity. If the patient was improperly rewarmed, he may show signs of shock.

A patient with severe hypothermia—a core body temperature of 77° to 82.4° F (25° to 28° C)—appears dead, with no palpable pulse and no audible heart sounds. His pupils may be dilated, and he may appear to be in a state of rigor mortis. Ventricular fibrillation and a loss of deep tendon reflexes commonly occur.

A patient with a body temperature below 77° F (25° C) will suffer cardiopulmonary arrest.

DIAGNOSTIC TESTS

In frostbite, technetium 99m pertechnetate scanning shows perfusion defects and deep tissue damage and can identify nonviable bone. Doppler and plethysmographic studies help determine the extent of frostbite after thawing.

Electrocardiogram findings can help establish a diagnosis of hypothermia. Essential laboratory tests during treatment of moderate or severe hypothermia include urine volume, pH, and serum amylase, electrolyte, hemoglobin, blood glucose, and arterial blood gas levels.

TREATMENT

For frostbite injuries, treatment consists of rapidly rewarming the injured part to slightly above ideal body temperature to preserve viable tissue. Slow rewarming may increase tissue damage. Treatment also includes administration of antibiotics and tetanus prophylaxis, as needed, and narcotic analgesics to relieve pain when the affected part begins to rewarm.

After rewarming, the affected part is kept elevated and uncovered at room temperature. A regimen of whirlpool treatments for 3 or more weeks cleans the skin and debrides sloughing tissue. After the early stage, active range-of-motion exercises restore mobility. Surgery usually isn't required; however, if gangrene develops, amputation may be necessary.

Treatment for hypothermia consists of supportive measures and specific rewarming techniques, including:
• passive rewarming (the patient rewarms on his own)
• active external rewarming with heating blankets, warm water immersion, heated objects such as water bottles, and radiant heat
• active core rewarming with heated I.V. fluids, genitourinary tract irrigation, peritoneal dialysis, hemodialysis, and extracorporeal rewarming.

Any arrhythmias that may develop usually convert to normal sinus rhythm with rewarming. If the patient has no pulse or respirations, he'll need cardiopulmonary resuscitation (CPR) until he's been rewarmed to a core temperature of at least 89.6° F (32° C).

Administration of oxygen, endotracheal intubation, controlled ventilation, and I.V. fluids and treatment of metabolic acidosis depend on test results and careful patient monitoring.

NURSING DIAGNOSES AND PATIENT OUTCOMES

Altered tissue perfusion (cardiopulmonary, cerebral, renal, gastrointestinal, and peripheral) related to decreased blood flow. Based on this nursing diagnosis, you'll establish these patient outcomes. The patient will:
• regain and maintain normal organ function
• demonstrate no residual damage upon resolution of cold injury.

Decreased cardiac output related to cold-induced arrhythmias. Based on this nursing diagnosis, you'll establish these patient outcomes. The patient will:
• maintain hemodynamic stability exhibited by normal vital signs and relief of cold signs and symptoms
• show resolution of arrhythmias on an electrocardiogram (ECG)
• recover and maintain normal cardiac output.

Hypothermia related to exposure to cold. Based on this nursing diagnosis, you'll establish these patient outcomes. The patient will:
• regain normal body temperature
• cease shivering
• show no complications associated with hypothermia, such as soft-tissue injury or hypovolemic shock if warmed too quickly.

NURSING INTERVENTIONS

• If the patient has a localized cold injury, remove all constrictive clothing.
• When the affected part begins to rewarm, give analgesics (as ordered) to relieve any pain. Check for a pulse. Be careful not to rupture any blebs. If the injury is on the foot, place cotton or gauze sponges between the toes to prevent maceration. Instruct him not to walk.
• If the injury has caused an open skin wound, give antibiotics and tetanus prophylaxis, as ordered.
• Rewarm the affected part by immersing it in tepid water (about 108° F [42.2° C]) for 20 minutes or until a distal flush is visible. Water

at this temperature feels warm but not hot to the normal hand.

▲ NURSING ALERT. *Never* rub the injured area— this aggravates tissue damage.

• If the patient has systemic hypothermia, first check for a pulse and respirations. If you can't detect them, begin CPR immediately. Continue CPR until the patient's core body temperature rises to at least 89.6° F (32° C). Keep in mind that hypothermia helps protect the brain from anoxia, which normally accompanies prolonged cardiopulmonary arrest. So even if the patient has been unresponsive for a long time, CPR may resuscitate him, especially after a cold-water near drowning.

• Assist with rewarming techniques as necessary. In moderate to severe hypothermia, aggressive rewarming should be attempted only by experienced personnel.

• During rewarming, provide supportive measures as ordered. These include mechanical ventilation and warm, humidified therapy to maintain tissue oxygenation, and I.V. fluids that have been warmed with a warming coil to correct hypotension and maintain urine output.

• Insert an indwelling urinary catheter as ordered.

• Allow the patient to express his anxiety and concerns, especially if amputation of a body part is required. Referral to a rehabilitation counselor may be necessary.

• Refer a patient who has developed cold injuries because of inadequate clothing or housing to a community social service agency.

Monitoring

• Frequently monitor the patient's core body temperature and other vital signs during and after initial rewarming. Continuously monitor his cardiac status, including ECG.

• Frequently check exposed extremities for pulse, temperature, and color changes.

• Be alert for signs and symptoms of complications. Review laboratory values, such as blood glucose level and renal function studies, for abnormalities.

• Monitor intake and urine output hourly in patients with systemic hypothermia.

• Assess the patient's pain level and the effectiveness of any administered analgesics.

• Evaluate the patient's emotional response to cold injury and to any lasting effects.

Patient teaching

• To prevent cold injuries in cold weather, teach the patient to wear mittens—not gloves; windproof, water-resistant, many-layered clothing; two pairs of socks (cotton next to the skin and then wool); a scarf; and a hat that covers the ears (to avoid substantial heat loss through the head).

• Before anticipated prolonged exposure to cold, advise the patient not to drink alcohol or smoke and to get adequate food and rest. If he gets caught in severe cold weather, he should find shelter early or increase physical activity to maintain body warmth.

ELECTRIC SHOCK

When an electric current passes through the body, the resultant damage depends on the intensity of the current (amperes, milliamperes, or microamperes), the resistance of the tissues it passes through, the kind of current (AC, DC, or mixed), and the frequency and duration of current flow.

Mild electric shock can cause a local, unpleasant tingling or a painful sensation. Severe electric shock can cause ventricular fibrillation, respiratory paralysis, burns, and even death. Even the smallest electric current—if it passes through the heart—may induce ventricular fibrillation or another arrhythmia that progresses to fibrillation or myocardial infarction.

In North America, about 1,000 persons die of electric shock each year. Electric shock is a particular hazard in the hospital. (See *Preventing electric shock.*)

The greatest threats to life from electric shock include cardiac arrhythmias, renal failure secondary to the precipitation of myoglobin and hemoglobin in the kidneys, and electrolyte imbalances, such as hyperkalemia and hypocalcemia from massive muscle breakdown.

The prognosis depends on the site and extent of damage, the patient's state of health, and the speed and adequacy of treatment. Dry, calloused, unbroken skin offers more resistance to electric current than mucous membrane, an open wound, or thin, moist skin.

CAUSES

Electric shock usually follows accidental contact with an exposed part of an electrical appliance or wiring. It also may result from lightning or the flash of electric arcs from high-voltage power lines or machines.

The current can cause a true electrical injury if it passes through the body. If it doesn't pass through the body, it can cause arc or flash burns. Thermal surface burns can result from associated heat and flames.

COMPLICATIONS

Although complications can occur in almost any part of the body, the most common complications include sepsis; neurologic, cardiac, or psychiatric dysfunction; renal failure; and electrolyte abnormalities.

ASSESSMENT

The patient's history reveals the source of the electric current and the approximate length of exposure. Varying signs and symptoms depend on the amount and type of current, the duration and area of exposure, and the pathway the current took through the body. If the shock was severe, the patient or an observer may report that the patient lost consciousness. After regaining consciousness, the patient may complain of muscle pain, fatigue, headache, and nervous irritability.

When electric shock results from a high-frequency current (which generates more heat in tissues than a low-frequency current), inspection usually reveals burns and local tissue coagulation and necrosis. Electric shock resulting from low-frequency current may produce serious burns if contact is concentrated in a small area (for example, when a toddler bites into an electric cord). When the electric current passes through the patient's body, inspection reveals entrance and exit in-

Preventing electric shock

Take these steps to help prevent electric shock in the hospital.

Check connections
• Check for cuts, cracks, or frayed insulation on electric cords, call buttons (also check for warm call buttons), and electrical devices attached to the patient's bed. Report any problems to maintenance personnel.
• Avoid using extension cords because they may circumvent the ground; if they're necessary, don't place them under carpeting or where they'll be walked on.
• Make sure ground connections on electrical equipment are intact. Electric cord plugs should have three prongs; the prongs should be straight and firmly fixed. Check that prongs fit wall outlets properly and that outlets aren't loose or broken. Don't use adapters on plugs.

Handle with care
• Keep all electrical devices away from hot or wet surfaces and sharp corners. Also, don't set glasses of water, damp towels, or other wet items on electrical equipment. Wipe up accidental spills before they leak into electrical equipment.
• If a machine sparks, smokes, seems unusually hot, or gives you or your patient a slight shock, unplug it immediately, if doing so won't endanger the patient's life. Promptly report such faulty equipment to maintenance personnel. Also, check inspection labels, and report equipment overdue for inspection.
• Be especially careful when using electrical equipment near a patient with a pacemaker or direct cardiac line because a cardiac catheter or pacemaker can create a direct, low-resistance path to the heart; even a small shock may cause ventricular fibrillation.
• Make sure defibrillator paddles are free of dry, caked gel before applying fresh gel. Otherwise, the patient may suffer burns from poor electrical contact. Also, don't apply too much gel. If the gel runs over the edge of the paddle and touches your hand, you'll receive some of the defibrillator shock, and the patient will lose some of the energy in the discharge.

juries that appear as round or oval yellow-brown lesions.

Depending on the action of the current, inspection and palpation also may reveal contusions, evidence of fractures, and other injuries that can result from violent muscle contractions or falls during the shock. If ventricular fibrillation occurs, you won't be able to palpate the pulse or auscultate heart sounds, and the patient will be unconscious. Respirations may continue for a short time and then cease.

If respiratory failure occurs, inspection discloses cyanosis, absent respirations, markedly decreased blood pressure, cold skin, and unconsciousness. Pulses, however, can still be palpated.

Neurologic examination may reveal numbness or tingling or sensorimotor deficits.

DIAGNOSTIC TESTS

An electrocardiogram (ECG), arterial blood gas (ABG) analysis, urine myoglobin tests, and X-rays of injured areas are used to evaluate internal damage and guide treatment.

TREATMENT

The first step in treatment involves separating the victim from the current source by turning it off or unplugging it. If this isn't possible, the victim is pulled free with a nonconductive device, such as a loop of dry cloth or rubber, a dry rope, or a leather strap.

After interrupting the current source, perform emergency measures, including assessing vital functions and instituting cardiopulmonary resuscitation (CPR) if the patient has no respirations or pulse. When the patient is revived, treatment includes:
• assessment for shock, acid-base imbalance, cardiac arrhythmias, hemorrhage, myoglobinuria, traumatic injury, and neurologic damage
• use of a cardiac monitor to permit rapid identification and treatment of arrhythmias
• use of a cervical collar and backboard until spinal injury has been ruled out
• vigorous fluid replacement using lactated Ringer's solution, along with central venous pressure and urine output monitoring

• administration of an osmotic diuretic (mannitol) for myoglobinuria once intravascular volume has been replaced
• administration of tetanus prophylaxis
• if necessary, referral to a burn center for further treatment.

KEY NURSING DIAGNOSES AND PATIENT OUTCOMES

Decreased cardiac output related to cardiac arrhythmias caused by electric shock. Based on this nursing diagnosis, you'll establish these patient outcomes. The patient will:
• attain hemodynamic stability, evidenced by normal vital signs and resolution of arrhythmia on the ECG
• recover and maintain normal cardiac output.

High risk for injury related to precipitation of myoglobin and hemoglobin in the kidneys caused by electric shock. Based on this nursing diagnosis, you'll establish these patient outcomes. The patient will:
• maintain a normal urine output of at least 30 ml/hour
• exhibit values within the normal range on all renal function studies
• show no signs or symptoms of acute renal failure.

Inability to sustain spontaneous ventilation related to respiratory failure caused by electric shock. Based on this nursing diagnosis, you'll establish these patient outcomes. The patient will:
• recover from lung tissue damage
• resume spontaneous ventilation with treatment
• regain and maintain normal ABG values.

NURSING INTERVENTIONS

• If it hasn't already been done, separate the victim from the current source and then begin emergency treatment. If necessary, start CPR at once. Continue until vital signs return or emergency help arrives with a defibrillator and other life-support equipment.
• Assist with intubation or emergency tracheostomy if spontaneous respirations are absent or inadequate. Provide the supportive care needed with mechanical ventilation.

• Once the patient has received emergency treatment, obtain a 12-lead ECG.
• Because internal tissue destruction may be much greater than skin damage suggests, give I.V. lactated Ringer's solution, as ordered, to maintain a urine output of 50 to 100 ml/hour. Insert an indwelling urinary catheter and send the first specimen to the laboratory.
• To prevent renal shutdown, give mannitol as ordered.
• If necessary, institute seizure precautions, according to hospital policy.
• Immobilize the patient's spine until fractures have been ruled out.
• Elevate any injured extremities.
• Care for the burned area as indicated. If ordered, apply a sterile dressing and administer topical and systemic antibiotics to help reduce the risk of infection.
• Take steps to prevent electric shock in the hospital.

Monitoring

• Assess the patient's vital signs closely for deviations from normal.
• Check the patient's cardiac status, including cardiac rhythm, continuously. Also monitor respiratory status—rate, pattern, and breath sounds. Alert the doctor immediately if the patient's condition deteriorates.
• Measure intake and output hourly and watch for tea- or port wine–colored urine, which occurs when coagulation necrosis and tissue ischemia liberate myoglobin and hemoglobin. These proteins can precipitate in the renal tubules, causing tubular necrosis and renal shutdown.
• Frequently assess the patient's neurologic status because central nervous system damage may result from ischemia or demyelination.
• Because a spinal cord injury may follow cord ischemia or a compression fracture, continue to watch for sensorimotor deficits.
• Check for neurovascular damage in the extremities by assessing peripheral pulses and capillary refill and by asking the patient about numbness, tingling, and pain.
• Monitor electrolyte levels, renal function studies, and ABG values as ordered.

Patient teaching

• Reinforce the doctor's explanation of all treatments and procedures. Encourage the patient to discuss his experience with you to help decrease his anxiety.
• Tell the patient how to avoid electrical hazards at home and at work. Warn him not to use electrical appliances while showering or wet. Also warn him *never* to touch electrical appliances while touching faucets or cold water pipes in the kitchen; these pipes may provide the ground for all circuits in the house.
• If the patient is a young child, advise his parents to put safety guards on all electrical outlets and to keep him away from electrical devices.

POISONING

Inhalation, ingestion, or injection of, or skin contamination from, any harmful substance is a common problem. In the United States, about 10 million people are poisoned annually, 4,000 of them fatally. The prognosis depends on the amount of poison absorbed, its toxicity, and the time interval between poisoning and treatment.

CAUSES

Because of their curiosity and ignorance, children are the most common poison victims. In fact, accidental poisoning—usually from the ingestion of salicylates (aspirin), cleaning agents, insecticides, paints, cosmetics, and plants—is the fourth leading cause of death in children.

In adults, poisoning is most common among chemical company employees, particularly those in companies that use chlorine, carbon dioxide, hydrogen sulfide, nitrogen dioxide, and ammonia, and in companies that ignore safety standards. Other causes of poisoning in adults include improper cooking, canning, and storage of food; ingestion of, or skin contamination from, plants (for example, dieffenbachia, mistletoe, azalea, and philodendron); and accidental or intentional drug

Identifying poison's effects

Use the list below to help match your patient's signs and symptoms with the possible toxin.

Agitation, delirium
Alcohol, amphetamines, atropine, barbiturates, physostigmine, scopolamine

Coma
Atropine, barbiturates, bromide, carbon monoxide, chloral hydrate, ethanol, ethchlorvynol, paraldehyde, salicylates, scopolamine

Constricted pupils
Barbiturates, chloral hydrate, morphine, propoxyphene

Diaphoresis
Alcohol, fluoride, insulin, physostigmine

Diarrhea, nausea, vomiting
Alcohol (ethanol, methanol, ethylene glycol), digitalis glycosides, heavy metals (lead, arsenic), morphine and its analogues, salicylates

Dilated pupils
Alcohol, amphetamines, belladonna alkaloids (such as atropine and scopolamine), botulin toxin, cocaine, cyanide, ephedrine, glutethimide, meperidine, parasympatholytics, sympathomimetics

Dry mouth
Antihistamines, belladonna alkaloids, botulin toxin, morphine, phenothiazines, tricyclic antidepressants

Extrapyramidal tremor
Phenothiazines

Hematemesis
Fluoride, mercuric chloride, phosphorus, salicylates

Seizures
Alcohol (ethanol, methanol, ethylene glycol), amphetamines, carbon monoxide, cholinesterase inhibitors, hydrocarbons, phenothiazines, propoxyphene, salicylates, strychnine

overdose (usually barbiturates) or chemical ingestion.

COMPLICATIONS
Depending on the poison, possible complications vary widely but can include hypotension, cardiac arrhythmias, and seizures.

ASSESSMENT
The patient's history should reveal the source of poison and the form of exposure (ingestion, inhalation, injection, or skin contact). Assessment findings vary according to the poison. (See *Identifying poison's effects*.)

DIAGNOSTIC TEXTS
Toxicologic studies (including drug screens) of poison levels in the mouth, vomitus, urine, feces, or blood or on the victim's hands or clothing confirm the diagnosis. If possible, have the family or patient bring the container holding the poison to the emergency department for comparable study. In inhalation poisoning, chest X-rays may show pulmonary infiltrates or edema; in petroleum distillate inhalation, X-rays may show aspiration pneumonia.

Arterial blood gas (ABG) studies are used to evaluate oxygenation, ventilation, and the metabolic status of seriously poisoned patients.

TREATMENT
Initial treatment includes emergency resuscitation; support for the patient's airway, breathing, and circulation; and prevention of further absorption of poison. After this, treatment consists of continuing supportive or symptomatic care and, when possible, administration of a specific antidote.

A poisoning victim who exhibits an altered level of consciousness (LOC) routinely receives oxygen, glucose, and naloxone. Activated charcoal has proved effective in eliminating many toxic substances. The specific treatment depends on the poison.

KEY NURSING DIAGNOSES AND PATIENT OUTCOMES

High risk for aspiration related to absence of protective mechanisms. Based on this nursing diagnosis, you'll establish these patient outcomes. The patient will:
• show no sign of aspiration
• exhibit a normal temperature, normal white blood cell count, and clear, odorless respiratory secretions
• maintain normal breath sounds.

High risk for injury related to poison's effects within the body. Based on this nursing diagnosis, you'll establish these patient outcomes. The patient will:
• regain and maintain normal body function
• not exhibit residual damage or deficits as a result of the poisoning.

Ineffective breathing pattern related to respiratory depression as a result of the poison's effect on the central nervous system. Based on this nursing diagnosis, you'll establish these patient outcomes. The patient will:
• regain and maintain a normal respiratory rate and pattern
• report breathing comfort
• exhibit normal ABG and oxygen saturation values.

NURSING INTERVENTIONS

• If necessary, begin cardiopulmonary resuscitation.
• Depending on the poison, prevent further absorption of ingested poison by inducing emesis, using syrup of ipecac, or by administering gastric lavage and cathartics (magnesium sulfate). The treatment's effectiveness depends on the speed of absorption and the time elapsed between ingestion and removal. With syrup of ipecac, give warm water (usually less than 1 qt [less than 1 liter]) until vomiting occurs, or give another dose of ipecac as ordered.
• Never induce emesis if you suspect corrosive acid poisoning, if the patient is unconscious or has seizures, or if the gag reflex is impaired— even in a conscious patient. Instead, neutralize the poison by instilling the appropriate antidote by nasogastric (NG) tube. Common an-

tidotes include milk, magnesium salts (milk of magnesia), activated charcoal, or other chelating agents (such as deferoxamine or edetate disodium).

When possible, add the antidote to water or juice.

♦ NURSING ALERT. Methods of removing a poisonous hydrocarbon are controversial. In the conscious patient, because of a lower risk of aspiration with ipecac-induced emesis than with lavage, emesis may be the preferred treatment. However, some doctors still use lavage. Also, some believe that because of poor absorption, kerosene (a hydrocarbon) doesn't require removal from the GI tract; others believe that removal depends on the amount ingested.
• When you do want to induce emesis and the patient has already taken syrup of ipecac, don't give activated charcoal to neutralize the poison until *after* emesis; activated charcoal absorbs ipecac.
• To perform gastric lavage, instill 30 ml of fluid by NG tube; then aspirate the liquid. Repeat until the aspirate is clear. Save vomitus and aspirate for analysis. (To prevent aspiration in the unconscious patient, an endotracheal tube should be in place before lavage.)
• If several hours have passed since the patient ingested the poison, use large quantities of I.V. fluids to diurese the patient. The kind of fluid you'll use depends on the patient's acid-base balance and cardiovascular status and on the flow rate necessary for effective diuresis of poison.
• If ingested poisoning is severe and peritoneal dialysis or hemodialysis is necessary, assist as needed.
• To prevent further absorption of inhaled poison, remove the patient to fresh or uncontaminated air. Alert the anesthesia department, and provide supplemental oxygen. Some patients may require intubation. To prevent further absorption from skin contamination, remove the clothing covering the contaminated skin, and immediately flush the area with large amounts of water.
• If the patient is in severe pain, give analgesics as ordered.

• Keep the patient warm, and provide support in a quiet environment.
• If the poison was ingested intentionally, refer the patient for counseling to prevent future suicide attempts.
• For more specific treatment, contact your local poison center or a national center, such as the Arizona Poison and Drug Information Center.

Monitoring

• Carefully monitor the patient's vital signs and LOC.
• Monitor fluid intake and output. Also measure and evaluate vomitus and liquid stools.
• Closely monitor the patient's cardiopulmonary status.
• Evaluate the effectiveness of treatment measures.
• Assess the patient's pain level and the effectiveness of administered analgesics.
• Check for complications or residual damage or deficits.

Patient teaching

• To prevent accidental poisoning, instruct the patient to read the label before he takes medication. Instruct him to store all medications and household chemicals properly, keep them out of the reach of children, and discard old medications. Warn him not to take medications prescribed for someone else, not to transfer medications from their original containers to other containers without labeling them properly, and never to transfer poisons to food containers. Parents should avoid taking medication in front of young children or calling medication "candy" to get children to take it.
• Tell the patient to keep syrup of ipecac available. Emphasize the importance of understanding the directions for proper use.
• Advise parents to use childproof caps on medication containers.
• Stress the importance of using toxic sprays only in well-ventilated areas and of following instructions carefully. Teach the patient to use pesticides carefully and to keep the number of his poison control center handy.

2

Infection

Despite potent antibiotics, rigorous immunization schedules, and modern sanitation, infection remains a common cause of fatal illnesses, even in highly industrialized countries such as the United States and Canada. In developing countries, infection remains one of the most urgent health problems and carries a much higher mortality.

Although most infections are mild, they can become life-threatening if they are severe or result in septic shock, a condition characterized by hypotension and inadequate organ perfusion.

Your assessment skills and supportive care are vital to the patient with a life-threatening infection. Assessment allows you to judge the patient's response to the prescribed antibiotics and to check for early signs of a worsening condition or septic shock. Supportive care, such as cooling measures to combat hyperthermia and fluid replacements to prevent dehydration, can help prevent serious complications and promote patient comfort.

This section provides the information you need to care for a patient with one of the following life-threatening infections: septic shock, tetanus, botulism, gas gangrene, and Rocky Mountain spotted fever.

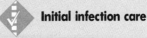
Check for:
- □ immunization history
- □ recent invasive tests or procedures
- □ recent trauma
- □ food intake over the past 36 hours
- □ medical conditions, especially those associated with infection, such as diabetes mellitus
- □ drug history, especially recent antibiotic or immunosuppressive therapy
- □ history of fever and chills
- □ potential sources of infection, such as indwelling catheters or tubes
- □ changes in vital signs
- □ chills
- □ seizures
- □ altered mental status
- □ signs of infection
- □ signs of dehydration
- □ changes in skin color and temperature
- □ neuromuscular abnormalities
- □ changes in organ function.

Intervene by:
- □ notifying the doctor
- □ obtaining blood cultures
- □ starting an I.V. line
- □ rechecking known drug allergies
- □ taking seizure precautions.

Prepare for:
- □ antibiotic administration
- □ antipyretic administration
- □ use of a cooling blanket
- □ invasive procedures, such as surgery
- □ fluid resuscitation measures
- □ oxygen administration
- □ hemodynamic monitoring.

SEPTIC SHOCK

Low systemic vascular resistance and an elevated cardiac output characterize septic shock. The disorder is thought to occur in response to infections that release microbes or one of the immune mediators. (See *What happens in septic shock.*)

Septic shock is usually a complication of another disorder or invasive procedure and has a mortality as high as 25%. The incidence of septic shock approaches 500,000 cases annually.

CAUSES

Any pathogenic organism can cause septic shock. Gram-negative bacteria, such as *Escherichia coli, Klebsiella pneumoniae, Serratia, Enterobacter,* and *Pseudomonas,* rank as the most common causes and account for up to 70% of all cases. Opportunistic fungi cause about 3% of cases. Rare causative organisms include mycobacteria and some viruses and protozoa.

Many organisms that are normal flora on the skin and in the intestines are beneficial and pose no threat. But when they spread throughout the body by way of the bloodstream, they can progress to overwhelming infection unless body defenses destroy them. The organisms may gain entry through any alteration in the body's normal defenses or through artificial devices that penetrate the body, such as I.V., intra-arterial, and urinary catheters and knife or bullet wounds.

Initially, these defenses activate chemical mediators in response to the invading organisms. The release of these mediators results in low systemic vascular resistance and increased cardiac output. Blood flow is unevenly distributed in the microcirculation, and plasma leaking from capillaries causes functional hypovolemia. Eventually, cardiac output falls, and poor tissue perfusion and hypotension cause multisystem organ failure and death.

Septic shock can occur in any person with impaired immunity, but elderly people are at greatest risk. About two-thirds of septic shock cases occur in hospitalized patients, most of whom have underlying diseases. Those at high risk include patients with burns; chronic cardiac, hepatic, or renal disorders; diabetes mellitus; immunosuppression; malnutrition; stress; and excessive antibiotic use. Also at risk are patients who have had invasive diagnostic or therapeutic procedures, surgery, or traumatic wounds.

COMPLICATIONS

In septic shock, complications include disseminated intravascular coagulation, renal failure, heart failure, GI ulcers, and abnormal liver function.

ASSESSMENT

The patient's history may include a disorder or treatment that can cause immunosuppression. Or it may include a history of invasive tests or treatments, surgery, or trauma. It may also reveal a current history of an infection, especially arising from the urinary, biliary, or GI tract or the presence of a common infection source, such as an indwelling catheter or tube. At onset, the patient may have fever and chills, although 20% of patients may be hypothermic. For more information, see *Nursing care in septic shock,* pages 22 and 23.

The patient's signs and symptoms will reflect either the *hyperdynamic* or *warm phase* of septic shock (increased cardiac output, peripheral vasodilation, and decreased systemic vascular resistance) or the *hypodynamic* or *cold phase* (decreased cardiac output, peripheral vasoconstriction, increased systemic vascular resistance, and inadequate tissue perfusion).

In the hyperdynamic phase, the patient's skin may appear pink and flushed. His altered level of consciousness (LOC) is reflected in agitation, anxiety, irritability, and shortened attention span. Respirations will be rapid and shallow. Urine output is below normal.

Palpation of peripheral pulses may detect a rapid, full, bounding pulse. The skin may feel warm and dry. Blood pressure may be normal or slightly elevated.

In the hypodynamic phase, the patient's skin may appear pale and, possibly, cyanotic.

What happens in septic shock

Massive infection, most commonly from gram-negative bacteria, is the cause of septic shock. As the body fights the infection, the bacteria die, releasing endotoxins. These endotoxins, through as-yet-unknown mechanisms, impair cell metabolism and damage surrounding tissues. The damaged cells release lysosomal enzymes and histamine. The lysosomal enzymes travel through the bloodstream to other tissues, causing more cell damage. They also trigger the release of bradykinin, a powerful vasoactive substance. Combined with histamine from the damaged cells, bradykinin causes massive peripheral vasodilation and increased capillary permeability (the so-called warm stage of septic shock). This leads to increased third-space fluid shifting and relative hypovolemia. The heart's preload, afterload, and stroke volume all decrease, triggering compensation (the cool stage) in an attempt to stave off decompensation (the cold stage) and death.

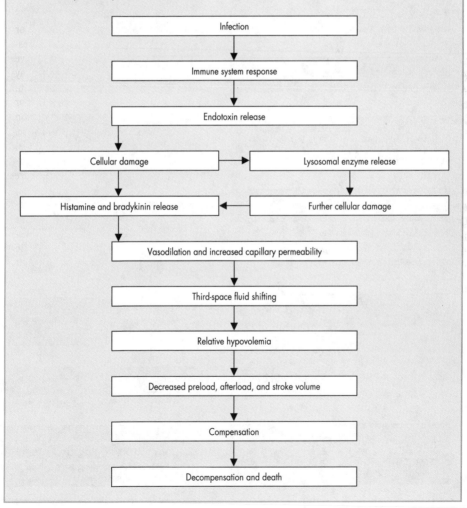

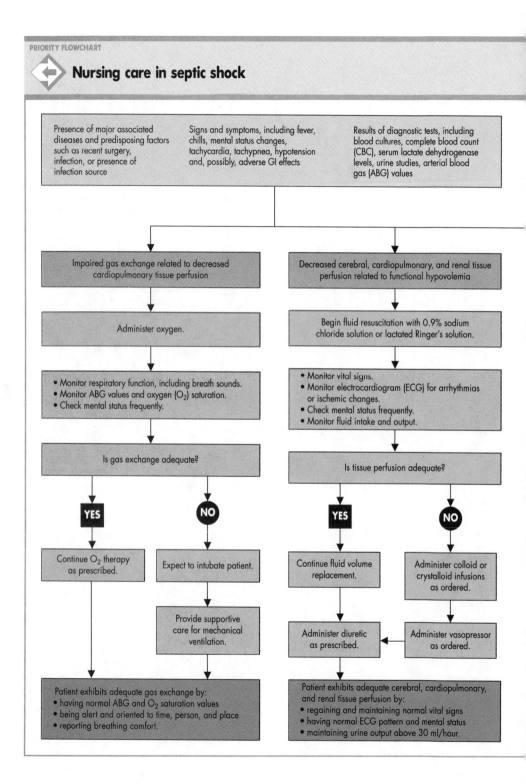

PRIORITY FLOWCHART

Nursing care in septic shock

Presence of major associated diseases and predisposing factors such as recent surgery, infection, or presence of infection source

Signs and symptoms, including fever, chills, mental status changes, tachycardia, tachypnea, hypotension and, possibly, adverse GI effects

Results of diagnostic tests, including blood cultures, complete blood count (CBC), serum lactate dehydrogenase levels, urine studies, arterial blood gas (ABG) values

Impaired gas exchange related to decreased cardiopulmonary tissue perfusion

Decreased cerebral, cardiopulmonary, and renal tissue perfusion related to functional hypovolemia

Administer oxygen.

Begin fluid resuscitation with 0.9% sodium chloride solution or lactated Ringer's solution.

• Monitor respiratory function, including breath sounds.
• Monitor ABG values and oxygen (O_2) saturation.
• Check mental status frequently.

• Monitor vital signs.
• Monitor electrocardiogram (ECG) for arrhythmias or ischemic changes.
• Check mental status frequently.
• Monitor fluid intake and output.

Is gas exchange adequate?

Is tissue perfusion adequate?

YES

NO

YES

NO

Continue O_2 therapy as prescribed.

Expect to intubate patient.

Continue fluid volume replacement.

Administer colloid or crystalloid infusions as ordered.

Provide supportive care for mechanical ventilation.

Administer diuretic as prescribed.

Administer vasopressor as ordered.

Patient exhibits adequate gas exchange by:
• having normal ABG and O_2 saturation values
• being alert and oriented to time, person, and place
• reporting breathing comfort.

Patient exhibits adequate cerebral, cardiopulmonary, and renal tissue perfusion by:
• regaining and maintaining normal vital signs
• having normal ECG pattern and mental status
• maintaining urine output above 30 ml/hour.

Peripheral areas may be mottled. His LOC may be decreased; obtundation and coma may be present. Respirations may be rapid and shallow, and urine output less than 25 ml/hour or absent.

Palpation of peripheral pulses may reveal no pulse or a rapid pulse that's weak or thready. It may also be irregular if arrhythmias are present. The skin may feel cold and clammy.

Auscultation of blood pressure may reveal hypotension, usually with a systolic pressure below 90 mm Hg or 50 to 80 mm Hg below the patient's previous level. Auscultation of the lungs may reveal crackles or rhonchi if pulmonary congestion is present.

If central pressures are being monitored, the pulmonary artery wedge pressure will be reduced or normal and cardiac output will be moderately to severely increased or normal. Rarely, cardiac output will be decreased.

DIAGNOSTIC TESTS

The following are characteristic laboratory findings:

• *Blood cultures* are positive for the offending organism.

• *Complete blood count (CBC)* shows the presence or absence of anemia and leukopenia, severe or absent neutropenia, and usually the presence of thrombocytopenia.

• *Serum lactate dehydrogenase levels* are elevated with metabolic acidosis.

• *Urine studies* show increased specific gravity (more than 1.020) and osmolality and decreased sodium.

• *Arterial blood gas (ABG) analysis* demonstrates elevated blood pH and partial pressure of oxygen and decreased partial pressure of carbon dioxide with respiratory alkalosis in early stages.

TREATMENT

Location and treatment of the underlying sepsis is essential to treating septic shock. If any I.V., intra-arterial, or urinary drainage catheters are in place, they should be removed. Aggressive antimicrobial therapy appropriate for the causative organism must be initiated immediately. Culture and sensitivity tests help

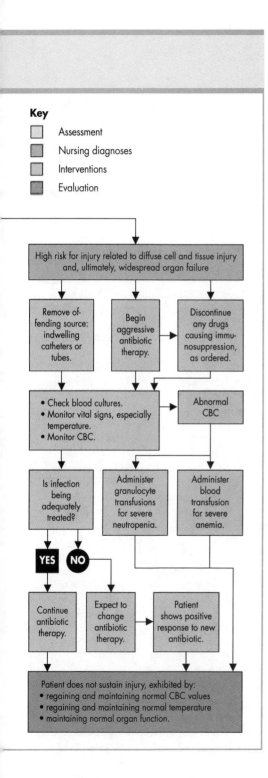

Key

☐ Assessment
▨ Nursing diagnoses
☐ Interventions
▦ Evaluation

High risk for injury related to diffuse cell and tissue injury and, ultimately, widespread organ failure

Remove offending source: indwelling catheters or tubes.

Begin aggressive antibiotic therapy.

Discontinue any drugs causing immunosuppression, as ordered.

• Check blood cultures.
• Monitor vital signs, especially temperature.
• Monitor CBC.

Abnormal CBC

Is infection being adequately treated?

Administer granulocyte transfusions for severe neutropenia.

Administer blood transfusion for severe anemia.

YES   NO

Continue antibiotic therapy.

Expect to change antibiotic therapy.

Patient shows positive response to new antibiotic.

Patient does not sustain injury, exhibited by:
• regaining and maintaining normal CBC values
• regaining and maintaining normal temperature
• maintaining normal organ function.

determine the most effective antimicrobial drug.

In patients who are immunosuppressed because of drug therapy, drugs should be discontinued or reduced. Granulocyte transfusions may be used in patients with severe neutropenia.

Oxygen therapy should be initiated to maintain arterial oxygen saturation above 95%. Mechanical ventilation may be required if respiratory failure occurs.

Colloid or crystalloid infusions are given to increase intravascular volume and raise blood pressure. After sufficient fluid volume has been replaced, diuretics such as furosemide can be given to maintain urine output greater than 30 ml/hour. If fluid resuscitation fails to increase blood pressure, a vasopressor such as dopamine can be started. Blood transfusion may be needed if anemia is present.

KEY NURSING DIAGNOSES AND PATIENT OUTCOMES

Altered tissue perfusion (cerebral, cardiopulmonary, and renal) related to functional hypovolemia. Based on this nursing diagnosis, you'll establish these patient outcomes. The patient will:
• regain and maintain adequate cardiac output
• regain and maintain stable vital signs, normal mental status, and urine output greater than 30 ml/hour
• remain free of chest pain and arrhythmias.

High risk for injury related to potential complications of septic shock. Based on this nursing diagnosis, you'll establish these patient outcomes. The patient will:
• regain and maintain a normal temperature and CBC
• maintain normal organ function
• show no permanent adverse effects from septic shock.

Impaired gas exchange related to decreased cardiopulmonary tissue perfusion. Based on this nursing diagnosis, you'll establish these patient outcomes. The patient will:
• regain and maintain normal ABG and oxygen saturation values

• remain alert and oriented to time, person, and place
• report breathing comfort.

NURSING INTERVENTIONS

• Remove any I.V., intra-arterial, or urinary drainage catheters and send them to the laboratory to culture for the presence of the causative organism. New catheters can be reinserted in the intensive care unit.
• Start an I.V. infusion with 0.9% sodium chloride or lactated Ringer's solution, using a large-bore (14G to 18G) catheter, which allows easier administration of later blood transfusions.

◆ NURSING ALERT. When the patient's blood pressure drops below 80 mm Hg, increase the oxygen flow rate and the I.V. infusion rate and notify the doctor immediately. A progressive drop in blood pressure accompanied by a thready pulse generally signals inadequate cardiac output from reduced intravascular volume.
• Administer appropriate antimicrobial drugs I.V. to achieve effective blood levels rapidly.
• If urine output falls below 30 ml/hour, increase the fluid infusion rate. Notify the doctor if urine output doesn't improve. A diuretic may be ordered to increase renal blood flow and urine output.
• Draw an arterial blood sample to measure ABG levels. Administer oxygen by face mask or airway to ensure adequate tissue oxygenation. Adjust the oxygen flow rate to a higher or lower level, as ABG measurements indicate.
• Provide emotional support to the patient and his family.
• Document the occurrence of a nosocomial infection and report it to the infection-control nurse. Investigation of all hospital-acquired infections can help identify their sources and prevent future infections.

Monitoring

• Record the patient's blood pressure, pulse and respiratory rates, and peripheral pulses every 1 to 5 minutes until he is stabilized. Record hemodynamic pressure readings every 15 minutes. Monitor cardiac rhythm continuously. Systolic blood pressure below

80 mm Hg usually results in inadequate coronary artery blood flow, cardiac ischemia, arrhythmias, and further complications of low cardiac output.
• Measure the patient's hourly urine output. Watch for signs of fluid overload, such as an increase in pulmonary artery wedge pressure.
• Monitor ABG values. Perform cardiopulmonary assessment frequently.
• Watch for complications associated with septic shock.

Patient teaching
• Explain all procedures and their purpose to ease the patient's anxiety.
• Explain the risks associated with blood transfusions to the patient and his family, and answer their questions.

TETANUS

Also referred to as lockjaw, tetanus is an acute exotoxin-mediated infection caused by the anaerobic, spore-forming, gram-positive bacillus *Clostridium tetani*. The infection usually is systemic, but it may be localized. Tetanus is a life-threatening infection. It is fatal in up to 60% of nonimmunized people, often within 10 days of onset. The disease's incubation period ranges from 3 to 4 weeks in mild tetanus to under 2 days in severe tetanus. When symptoms develop within 3 days of exposure, the prognosis is poor. In North America, about 75% of all cases occur between April and September.

Tetanus occurs worldwide, but it's more prevalent in agricultural regions and developing countries that lack mass immunization programs.

Once *C. tetani* enters the body, it causes local infection and tissue necrosis. It also produces toxins that enter the bloodstream and lymphatics and eventually spread to central nervous system tissue.

CAUSES
Transmission occurs through a puncture wound that is contaminated by soil, dust, or animal excreta containing *C. tetani*, or by way of burns or minor wounds.

COMPLICATIONS
Atelectasis, pneumonia, pulmonary emboli, acute gastric ulcers, flexion contractures, and cardiac arrhythmias can result from tetanus.

ASSESSMENT
The patient's history may reveal inadequate immunization, and the patient may report a recent skin wound or burn. He may complain of pain or paresthesia at the site of injury and recall early complaints of difficulty chewing or swallowing food. He usually has a normal body temperature or a slight fever in the early stages, but his fever may rise as the disease progresses.

If the tetanus remains localized, your assessment may disclose signs of spasm and increased muscle tone near the wound.

If the tetanus becomes systemic, your assessment may reveal an irregular heartbeat, marked muscle hypertonicity, hyperactive deep tendon reflexes, tachycardia, profuse sweating, low-grade fever, and painful, involuntary muscle contractions. Specific findings may include:
• rigid neck and facial muscles (especially cheek muscles), resulting in lockjaw (trismus) and a grotesque, grinning expression called risus sardonicus
• rigid somatic muscles, causing arched-back rigidity (opisthotonos); palpation reveals boardlike abdominal rigidity
• intermittent tonic seizures that last for several minutes and may result in cyanosis and sudden death by asphyxiation.

Despite such pronounced neuromuscular symptoms, assessment shows normal cerebral and sensory function.

Identifying antitoxin dosage in tetanus

In emergency treatment of tetanus for patients with no previous history of immunization, give an adult 10,000 to 20,000 units of equine tetanus antitoxin injected into the wound. Give an additional 40,000 to 100,000 units I.V.

DIAGNOSTIC TESTS

Blood cultures and tetanus antibody tests commonly are negative; only one-third of patients have a positive wound culture. Cerebrospinal fluid pressure may rise above normal.

TREATMENT

Within 72 hours of a puncture wound, a patient with no previous history of tetanus immunization first requires tetanus immune globulin or tetanus antitoxin to confer temporary protection. (See *Identifying antitoxin dosage in tetanus.*) Next, he needs active immunization with tetanus toxoid. A patient who hasn't received tetanus immunization within 5 years needs a booster injection of tetanus toxoid.

If tetanus develops despite immediate post-injury treatment, the patient will require airway maintenance and a muscle relaxant such as diazepam to decrease muscle rigidity and spasm. If muscle contractions aren't relieved by muscle relaxants, a neuromuscular blocker may be needed.

The patient with tetanus also requires high-dose antibiotics – preferably penicillin (administered I.V.), if he's not allergic to it. If he is allergic to penicillin, tetracycline can be substituted.

KEY NURSING DIAGNOSES AND PATIENT OUTCOMES

High risk for injury related to intermittent tonic seizures that may result in cyanosis and asphyxiation. Based on this nursing diagnosis, you'll establish these patient outcomes. The patient will:

• have seizure activity identifed immediately and treated promptly
• exhibit normal neurologic function following each seizure.

Ineffective airway clearance related to rigid neck muscles. Based on this nursing diagnosis, you'll establish these patient outcomes. The patient will:

• maintain a patent airway
• not have dyspnea or a change in respiratory pattern
• maintain adequate ventilation, as evidenced by clear breath sounds and normal arterial blood gas values.

Pain related to intense muscle rigidity and spasms. Based on this nursing diagnosis, you'll establish these patient outcomes. The patient will:

• identify activities and body movements that precipitate or increase pain, and make nurses aware of them
• adhere to activity restrictions to decrease or prevent painful muscle spasms
• report pain relief following administration of a muscle relaxant.

NURSING INTERVENTIONS

• Before tetanus develops, thoroughly debride and clean the injury site with 3% hydrogen peroxide and check the patient's immunization history. Record the cause of the injury. If it was caused by an animal bite, report the case to local public health authorities.
• Before giving penicillin and tetanus immune globulin, antitoxin, or toxoid, obtain an accurate history of the patient's allergies to immunizations or penicillin. If the patient has a history of any allergies, keep epinephrine 1:1,000 (for subcutaneous injection) and emergency airway equipment available.
• After tetanus develops, maintain an adequate airway and ventilation to prevent pneumonia and atelectasis. Suction as needed.
• Insert an artificial airway, if necessary, to prevent tongue injury and maintain the airway during spasms.
• Keep emergency airway equipment on hand because the patient may require artificial ventilation or oxygen administration. Have endotracheal and tracheotomy equipment on

hand. In an emergency, the doctor may perform a tracheotomy if the patient becomes extremely rigid.
• Be prepared to resuscitate the patient and initiate life support.
• Administer I.V. therapy as prescribed.
• Because even minimal external stimulation provokes muscle spasms, keep the patient's room dark and quiet. Warn visitors not to upset or overly stimulate the patient.
• Turn the patient frequently to prevent contractures, pressure ulcers, and pulmonary stasis. Perform range-of-motion exercises to maintain flexibility.
• Place the patient on an air mattress, and use other skin protective measures as warranted.
• Perform all activities of daily living for the sedated patient.
• Give muscle relaxants and sedatives, as ordered, and schedule patient care to coincide with heaviest sedation.
• If urine retention develops, insert an indwelling urinary catheter.
• Provide adequate nutrition to meet the patient's increased metabolic needs. He may need nasogastric feedings or total parenteral nutrition.

Monitoring
• Evaluate the patient's respiratory status continuously, and watch for signs of respiratory distress.
• Monitor intake and output.
• Frequently check the patient's electrocardiogram for arrhythmias. Also monitor vital signs.
• Check the patient's skin for signs of pressure ulcers.
• Monitor the patient's nutritional status. Watch for signs of rapid weight loss and nutritional deficits because of the patient's increased metabolic needs.
• Assess the patient for increased muscle spasms and rigidity and for the effectiveness of administered muscle relaxants.

Patient teaching
• During the patient's convalescence, encourage gradual active exercises.
• Institute a bladder retraining program if the patient was catheterized.
• Stress the importance of maintaining active immunization with a booster dose of tetanus toxoid every 10 years.
• Inform the patient with a skin injury or burn that he should receive tetanus prophylaxis.

BOTULISM

This life-threatening paralytic illness results from an exotoxin produced by the gram-positive, anaerobic bacillus *Clostridium botulinum*. It occurs as botulism food poisoning or wound botulism.

Botulism occurs worldwide and affects adults more often than children. The incidence of botulism in the United States had been declining, but the current trend toward home canning has resulted in an upswing in recent years.

The mortality rate is about 25%, with death most often caused by respiratory failure during the first week of illness. Onset within 24 hours of ingestion signals critical and potentially fatal illness.

CAUSES
Botulism usually results from eating improperly preserved foods, such as home-canned fruits and vegetables, sausages, and smoked or preserved fish or meat. Rarely, it results from wound infection with *C. botulinum*.

COMPLICATIONS
Botulism can result in respiratory failure and paralytic ileus.

ASSESSMENT
The patient may report having eaten home-canned food 12 to 36 hours before the onset of symptoms.

The patient may complain of vertigo, dry mouth, sore throat, weakness, nausea, vomiting, and constipation or diarrhea. Concur-

Identifying antitoxin dosage in botulism

For emergency treatment of botulism, give an adult 1 vial I.V. stat and then every 4 hours p.r.n. until the patient's condition improves. Dilute the antitoxin 1:10 in dextrose 5% or 10% in water or 0.9% sodium chloride solution. Give the first 10 ml of dilution over 5 minutes; after 15 minutes, the rate may be increased.

rently or up to 3 days later, he may report diplopia, blurred vision, dysarthria, and dysphagia from cranial nerve impairment. Later, he may experience dyspnea from muscle weakness or paralysis. His body temperature remains normal.

The patient may appear alert and oriented on inspection. Ocular signs may include ptosis and dilated, nonreactive pupils. Oral mucous membranes commonly appear dry, red, and crusted.

Palpation may reveal abdominal distention with absent bowel sounds.

Further assessment may disclose descending weakness or paralysis of muscles in the extremities or trunk—the major physical finding in botulism. The patient's deep tendon reflexes may be intact, diminished, or absent. He won't have pathologic reflexes or sensory impairment.

DIAGNOSTIC TESTS
Identification of the exotoxin in the patient's serum, stool, or gastric contents or in the suspected food confirms the diagnosis. An electromyogram showing diminished muscle action potential after a single supramaximal nerve stimulus also is diagnostic.

Diagnosis must rule out conditions often confused with botulism, such as Guillain-Barré syndrome, myasthenia gravis, cerebrovascular accident, staphylococcal food poisoning, tick paralysis, chemical intoxication, carbon monoxide poisoning, fish poisoning, trichinosis, and diphtheria.

TREATMENT
Appropriate treatment consists of I.V. or I.M. administration of botulinum antitoxin, which is available through the Centers for Disease Control and Prevention. (See *Identifying antitoxin dosage in botulism.*)

Early elective tracheotomy and ventilatory assistance can be lifesaving in respiratory failure. The patient will need nasogastric suctioning and total parenteral nutrition (TPN) if he develops significant paralytic ileus.

KEY NURSING DIAGNOSES AND PATIENT OUTCOMES
Anxiety related to the threat of death. Based on this nursing diagnosis, you'll establish these patient outcomes. The patient will:
• state feelings of anxiety
• use support systems to assist with coping
• demonstrate abated physical symptoms of anxiety.

High risk for aspiration related to muscle weakness and dysphagia. Based on this nursing diagnosis, you'll establish these patient outcomes. The patient will:
• show no signs of aspiration
• maintain clear and odorless respiratory secretions
• exhibit normal breath sounds.

Ineffective breathing pattern related to decreased respiratory muscle function. Based on this nursing diagnosis, you'll establish these patient outcomes. The patient will:
• maintain adequate ventilation
• maintain normal arterial blood gas (ABG) values
• recover and maintain normal breathing pattern.

NURSING INTERVENTIONS
• If you suspect the patient ate contaminated food, obtain a careful history of his food intake for the past several days. Determine if other family members exhibit similar symptoms and ate the same food.
• If the patient ate the food within the last several hours, induce vomiting, begin gastric lavage, and give a high enema to purge any unabsorbed toxin from the bowel. Family mem-

bers or friends who ate the same food also should receive this treatment.

• If clinical signs of botulism appear, have the patient admitted to the intensive care unit (isolation isn't required).

• Before giving the antitoxin, obtain an accurate patient history of allergies, especially to horses, and perform a skin test. Then administer botulinum antitoxin, as ordered, to neutralize any circulating toxin. Keep epinephrine 1:1,000 (for subcutaneous administration) and emergency airway equipment available.

• If the patient has difficulty swallowing, initiate nasogastric tube feedings or TPN, as ordered. Suction the patient as needed.

• Administer I.V. fluids as ordered.

• Turn the patient often, and encourage deep-breathing exercises. Position him in proper alignment, and assist with range-of-motion exercises.

• If the patient has difficulty speaking, try to anticipate his needs. Assure him that this symptom will pass, and establish an alternative method of communication.

• Because botulism sometimes is fatal, keep the patient and family informed about the course of the disease. Also provide opportunities for the patient and family to express anxieties and concerns.

• Immediately report all cases of botulism to local public health authorities.

Monitoring

• Monitor cardiac and respiratory function carefully. Assess vital capacity frequently; report reduced vital capacity, reduced inspiratory effort, or respiratory distress.

• If the patient is on mechanical ventilation, monitor his ABG values to detect signs of hyperventilation or hypoventilation.

• Observe the patient carefully for abnormal neurologic signs.

• Closely assess and record the patient's neurologic function, including bilateral motor status (reflexes and ability to move his arms and legs). Check the patient's cough and gag reflexes.

• Monitor intake and output.

• After administering botulinum antitoxin, watch for anaphylaxis or other hypersensitivity reactions as well as serum sickness.

Patient teaching

• If ingestion of contaminated food is suspected but the patient returns home before neurologic symptoms occur, advise him and his family to watch for such signs as weakness, blurred vision, and slurred speech. Tell them to return the patient to the hospital immediately if such signs appear.

• To help prevent botulism in the future, encourage the patient and his family to use proper techniques in processing and preserving foods. Warn them to avoid even *tasting* food from a bulging can or one with a peculiar odor and to sterilize by boiling any utensil that contacts suspected food. Explain that eating even a small amount of food contaminated with botulism toxin can prove fatal.

GAS GANGRENE

This rare condition is caused by local infection with the anaerobic, spore-forming, gram-positive, rod-shaped bacillus *Clostridium perfringens* or another clostridial species. It occurs in devitalized tissues and results from compromised arterial circulation after trauma or surgery. The usual incubation period is 1 to 4 days but can vary from 3 hours to 6 weeks or longer.

Gas gangrene carries a high mortality unless therapy begins immediately. With prompt treatment, 80% of patients with gas gangrene of the extremities survive; the prognosis is poorer for gas gangrene in other sites, such as the abdominal wall or the bowel.

CAUSES

The organism most often responsible, *C. perfringens,* is a normal inhabitant of the GI tract and of the female genitourinary tract; it's also prevalent in soil. Transmission occurs when the organism enters the body during trauma or surgery.

Because *C. perfringens* is anaerobic, gas gangrene occurs most frequently in deep

Effects of *Clostridium perfringens*

When *C. perfringens* invades a closed wound, it destroys cell walls and causes hemolysis, local tissue death, and increasing edema.

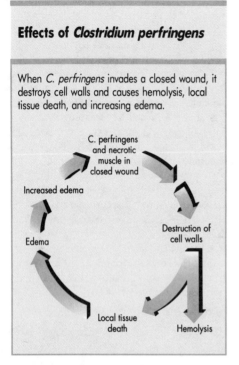

typically complains of sudden, severe pain at the wound site.

Your assessment in the early stages may show a normal body temperature, followed by a moderate rise, usually not above 101° F (38.3° C). Other assessment findings may include hypotension, tachycardia, and tachypnea, all signs of toxemia.

Inspection may reveal localized swelling and discoloration (often dusky brown or reddish), with formation of bullae and necrosis within 36 hours from the onset of symptoms. Soon the skin over the wound may rupture, revealing dark red or black necrotic muscle, accompanied by a foul-smelling, watery or frothy discharge. The patient may appear pale, prostrate, and motionless because of systemic toxicity but usually remains alert and oriented and is extremely apprehensive.

Palpation may detect subcutaneous emphysema (the presence of gas in the soft tissues), the hallmark of gas gangrene.

In later stages, the patient's level of consciousness may deteriorate to delirium and coma.

DIAGNOSTIC TESTS

Several tests confirm the diagnosis of gas gangrene:
• *Anaerobic cultures* of wound drainage show *C. perfringens.*
• *A Gram stain* of wound drainage discloses large, gram-positive, rod-shaped bacteria.
• *X-rays* reveal gas in tissues.
• *Blood studies* show leukocytosis and, later, hemolysis.

Diagnostic tests must rule out synergistic gangrene and necrotizing fasciitis. Unlike gas gangrene, both of these disorders anesthetize the skin around the wound.

wounds, especially those in which tissue necrosis further reduces the oxygen supply. When *C. perfringens* invades soft tissues, it produces thrombosis of regional blood vessels, tissue necrosis, and localized edema. Such necrosis releases both carbon dioxide and hydrogen subcutaneously, producing interstitial gas bubbles.

Gas gangrene occurs most commonly in the extremities and in abdominal wounds and less often in the uterus. (See *Effects of* Clostridium perfringens.)

COMPLICATIONS

Possible complications include renal failure, hypotension, hemolytic anemia, and tissue death, requiring amputation of the affected body part.

ASSESSMENT

The patient's medical history may reveal recent surgery (within 72 hours), traumatic injury, septic abortion, or delivery. The patient

TREATMENT

Appropriate treatment includes careful observation for signs of myositis and cellulitis. The patient needs *immediate treatment* if these signs appear and *immediate* wide surgical excision of all affected tissues and necrotic muscle in myositis. Delayed or inadequate surgical excision is fatal.

The patient also needs I.V. administration of high-dose penicillin and, after adequate debridement, hyperbaric oxygenation, if available. For 1 to 3 hours every 6 to 8 hours, the patient is placed in a hyperbaric chamber and exposed to pressures designed to increase oxygen tension and prevent multiplication of the anaerobic clostridia. Surgery may take place within the hyperbaric chamber if the chamber is large enough.

KEY NURSING DIAGNOSES AND PATIENT OUTCOMES

Fear related to threat of death or loss of a body part caused by gas gangrene. Based on this nursing diagnosis, you'll establish these patient outcomes. The patient will:
• identify sources of fear
• state understanding of procedures being used to save the affected extremity or his life or both
• use available support systems to assist in coping with fear.

High risk for peripheral neurovascular dysfunction related to thrombosis of regional blood vessels and tissue necrosis. Based on this nursing diagnosis, you'll establish these patient outcomes. The patient will:
• maintain circulation in extremities
• express understanding of risk for altered neurovascular status and the need to report symptoms of impaired circulation to the nurse immediately
• not experience disability related to peripheral neurovascular dysfunction after injury or treatment.

Impaired tissue integrity related to tissue necrosis. Based on this nursing diagnosis, you'll establish these patient outcomes. The patient will:
• maintain adequate fluid and nutritional intake for tissue building
• express feelings of comfort
• maintain adequate circulation at site of injury.

NURSING INTERVENTIONS

• Provide the patient with adequate fluid replacement throughout his illness.
• Maintain a patent airway and ensure ventilation.

• To prevent skin breakdown and further infection, provide good skin care. Place the patient on an air mattress or an air-fluidized bed.
• After surgery, provide meticulous wound care.
• Deodorize the room to control foul odor from the wound. Prepare the patient emotionally for a large wound after surgical excision and for possible daily debridement. The wound usually is left open and requires frequent dressing changes and soaks.
• Institute wound precautions. Dispose of drainage material properly (double-bag dressings in plastic bags for incineration), and wear sterile gloves when changing dressings. No special cleaning measures are required after the patient is discharged.
• After recovery, refer the patient for physical rehabilitation as necessary.
• For the patient who won't survive, psychological support is critical. The patient may remain alert until death, knowing that death is imminent and unavoidable.
• To prevent gas gangrene, routinely take precautions to prevent the growth of clostridia at wound sites by attempting to keep granulation tissue viable. Adequate debridement is imperative to reduce anaerobic growth conditions. Be alert for devitalized tissues, and promptly tell the surgeon if you notice any. Position the patient to facilitate drainage, and eliminate all dead spaces in closed wounds.

Monitoring

• Assess vital signs, intake and output, and central venous pressure, and monitor pulmonary and cardiac function often to detect impending complications or changes in the patient's condition.
• Before penicillin administration, obtain a patient history of allergies. Afterward, watch closely for signs of a hypersensitivity reaction.
• Assess the affected site regularly for evidence of deterioration in circulation and neurovascular function.
• Monitor the patient's and the family's emotional state throughout treatment.

Patient teaching

• Instruct any patient who reports sudden, severe, and persistent pain at a wound site to consult a doctor immediately.

ROCKY MOUNTAIN SPOTTED FEVER

An acute infectious, febrile, and rash-producing illness, Rocky Mountain spotted fever is associated with outdoor activities, such as camping and hiking. Endemic throughout the continental United States, the disease is particularly prevalent in the southeastern, southwestern, southern, and eastern states. As outdoor activities increase in popularity, so does the risk of contracting Rocky Mountain spotted fever—especially in the spring and summer months.

Without early and appropriate treatment, the disease can be fatal (with mortality up to 40%). Appropriate treatment reduces the risk of death to less than 10%. The usual incubation period is 7 days, but it can range from 2 to 12 days. As a rule, the shorter the incubation time, the more severe the infection.

CAUSES

The *Rickettsia rickettsii* organism causes Rocky Mountain spotted fever. Transmitted by the wood tick (*Dermacentor andersoni*) in the western United States and by the dog tick (*D. variabilis*) in the eastern United States, this rickettsial organism enters humans or small animals via the prolonged bite (4 to 6 hours) of an adult tick. Occasionally, this disease is acquired through inhalation or through contact of abraded skin with tick excreta or tissue juices. (This explains why people shouldn't crush ticks between their fingers when removing them from others.) In most tick-infested areas, 1% to 5% of the ticks harbor *R. rickettsii.*

COMPLICATIONS

Although uncommon, complications can include lobar pneumonia, pneumonitis, otitis media, parotitis, disseminated intravascular coagulation (DIC), shock, and renal failure.

ASSESSMENT

The patient's history may show recent exposure to ticks or tick-infested areas, or a known tick bite, although about 25% of patients with the disease have no history of a tick bite.

The patient typically complains of symptoms that began abruptly, including a persistent fever with temperature ranging between 102° and 104° F (38.9° to 40° C); generalized, excruciating headache; and aching in the bones, muscles, joints, and back. He also may report anorexia, nausea, vomiting, constipation, and abdominal pain.

Inspection may disclose the tongue covered with a thick white coating that gradually turns brown as the fever persists and the patient's temperature rises. The skin initially may appear flushed, but in 2 to 5 days, eruptions begin at the wrists, ankles, or forehead and spread centrally. Within 2 days, the rash covers the entire body (including the scalp, palms, and soles). It consists of erythematous macules 1 to 5 mm in diameter that blanch on pressure. Untreated, the rash may become petechial and maculopapular. By the third week, the skin peels off; sometimes gangrene develops over the elbows, fingers, and toes.

The patient may have a bronchial cough, a rapid respiratory rate (up to 60 breaths/minute), insomnia, restlessness and, in extreme cases, delirium and circulatory collapse. Urine output decreases considerably, and the urine, which appears dark, contains albumin.

At disease onset, palpation may reveal a strong pulse, which gradually becomes rapid (possibly reaching 150 beats/minute) and thready. The rapid pulse rate and hypotension (below 90 mm Hg systolic) herald imminent death from vascular collapse. Additionally, you may detect hepatomegaly, splenomegaly, and generalized pitting edema. Postauricular adenopathy may be palpated on one side if the tick bit the patient's head.

DIAGNOSTIC TESTS

Blood cultures to isolate the rickettsial organism can confirm the diagnosis. Some laboratories conduct direct immunofluorescence of cutaneous tissue to detect *R. rickettsii.*

Serologic tests performed during the patient's convalescence can confirm the diagnosis retrospectively. Four tests are performed together (separately, test findings are nonspecific). Diagnostically significant findings include:
• complement fixation titer – 1:16 or more
• indirect hemagglutination titer – 1:128 or more
• indirect immunofluorescence titer – 1:64 or more
• latex agglutination titer – 1:64 or more.

Other laboratory test findings may include a decreased platelet count, white blood cell count, and fibrinogen levels; prolonged prothrombin time and partial thromboplastin time; decreased serum protein levels, especially albumin; hyponatremia and hypochloremia associated with increased aldosterone excretion; and abnormal hepatic function.

Mild mononuclear pleocytosis with slightly elevated protein content in cerebrospinal fluid is common.

TREATMENT

In Rocky Mountain spotted fever, treatment requires careful removal of the tick and administration of antibiotics, such as tetracycline or chloramphenicol, until 3 days after the fever subsides. Treatment also involves measures to relieve symptoms. If DIC occurs, treatment includes heparin administration and platelet transfusion.

KEY NURSING DIAGNOSES AND PATIENT OUTCOMES

Decreased cardiac output related to tachycardia and hypotension caused by Rocky Mountain spotted fever. Based on this nursing diagnosis, you'll establish these patient outcomes. The patient will:
• maintain hemodynamic stability
• regain and maintain adequate cardiac output reflected by a normal heart rate and blood pressure
• exhibit no profound signs and symptoms of circulatory collapse as a result of decreased cardiac output.

Hyperthermia related to the inflammatory process caused by Rocky Mountain spotted fever. Based on this nursing diagnosis, you'll establish these patient outcomes. The patient will:
• regain and maintain a normal temperature
• not have signs and symptoms of complications associated with hyperthermia, such as seizures or dehydration.

Ineffective breathing pattern related to extreme tachypnea caused by the infectious process of Rocky Mountain spotted fever. Based on this nursing diagnosis, you'll establish these patient outcomes. The patient will:
• regain and maintain a normal respiratory rate
• maintain adequate gas exchange exhibited by normal arterial blood gas and oxygen saturation values
• not show signs and symptoms of hypoxia.

NURSING INTERVENTIONS

• Administer analgesics as ordered. Avoid giving aspirin, which increases the patient's risk of bleeding.
• Give antipyretic medications, as ordered, and tepid sponge baths to reduce fever.
• Administer antibiotics at ordered administration times.
• Be prepared to provide oxygen therapy and assisted ventilation for pulmonary complications.
• Adjust the I.V. fluid infusion rate hourly, as prescribed. Deliver enough fluids to prevent dehydration, provided the patient has adequate urine output.
• Provide meticulous mouth and skin care. Offer mentholated lotions to soothe itching resulting from the rash.
• Frequently turn the patient to prevent pressure sores and pneumonia. Encourage incentive spirometry and deep breathing to reduce the patient's risk of atelectasis.
• Plan care to promote adequate rest periods.

• Provide frequent, small, high-protein, high-calorie meals, or administer tube feedings if needed.
• Closely supervise the patient. Use restraining devices only if necessary. Administer sedatives, as ordered. Implement any safety measures needed to prevent patient injury.

Monitoring

• Assess vital signs, and watch for profound hypotension and shock.
• Record intake and output. Watch closely for decreased urine output – a possible indicator of renal failure.
• Observe for petechiae.
• Monitor the patient for complications of the disease and for adverse effects of medications.
• Evaluate the patient's daily nutritional intake. Weigh him regularly.

Patient teaching

• Instruct the patient to report any recurrent symptoms to the doctor at once so that treatment can resume promptly.
• To prevent Rocky Mountain spotted fever, advise the patient to avoid tick-infested areas. If he does frequent these areas, instruct him to inspect his entire body (including his scalp) every 3 to 4 hours for attached ticks. Remind him to wear protective clothing, such as a long-sleeved shirt and slacks that are firmly tucked into laced boots. Tell him to apply insect repellant to clothes and exposed skin.
• Teach patients and caregivers how to correctly remove ticks with tweezers or forceps and steady traction. Show them how to avoid leaving mouth parts in skin. Instruct them not to handle the tick or tick fragments.

3
Immune and hematologic disorders

Although most immune and hematologic disorders are chronic, some may be acute and life-threatening. For instance, anaphylaxis reflects a fulminating immune response to an antigen. Another perilous condition, disseminated intravascular coagulation (DIC), occurs as a life-threatening complication of another disease or condition. Yet another, sickle cell crisis, a complication of sickle cell anemia, constitutes a medical emergency. These three disorders—discussed in this section—are frequently fatal if not recognized and treated early.

Because anaphylaxis, DIC, and sickle cell crisis can strike rapidly, you may be the one to detect them. Your astute assessment skills coupled with effective interventions can help halt the progression or reduce the severity of the disorder. Afterward, giving supportive care—including fluid, blood, and medication administration—can help prevent complications.

Check for:
- □ history of immune or hematologic disorders
- □ recent infection, illness, cold exposure, or stress
- □ recent unexplained bruises, hematomas, epistaxis, or other bleeding
- □ recent surgery or other invasive procedures
- □ history of allergies
- □ family history of immune or hematologic disorders
- □ changes in vital signs
- □ altered mental status
- □ neurologic deficits
- □ changes in skin color and temperature
- □ presence and severity of pain
- □ urticaria and angioedema
- □ dyspnea
- □ decreased urine output.

Intervene by:
- □ notifying the doctor
- □ obtaining emergency drugs and equipment
- □ initiating cardiopulmonary resuscitation, if indicated
- □ starting an I.V. line with a large-gauge needle
- □ trying to stop uncontrolled bleeding, if present.

Prepare for:
- □ emergency drug administration
- □ rapid blood or fluid replacement therapy or both
- □ oxygen administration
- □ hemodynamic monitoring.

ANAPHYLAXIS

A dramatic, acute atopic reaction, anaphylaxis is marked by the sudden onset of rapidly progressive urticaria and respiratory distress. A severe reaction may initiate vascular collapse, leading to systemic shock and possibly death.

CAUSES

Anaphylactic reactions result from systemic exposure to sensitizing drugs or other specific antigens. Such substances may be serums (usually horse serum), vaccines, allergen extracts (such as pollen), enzymes (L-asparaginase), hormones, penicillin and other antibiotics, sulfonamides, local anesthetics, salicylates, polysaccharides (such as iron dextran), diagnostic chemicals (sodium dehydrocholate, radiographic contrast media), foods (legumes, nuts, berries, seafood, egg albumin) and sulfite-containing food additives, insect venom (honeybees, wasps, hornets, yellow jackets, fire ants, and certain spiders) and, rarely, a ruptured hydatid cyst.

The most common anaphylaxis-causing antigen is penicillin. This drug induces a reaction in 1 to 4 of every 10,000 patients treated with it. Penicillin is most likely to induce anaphylaxis after parenteral administration or prolonged therapy.

After initial exposure to an antigen, the immune system responds by producing specific immunoglobulin (Ig) antibodies in the lymph nodes. Helper T cells enhance the process. These antibodies (IgE) then bind to membrane receptors located on mast cells (found throughout connective tissue) and basophils.

Once the body reencounters the antigen, the IgE antibodies, or cross-linked IgE receptors, recognize the antigen as foreign. This activates a series of cellular reactions that, if left unchecked, will lead to rapid vascular collapse and, ultimately, hemorrhage, disseminated intravascular coagulation, and cardiopulmonary arrest. (For more information on this process, see *What happens in an anaphylactic reaction,* pages 38 and 39.)

COMPLICATIONS

Untreated anaphylaxis causes respiratory obstruction, systemic vascular collapse, and death minutes to hours after the first symptoms (although a delayed or persistent reaction may occur for as long as 24 hours).

ASSESSMENT

The patient, a relative, or another responsible person will report the patient's exposure to an antigen. Immediately after exposure, the patient may complain of a feeling of impending doom or fright, weakness, sweating, sneezing, dyspnea, nasal pruritus, and urticaria. He may impress you as extremely anxious. Keep in mind that the sooner signs and symptoms begin after exposure to the antigen, the more severe the anaphylaxis.

On inspection, the patient's skin may display well-circumscribed, discrete cutaneous wheals with erythematous, raised, serpiginous borders and blanched centers. They may coalesce to form giant hives.

Angioedema may cause the patient to complain of a "lump" in his throat, or you may hear hoarseness or stridor. Wheezing, dyspnea, and complaints of chest tightness suggest bronchial obstruction. These are early signs of impending, potentially fatal respiratory failure.

Other effects may follow rapidly. The patient may report GI and genitourinary effects, including severe stomach cramps, nausea, diarrhea, and urinary urgency and incontinence. Neurologic effects include dizziness, drowsiness, headache, restlessness, and seizures. Cardiovascular effects include hypotension, shock and, sometimes, cardiac arrhythmias, which may precipitate vascular collapse if untreated.

DIAGNOSTIC TESTS

No tests are required to identify anaphylaxis. The patient's history and signs and symptoms establish the diagnosis. If signs and symptoms occur without a known allergic stimulus, other possible causes of shock, such as acute myocardial infarction, status asthmaticus, or congestive heart failure, must be ruled out.

Skin testing may help to identify a specific allergen. However, because skin tests can cause serious reactions, a scratch test should be done first in high-risk situations.

TREATMENT

Always an emergency, anaphylaxis requires an *immediate* injection of epinephrine. In the early stages of anaphylaxis, when the patient remains conscious and normotensive, give epinephrine I.M. or subcutaneously. Speed it into circulation by massaging the injection site. In severe reactions, when the patient is unconscious and hypotensive, give the drug I.V., as ordered.

Other drugs commonly used in the treatment of anaphylaxis include diphenhydramine, hydrocortisone, aminophylline, and cimetidine. (For more information on epinephrine and these drugs, see *Drugs commonly used to treat anaphylactic shock,* page 40.)

Establish and maintain a patent airway. Watch for early signs of laryngeal edema (stridor, hoarseness, and dyspnea), which will probably require endotracheal tube insertion or a tracheotomy and oxygen therapy.

If cardiac arrest occurs, begin cardiopulmonary resuscitation. Assist with ventilation, closed-chest cardiac massage, and sodium bicarbonate administration as ordered.

Watch for hypotension and shock. As ordered, maintain circulatory volume with volume expanders (plasma, plasma expanders, 0.9% sodium chloride solution, and albumin) as needed. As ordered, administer I.V. vasopressors, norepinephrine, and dopamine to stabilize the patient's blood pressure. Monitor blood pressure, central venous pressure, and urine output.

KEY NURSING DIAGNOSES AND PATIENT OUTCOMES

Anxiety related to the rapid deterioration in body function and a feeling of impending doom. Based on this nursing diagnosis, you'll establish these patient outcomes. The patient will:
• express feelings of anxiety
• demonstrate diminished physical symptoms of anxiety following reassurance and support from health professionals and treatment of anaphylaxis.

Decreased cardiac output related to shock, hypotension, and vascular collapse. Based on this nursing diagnosis, you'll establish these patient outcomes. The patient will:
• attain hemodynamic stability, evidenced by normal vital signs and relief of anaphylactic signs and symptoms
• not exhibit cardiac arrhythmias
• recover and maintain normal cardiac output.

High risk for suffocation related to swelling and edema in respiratory tract caused by anaphylaxis. Based on this nursing diagnosis, you'll establish these patient outcomes. The patient will:
• maintain adequate ventilation
• experience relief of respiratory symptoms, indicating that respiratory tissues have returned to normal
• identify or seek to identify the offending allergen that precipitated anaphylaxis and take steps to prevent future episodes of anaphylaxis.

NURSING INTERVENTIONS

• Provide supplemental oxygen, and observe the patient's response. If hypoxia continues, prepare to help insert an artificial airway.
• Insert a peripheral I.V. line for administering emergency drugs and volume expanders.
• Administer ordered medications: epinephrine, corticosteroids, diphenhydramine, cimetidine, and aminophylline.

◆ NURSING ALERT. Be aware that rapid infusion of aminophylline may cause or aggravate severe hypotension in a patient experiencing an allergic reaction. If aminophylline must be used, administer it under the direct supervision of a doctor and monitor the patient's blood pressure continuously. Have emergency equipment close by.
• Continually reassure the patient, and explain all tests and treatments to reduce his fear and anxiety. If necessary, reorient the patient to the situation and surroundings.
• If the patient undergoes skin or scratch testing, keep emergency resuscitation equipment nearby during and after the test.

(Text continues on page 41.)

What happens in an anaphylactic reaction

An anaphylactic reaction requires previous sensitization or exposure to the specific antigen. These illustrations show what happens during the reaction.

Response to the antigen

Immunoglobulin M (IgM) and IgG recognize the antigen as a foreign substance and attach themselves to it.

The antigen destruction process, called the *complement cascade,* begins but can't finish either because of insufficient amounts of protein catalyst A or because the antigen rejects certain complement destruction enzymes. At this stage, the patient has no signs or symptoms.

Release of chemical mediators

The antigen's continued presence activates IgE (attached to basophils and mast cells). The activated IgE causes degranulation (cell membrane breakdown) of basophils and mast cells, causing mediators within these cells to leak. These mediators include histamine, serotonin, slow-reacting substance of anaphylaxis (SRS-A), eosinophil chemotactic factor of anaphylaxis (ECF-A), platelet-activating factor (PAF), prostaglandins, and bradykinins.

Histamine induces generalized vasodilation, increased vascular permeability, increased pulmonary secretions, and bronchoconstriction. *Serotonin,* found in large concentrations in the brain and GI tract, acts like histamine. *SRS-A* stimulates small-airway bronchoconstriction, vasodilation, increased vascular permeability, and wheal reactions. *ECF-A* causes cellular infiltration. *PAF* leads to decreased coronary blood flow, a negative inotropic effect, platelet aggregation and release, and pulmonary hypertension. *Prostaglandins* increase lung secretions and enhance histamine's effect on permeability. *Bradykinins* cause an increase in sweat and salivary gland secretions, bronchoconstriction, systemic

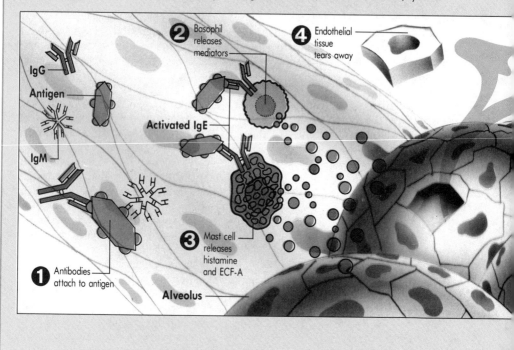

vasodilation, and increased vascular permeability.

Intensification of patient response

The activated IgE also stimulates mast cells located in connective tissue along the venule walls. The mast cells release more histamine and ECF-A. These substances produce disruptive lesions, which weaken the venules. The patient now has itchy red skin, wheals, and swelling.

Beginning of respiratory distress

In the lungs, histamine causes endothelial cells to break and endothelial tissue to tear away from surrounding tissue. Pulmonary compliance decreases as the alveoli fill with fluid and SRS-A prevents alveoli from expanding. During this stage, expect signs of respiratory distress — tachypnea, crowing, use of accessory breathing muscles, and cyanosis. The patient also may exhibit severe anxiety, an altered level of consciousness, and possibly seizures.

Deterioration in patient's condition

Meanwhile, basophils and mast cells secrete prostaglandins and bradykinins, along with histamine and serotonin. The combination of these secretions increases vascular permeability, causing fluids to leak from vessels. The patient may show evidence of rapid vascular collapse — shock; confusion; cool, pale skin; generalized edema; tachycardia; and hypotension.

Failure of compensatory mechanisms

Damage to endothelial cells causes basophils and mast cells to release heparin. Eosinophils release arylsulfatase B (to neutralize SRS-A), phospholipase D (to neutralize heparin), and cyclic adenosine monophosphate and prostaglandins E_1 and E_2 (to increase the metabolic rate). But this response can't reverse anaphylaxis. The patient may experience hemorrhage, disseminated intravascular coagulation, and cardiopulmonary arrest.

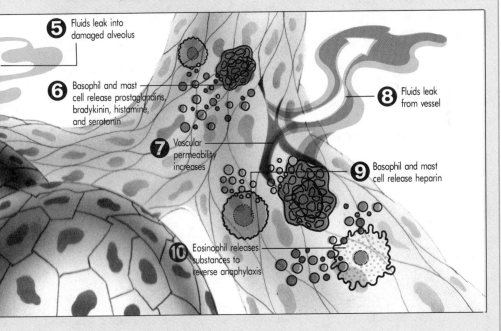

5 Fluids leak into damaged alveolus

6 Basophil and mast cell release prostaglandins, bradykinin, histamine, and serotonin

7 Vascular permeability increases

8 Fluids leak from vessel

9 Basophil and mast cell release heparin

10 Eosinophil releases substances to reverse anaphylaxis

Drugs commonly used to treat anaphylactic shock

DRUG	INDICATION, ROUTE, AND DOSAGES	ACTION	NURSING CONSIDERATIONS
Aminophylline Aminophyllin	Severe anaphylaxis I.V.: 5 to 6 mg/kg as loading dose, followed by 0.4 to 0.9 mg/kg/minute as infusion	• A xanthine derivative; causes bronchodilation • Stimulates respiratory drive • Dilates constricted pulmonary arteries • Causes diuresis • Strengthens cardiac contractions • Increases vital capacity • Causes coronary vasodilation	• Don't give cimetidine concurrently with aminophylline. They are incompatible. • Monitor blood pressure, electrocardiogram, pulse, and respirations. • Monitor intake and output, hydration status, and serum aminophylline and electrolyte levels. • Use I.V. controller to reduce risk of overdose. • Maintain serum levels at 10 to 20 mcg/ml.
Cimetidine Tagamet	Severe anaphylaxis I.V.: 600 mg diluted in dextrose 5% in water (D_5W) and administered over 20 minutes	• An antihistamine; competes with histamine for histamine$_2$ receptors • Prevents laryngeal edema	• Don't administer aminophylline concurrently with cimetidine; they are incompatible. • Reduce dosage for patients with impaired renal or hepatic function as ordered.
Diphenhydramine Benadryl	Mild anaphylaxis P.O.: 25 to 100 mg t.i.d. I.M. or I.V.: 25 to 50 mg q.i.d.	• An antihistamine; competes with histamine for histamine$_1$-receptor sites • Prevents laryngeal edema • Controls localized itching	• Administer I.V. doses slowly. • Monitor patient for hypotension. • Give oral fluids; drug causes dry mouth.
Epinephrine Adrenalin Chloride	Severe anaphylaxis (drug of choice) Initial infusion: 0.2 to 0.5 mg (0.2 to 0.5 ml of 1:1,000 strength diluted in 10 ml of 0.9% sodium chloride solution) given I.V. slowly over 5 to 10 minutes, followed by continuous infusion Continuous infusion: 1 to 4 mcg/minute. Mix 1 ml of 1:1,000 epinephrine in 250 ml of D_5W to yield concentration of 4 mcg/ml.	*Alpha-adrenergic effects* • Increases blood pressure • Reverses peripheral vasodilation and systemic hypotension • Decreases angioedema and urticaria • Improves coronary blood flow by raising diastolic pressure • Causes peripheral vasoconstriction *Beta-adrenergic effects* • Causes bronchodilation • Causes positive inotropic and chronotropic cardiac activity • Decreases synthesis and release of chemical mediators	• Choose large vein for infusion. • Use infusion controller to regulate drip. • Check blood pressure and heart rate. • Monitor patient for arrhythmias. • Check solution strength, dosage, and label before administering. • Watch for signs of extravasation at infusion site. • Monitor intake and output. • Assess color and temperature of extremities.
Hydrocortisone Solu-Cortef	Severe anaphylaxis I.V.: 100 to 200 mg every 4 to 6 hours	• A corticosteroid; prevents neutrophil and platelet aggregation • Inhibits synthesis of mediators • Decreases capillary permeability	• Monitor fluid and electrolyte balance, intake and output, and blood pressure closely. • Maintain ulcer regimen and antacids for prophylaxis.

• If the patient must receive a drug to which he's allergic, prevent a severe reaction by making sure he receives careful desensitization with gradually increasing doses of the antigen or with advance administration of corticosteroids. A person with a history of allergies should receive a drug with high anaphylactic potential only after cautious pretesting for sensitivity. Be sure you have resuscitation equipment and epinephrine on hand. When any patient takes a drug with high anaphylactic potential (particularly parenteral drugs), make sure he receives close medical observation.

Monitoring

• Continuously assess the patient's response to treatment. Monitor his vital signs and cardiopulmonary and neurologic function. Watch for complications associated with anaphylaxis, such as vascular collapse (shock, confusion, generalized edema, tachycardia, and hypotension) or acute respiratory insufficiency or obstruction (tachypnea, crowing, use of accessory muscles for breathing, and cyanosis).
• Closely observe a patient with a history of allergies for anaphylaxis when administering a drug with high anaphylactic potential, such as penicillin.
• Watch for signs and symptoms of serious allergic response in patients undergoing skin or scratch tests or diagnostic procedures that use radiographic contrast media, such as excretory urography, cardiac catheterization, and angiography. Notify the doctor immediately if you detect allergic signs and symptoms, including sudden nasal congestion, flushing, sweating, weakness, and anxiety, followed by itchy red skin, wheals, and swelling.

Patient teaching

• Teach the patient to avoid exposure to known allergens. If he has a food or drug allergy, instruct him not to consume the offending food or drug in any of its combinations and forms. If he's allergic to insect stings, he should avoid open fields and wooded areas during the insect season.
• Advise the patient to carry an anaphylaxis kit whenever he's outdoors. Urge him to familiar- ize himself with the kit and the directions before he needs them.
• Instruct the patient to wear medical identification at all times naming his allergy or allergies.

DISSEMINATED INTRAVASCULAR COAGULATION

Also known as consumption coagulopathy and defibrination syndrome, disseminated intravascular coagulation (DIC) complicates conditions that accelerate clotting, causing small-blood-vessel occlusion, organ necrosis, depletion of circulating clotting factors and platelets, and activation of the fibrinolytic system. This, in turn, can provoke severe hemorrhage.

Clotting in the microcirculation usually affects the kidneys and extremities but may occur in the brain, lungs, pituitary and adrenal glands, and GI mucosa. Other conditions, such as vitamin K deficiency, hepatic disease, and anticoagulant therapy, may cause a similar hemorrhage.

Although usually acute, DIC may be chronic in cancer patients. The prognosis depends on early detection and treatment, the severity of the hemorrhage, and treatment of the underlying condition.

CAUSES

DIC may result from:
• infection—gram-negative or gram-positive septicemia; viral, fungal, or rickettsial infection; protozoal infection
• obstetric complications—abruptio placentae, amniotic fluid embolism, retained dead fetus, eclampsia, septic abortion, postpartum hemorrhage
• neoplastic disease—acute leukemia, metastatic carcinoma, lymphomas
• disorders that produce necrosis—extensive burns and trauma, brain tissue destruction, transplant rejection, hepatic necrosis, anorexia nervosa

• other disorders and conditions – heatstroke, shock, poisonous snakebite, cirrhosis, fat embolism, incompatible blood transfusion, drug reactions, cardiac arrest, surgery necessitating cardiopulmonary bypass, giant hemangioma, severe venous thrombosis, purpura fulminans, adrenal disease, adult respiratory distress syndrome, diabetic ketoacidosis, pulmonary embolism, and sickle cell anemia.

Why such conditions and disorders lead to DIC is unclear. Regardless of how DIC begins, the typical accelerated clotting results in generalized activation of prothrombin and a consequent excess of thrombin. Excess thrombin converts fibrinogen to fibrin, producing fibrin clots in the microcirculation. This process consumes exorbitant amounts of coagulation factors (especially platelets, factor V, prothrombin, fibrinogen, and factor VIII), causing thrombocytopenia, deficiencies in factors V and VIII, hypoprothrombinemia, and hypofibrinogenemia.

Circulating thrombin activates the fibrinolytic system, which lyses fibrin clots into fibrinogen degradation products (FDPs). The hemorrhage that occurs may be due largely to the anticoagulant activity of FDPs, as well as to depletion of plasma coagulation factors.

COMPLICATIONS

DIC may be complicated by renal failure, hepatic damage, cerebrovascular accident, ischemic bowel, or respiratory distress. Hypoxia and anoxia can occur and can lead to severe striated muscle pain. Shock and coma can also result. After fibrinolysis, severe to fatal hemorrhaging of vital organs can occur without warning.

ASSESSMENT

The most significant clinical feature of DIC is abnormal bleeding *without* a history of a hemorrhagic disorder. Signs and symptoms are related to bleeding and thrombosis. Bleeding problems are usually more common than thrombotic problems unless coagulation occurs to a greater extent than fibrinolysis.

The patient history may include one of the causes of DIC. And although bleeding may oc-

cur from any site, the patient may report signs of bleeding into the skin, such as cutaneous oozing, petechiae, ecchymoses, and hematomas. If the patient is receiving treatment for another disorder when this problem occurs, he may also have bleeding from surgical or invasive procedure sites, such as incisions or venipuncture sites.

Other reported signs and symptoms may include nausea; vomiting; severe muscle, back, and abdominal pain; chest pain; hemoptysis; epistaxis; seizures; and oliguria.

Inspection may reveal petechiae and other signs of bleeding into the skin, acrocyanosis, and dyspnea. On palpation, you may detect reduced peripheral pulses. Auscultation may disclose decreased blood pressure, and neurologic assessment may reveal mental status changes, including confusion. (For a summary of assessment findings by body system, see *Physical findings in DIC.*)

DIAGNOSTIC TESTS

Abnormal bleeding in the absence of a known hematologic disorder suggests DIC. The following initial laboratory findings reflect coagulation deficiencies:

• platelet count – less than $100,000/mm^3$
• fibrinogen levels – less than 150 mg/dl
• prothrombin time – more than 15 seconds
• partial thromboplastin time – more than 60 seconds
• FDPs – often greater than 45 mcg/ml, or positive at less than 1:100 dilution
• D-dimer test (specific fibrinogen test for DIC) – positive at less than 1:8 dilution.

Other supportive data include prolonged thrombin time, positive fibrin monomers, diminished levels of factors V and VIII, fragmentation of red blood cells (RBCs), and decreased hemoglobin levels (less than 10 g/dl). Final confirmation of the diagnosis may be difficult because many of these test results also occur in other disorders (primary fibrinolysis, for example). However, the FDP and D-dimer tests are considered specific and diagnostic of DIC.

Physical findings in DIC

You may detect the following clinical abnormalities when assessing a patient with disseminated intravascular coagulation (DIC).

Skin
- Cool and moist
- Petechiae
- Ecchymoses
- Mottling

Eyes
- Blurred vision
- Intraocular hemorrhage

Nose and mouth
- Epistaxis
- Gangrene on tip of nose
- Bleeding gums

Ears
- Gangrene on earlobes
- Inner ear bleeding

Brain
- Confusion
- Irritability
- Headache
- Dizziness
- Fever
- Seizures
- Signs of increased intracranial pressure
- Hemiplegia
- Flat EEG (brain death)

Spinal cord
- Muscle weakness
- Diminished tendon reflex
- Fasciculations

- Diminished pain sensation
- Tremor

Heart
- Decreased blood return to heart (preload), as determined by pulmonary artery pressure (PAP) monitoring
- Increased pressure needed to pump against capillary clots (afterload), as determined by PAP monitoring
- Tachycardia
- Chest pain, irregular heartbeat, and decreased blood pressure from myocardial infarction or ischemia

Venous system
- Decreased blood pressure
- Bleeding from venipuncture sites or around I.V. insertion sites

Arterial system
- Absent or irregular pulse
- Bleeding from needles inserted into an artery

Lungs
- Hemoptysis
- Diffuse infiltrate on X-ray
- Chest pain (possibly indicating pulmonary embolism)
- Hypoxia
- Crackles
- Dyspnea
- Hemorrhage

GI system
- Occult blood in stool
- Severe pain and high-pitched bowel sounds, indicating mesenteric artery infarction
- Pain
- Nausea
- Vomiting

Kidneys
- Progressive oliguria
- Hematuria
- Failure

Genitalia
- Bleeding around indwelling catheters
- In a female, abnormally severe bleeding during menstruation and bleeding from vaginal mucous membranes

Fingers
- Cool, mottled skin
- Gangrene on fingertips
- Cyanosis

Legs
- Severe mottling of skin on lower legs
- Absent popliteal, posterior tibial, or pedal pulses
- Calf swelling
- Pain on foot dorsiflexion
- Blood pooling
- Acrocyanosis

Toes
- Cool, mottled skin
- Gangrene on tips of toes

Identifying heparin dosage in DIC

To treat disseminated intravascular coagulation (DIC), give an adult 50 to 100 units/kg I.V. every 4 hours. Discontinue the drug after 4 to 8 hours if no improvement occurs.

To treat venous thrombosis or pulmonary embolism, first give an adult 5,000 units as an I.V. bolus. Then give a continuous infusion of 20,000 to 40,000 units in 1,000 ml of 0.9% sodium chloride solution over 24 hours.

Or give 10,000 units as an I.V. bolus; then give an intermittent infusion of 5,000 to 10,000 units every 4 to 6 hours. Alternatively, give 5,000 units as an I.V. bolus; then give 10,000 to 20,000 units S.C. followed by 8,000 to 10,000 units every 8 hours or 15,000 to 20,000 units every 12 hours, or give a dosage based on the coagulation tests.

TREATMENT

Successful management of DIC requires prompt recognition and adequate treatment of the underlying disorder. Treatment may be supportive (when the underlying disorder is self-limiting, for example) or highly specific. If the patient isn't actively bleeding, supportive care alone may reverse DIC. Active bleeding may require administration of blood, fresh-frozen plasma, platelets, or packed RBCs to support hemostasis.

Heparin administration is controversial. It may be used early in the disorder to prevent microclotting but may be considered a last resort in the patient who is actively bleeding. If thrombosis occurs, heparin is usually mandatory. Typically, it's given with a transfusion.

KEY NURSING DIAGNOSES AND PATIENT OUTCOMES

Altered peripheral tissue perfusion related to small vessel occlusion. Based on this nursing diagnosis, you'll establish these patient outcomes. The patient will:
• demonstrate improved peripheral pulses

• not show changes in skin color and temperature in the extremities
• maintain tissue perfusion and cellular oxygenation in extremities.

Fluid volume deficit related to active bleeding. Based on this nursing diagnosis, you'll establish these patient outcomes. The patient will:
• have active bleeding detected and treated promptly
• regain and maintain adequate fluid volume as evidenced by equal intake and output volumes and stable vital signs.

Impaired gas exchange related to clotting in pulmonary microvascular system. Based on this nursing diagnosis, you'll establish these patient outcomes. The patient will:
• maintain adequate ventilation with or without supportive therapy
• regain normal arterial blood gas and oxygen saturation values
• exhibit normal respiratory function when DIC resolves.

NURSING INTERVENTIONS

• Administer prescribed analgesics for pain as necessary.
• Reposition the patient every 2 hours, and provide meticulous skin care to prevent skin breakdown.
• Administer oxygen as ordered.

◆ NURSING ALERT. To prevent clots from dislodging and causing fresh bleeding, don't vigorously rub these areas when washing. Use a 1:1 solution of hydrogen peroxide and water to help remove crusted blood.

• If bleeding occurs, use pressure, cold compresses, and topical hemostatic agents to control it; effective agents may include an absorbable gelatin sponge, a microfibrillar collagen hemostat, or thrombin. Administer heparin, as prescribed. (See *Identifying heparin dosage in DIC.*)
• After giving an injection or removing an I.V. catheter or needle, apply pressure to the injection site for at least 10 minutes. Alert other staff members to the patient's tendency to hemorrhage. Limit venipunctures whenever possible.

• Protect the patient from injury. Enforce complete bed rest during bleeding episodes. If the patient is very agitated, pad the bed rails.
• Perform bladder irrigations as ordered for genitourinary (GU) bleeding.
• If the patient can't tolerate activity because of blood loss, provide frequent rest periods.
• Inform the family of the patient's progress. Prepare them for his appearance (I.V. lines, nasogastric tubes, bruises, dried blood). Provide emotional support and encouragement, and listen to the patient's and family's concerns. As needed, enlist the aid of a social worker, chaplain, and other members of the health care team in providing such support.

Monitoring

• Monitor intake and output hourly in acute DIC, especially when administering blood products. Watch for transfusion reactions and signs of fluid overload.
• To measure blood loss, weigh dressings and linen and record drainage.
• Weigh the patient daily, particularly in renal involvement.
• Watch for bleeding from the GI and GU tracts. If you suspect intra-abdominal bleeding, measure the patient's abdominal girth at least every 4 hours, and observe closely for signs of shock.
• Monitor the results of serial blood studies (particularly hematocrit, hemoglobin levels, and coagulation times).
• Test all stools and urine for occult blood.
• Check all venipuncture sites frequently for bleeding.

Patient teaching

Explain the disorder to the patient and his family. Focus on early recognition of signs of abnormal bleeding, prompt treatment of the underlying disorders, and prevention of further bleeding.

SICKLE CELL CRISIS

Sickle cell crisis is a periodic exacerbation of sickle cell anemia. In this inherited, incurable form of anemia, defective hemoglobin molecules (hemoglobin S) reduce the oxygen-carrying capacity of red blood cells (RBCs) and induce intravascular removal of mutant RBCs.

During a sickle cell crisis, RBCs become sickle-shaped, causing vessel obstruction and serious clinical complications. Types of sickle cell crises include vaso-occlusive (the most common), anemic, aplastic, acute sequestration, and hemolytic.

Sickle cell crisis can be fatal if sufficient RBCs are dysfunctional and can't carry adequate oxygen — or when major thromboses occur.

CAUSES

Sickle cell crisis may be precipitated by several conditions or factors. (See *Common causes of sickle cell crisis,* page 46.)

During hypoxia, the abnormal hemoglobin S molecule becomes insoluble. RBCs then become rigid, rough, and elongated, forming a crescent or sickle shape. Sickled RBCs can't travel through the microcirculation and tend to plug the vessels, causing occlusion, pain, and tissue ischemia beyond the occlusion site. Sickling also may cause hemolysis.

The degree of hypoxia inducing this response, the percentage of sickled RBCs, and sickling reversibility differ from one person to another. Patients with severe disease may have sickling when the partial pressure of arterial oxygen (PaO_2) is 60 mm Hg, whereas others require a PaO_2 of 45 mm Hg. In some patients, many circulating RBCs sickle, whereas in others, only a few do. Sickling reversibility may depend partly on the degree and duration of hypoxia as well as on individual physiologic differences.

Sickled cells have the potential to revert to a normal state when oxygenation is restored. However, those with irreversible plasma membrane damage can't return to normal and subsequently are transported to the spleen and hemolyzed. Abnormal and excessive RBC hemolysis leads to anemia and hyperbilirubinemia. Reduced PaO_2 causes cellular hypoxia, stagnant blood flow, and blood hyperviscosity, resulting in the circulation of sickled RBCs. Cellular hypoxia triggers cellular acidosis and,

Common causes of sickle cell crisis

In a patient with sickle cell anemia, a crisis may result from conditions or precipitating factors that decrease arterial pH or oxygen tension, impair tissue perfusion, increase plasma osmolarity, or reduce plasma volume. This chart lists specific factors.

CAUSE	PRECIPITATING FACTORS
Decreased arterial oxygen tension	• High altitude • Respiratory infections • Chronic obstructive pulmonary disease • Pulmonary embolism • Anemia
Poor tissue perfusion	• Peripheral vascular disease • Cardiac disease (angina, myocardial infarction) • Hypotension • Vasoconstrictive drugs
Decreased arterial pH	• Septic shock • Drug overdose causing decreased respirations with hypercarbia • Obstructive lung disease • Neurologic disease resulting in reduced respiratory drive and hypoventilation with hypercarbia
Increased plasma osmolarity	• Dehydration • Excessive exercise • Diabetes insipidus • Hyperglycemia
Reduced plasma volume	• Hemorrhage • Excessive diuretics • Excessive heat

finally, tissue ischemia. Pain occurs from tissue ischemia and blood hyperviscosity.

COMPLICATIONS

Sickle cell crisis may lead to life-threatening thrombosis, hemorrhagic diathesis, uncontrolled infection (from circulatory stasis), and multisystem effects.

Less severe complications include frequent retinal thromboses, which may cause retinal hemorrhage or detachment and blindness; chronic hemolysis, which leads to gallstones with cholecystitis; and joint infarction

and arthritic changes, which may lead to aseptic necrosis (particularly of the head of the femur) or salmonella osteomyelitis of the joint.

ASSESSMENT

The patient's history usually reveals sickle cell anemia unless it has remained undetected. The patient in sickle cell crisis typically reports sudden, severe pain in the chest, abdomen, back, hand, or foot; headache and optical problems; aching joint pain; increased weakness; and dyspnea. He may also report a typical precipitating event, such as recent infection or illness, exposure to cold, or generalized life stress.

Inspection usually reveals yellow sclerae and pallor in the lips, tongue, palms, or nail beds. Lateral shifting of the point of maximal impulse from the fifth intercostal space to the midclavicular line may also be observed as well as elevated jugular vein pulsations (more than 3/4" [2 cm] above the clavicle) and peripheral edema if heart failure is present. The patient may appear lethargic, irritable, or sleepy. Fever, a productive cough, dyspnea, and tachypnea may be evident with infection.

Palpatation may disclose an enlarged liver or spleen. Auscultation may reveal heart gallops or murmurs, abnormal heart rate or rhythm, elevated blood pressure, and pulmonary crackles at end-inspiration. These findings signal heart failure and may become severe during sickle cell crisis. They also may occur in patients with repeated minor sickling episodes.

Distinct physical findings are associated with certain types of sickle cell crisis. For example, with vaso-occlusive crisis, you may detect jaundice, dark urine, and a low-grade fever. After the crisis subsides (4 days to several weeks), infection may develop, causing lethargy, sleepiness, fever, or apathy. Aplastic crisis (usually associated with infection) may cause pallor, lethargy, sleepiness, dyspnea, and possibly coma. With acute sequestration crisis, expect lethargy and pallor; with hemolytic crisis, expect increased jaundice and hepatomegaly.

DIAGNOSTIC TESTS

Diagnosis of sickle cell crisis is usually confirmed by a stained blood smear showing sickled RBCs. In a patient not previously diagnosed with sickle cell anemia, hemoglobin electrophoresis and arterial blood gas (ABG) analysis is ordered to evaluate oxygenation. (Pulse oximetry may yield inaccurate results because of the abnormal hemoglobin structure, circulating sickled cells, and tissue hypoxia.)

Serum lactate analysis also helps measure tissue oxygenation. Lactic acid forms during anaerobic metabolism in conditions of tissue hypoxia, such as RBC sickling.

◆ NURSING ALERT. Although arterial pH and bicarbonate values can identify acidosis, they won't reflect lactic acidosis caused by anaerobic metabolism.

A complete blood count (CBC) helps determine the severity of the crisis by evaluating hemoglobin levels, hematocrit, white blood cell count, RBC count, RBC morphology, and RBC indices. Other tests used for this purpose include a reticulocyte count and an erythrocyte sedimentation rate.

To check for organ damage, the doctor may measure levels of serum bilirubin, serum electrolytes (especially potassium, phosphate, and uric acid, which are all released from lysed cells), blood urea nitrogen, and creatinine, and may test liver function. Serum bilirubin commonly is elevated in sickle cell crisis, reflecting accelerated RBC turnover that exceeds the liver's ability to conjugate and remove bilirubin. Even patients without bilirubin elevations or visible jaundice may have increased urobilinogen in the urine and dark stools. Electrocardiography and chest X-ray also aid diagnosis of organ damage.

Because sickle cell crisis causes a wide spectrum of abnormal diagnostic results, assessing the severity of a crisis can be challenging. (See *Diagnostic findings in sickle cell crisis,* page 48.) However, the range of abnormalities and severity of pain don't necessarily reflect the severity of the crisis. Observing the patient for organ failure, thromboses, and hemorrhage is the best way to determine this.

TREATMENT

Oxygen is the key pharmacologic agent used to manage sickle cell crisis. Unless tissue oxygenation improves, sickling will persist. Oxygen therapy is initiated during emergency treatment and continues during recuperation until the patient's oxygen saturation exceeds 97%. Some patients return home with oxygen to use periodically or in emergencies.

Once the patient is somewhat stabilized, medical treatment involves managing fluid and circulatory status with fluid resuscitation measures such as crystalloid solutions. RBC transfusions usually aren't given until sickling is stabilized because they may increase blood viscosity and osmolarity, increasing sickling. However, the patient with significant RBC hemolysis or anemia (from loss of RBC mass) requires RBC transfusions. The doctor augments these with oral iron and folic acid supplements to enhance growth of functional RBCs, as needed.

During treatment, rapid RBC turnover may lead to elevated bilirubin levels, hyperkalemia, hyperphosphatemia, and signs of liver failure. The doctor may prescribe sodium polystyrene sulfonate for hyperkalemia and phosphate-binding agents for hyperphosphatemia. To prevent infection caused by stagnant blood flow and thromboses within organs, he may order broad-spectrum antibiotics.

Drug therapy includes analgesics for severe, prolonged pain. Although narcotics are preferred because they're highly effective against somatic pain, a patient with mild thromboses and coagulopathy may receive nonsteroidal anti-inflammatory drugs. These agents interfere with clotting, posing some risk of spontaneous bleeding. Acetaminophen is ordered rather than aspirin, which may promote acidosis and worsen sickling. Some patients also benefit from patient-controlled analgesia. Antisickling agents are still experimental.

If other treatment measures fail, therapeutic splenectomy may be performed on the patient with acute sequestration crisis or an enlarged, tender liver accompanied by coagu-

Diagnostic findings in sickle cell crisis

TEST	RESULT	CAUSE
Arterial blood gas analysis		
pH	Low	Microthrombi block circulation, promoting anaerobic metabolism and acidosis.
Partial pressure of arterial oxygen	Low	Abnormal hemoglobin causes red blood cell (RBC) lysis, decreasing oxygen-carrying capacity; microthrombi reduce oxygen circulation and gas exchange.
Bicarbonate	Low	Microthrombi block circulation, promoting anaerobic metabolism and acidosis.
Blood chemistry		
Bilirubin (indirect) level	Increased	Excessive indirect bilirubin (an RBC breakdown product) overwhelms the liver's conjugating mechanism.
Blood urea nitrogen level	Increased	Serum levels increase when RBCs (protein molecules) are lysed.
Creatinine level	Increased	Microthrombi block renal circulation, causing nephron damage and inability to clear creatinine.
Blood count		
Hematocrit and hemoglobin counts	Decreased	RBCs are sickled or permanently destroyed.
Mean corpuscular hemoglobin count	Decreased	Abnormal hemoglobin reduces hemoglobin concentration in RBCs.
Platelet count	Decreased	Platelets are destroyed by microthrombi in the microvasculature.
RBC count	Decreased	RBCs are sickled or permanently destroyed.
Reticulocyte count	Increased	Reticulocytes (early RBC precursors) are released from bone marrow early to compensate for RBC loss.
Other tests		
Erythrocyte sedimentation rate	Increased	Sickled cells don't settle in a column as rapidly as normal RBCs.
Total serum iron count	Increased	RBC hemolysis causes increased RBC turnover with resulting increases in free iron.

lopathy or thrombocytopenia. Extensive presurgical preparation can prevent the procedure and anesthetic from exacerbating the sickle cell crisis. For example, the doctor may order preoperative exchange transfusions to replace defective RBCs, or order additional oxygen and carefully regulate the patient's vascular volume status.

KEY NURSING DIAGNOSES AND PATIENT OUTCOMES

High risk for injury related to life-threatening complications associated with sickle cell crisis. Based on this nursing diagnosis, you'll establish these patient outcomes. The patient will:

• express an understanding of possible complications and report early warning signs immediately

• maintain vital functions throughout the crisis

• not exhibit signs and symptoms of organ dysfunctions or deficits after the crisis is resolved.

Impaired gas exchange related to altered oxygen-carrying capacity of the blood caused by sickling of RBCs. Based on this nursing diagnosis, you'll establish these patient outcomes. The patient will:

• report breathing comfort with oxygen therapy

• maintain adequate ventilation

• regain and maintain normal CBC and ABG values.

Pain related to tissue ischemia and blood hyperviscosity caused by sickle cell crisis. Based on this nursing diagnosis, you'll establish these patient outcomes. The patient will:

• report pain relief after analgesic administration

• articulate factors that intensify pain and modify behavior accordingly

• decrease the amount and frequency of pain medication as the crisis resolves.

NURSING INTERVENTIONS

• Administer oxygen therapy immediately, as prescribed. In a severe crisis, prepare to assist with endotracheal intubation and provide supportive care with mechanical ventilation.

• Establish I.V. access and expect to administer an isotonic solution, such as 0.9% sodium chloride solution, at an initial rate of 200 to 500 ml/hour. As the patient's volume status normalizes, taper the infusion as ordered.

• After fluid resuscitation, administer RBCs, as ordered, if the patient has lost RBC volume through sickling and removal by the liver or spleen.

• Administer ordered analgesics. Titrate dosages to the patient's reported pain level to reduce or eliminate pain, which may increase the sickling process.

• Promote tissue oxygenation through early mobility, coughing and deep breathing, frequent position changes, adequate rest periods, and optimal nutrition.

• Provide supportive care for organ decompensation or failure. For example, administer nitrates or vasodilators, as ordered, for a patient with chest pain, or give bronchodilators for respiratory distress.

• Take measures to prevent infection. If you suspect infection, notify the doctor immediately and expect to start antibiotic therapy.

• Provide emotional support, and take measures to reduce anxiety and stress, which can increase hypoxia and sickling and make breathing harder. Expect to administer anxiolytics (such as benzodiazepines), if ordered.

Monitoring

• Monitor the patient's arterial and tissue oxygenation status frequently through ABG analysis, pulse oximetry, serum lactate levels, and cardiopulmonary assessment. (See *Monitoring your patient during sickle cell crisis,* page 50.)

• Assess all body systems frequently for signs and symptoms of reduced oxygenation or circulatory impairment.

• To assess fluid status, closely monitor hematologic and serum electrolyte tests, intake and output, and daily weight. If a central venous line is in place, obtain central venous pressure measurements.

• Monitor the patient's pain level and response to analgesic therapy.

• Watch continuously for signs and symptoms of infection.

• Closely monitor renal function, and adjust antibiotic dosages as needed and ordered.

• Review potassium levels closely – hyperkalemia may occur during a sickle cell crisis. To assess the patient's response to therapy, monitor diagnostic tests that reveal continued sickling, such as reticulocyte count, RBC morphology, bilirubin measurement, and ABG analysis.

Patient teaching

• To compensate for abnormal hemoglobin production, the patient may need lifelong RBC precursor nutrients, such as B vitamins and iron. Promote compliance by explaining the

Monitoring your patient during sickle cell crisis

At the beginning of the crisis, you must assess the patient thoroughly to uncover early signs and symptoms of complications. The chart below shows the body systems at risk and how often you should check vital indicators within each.

BODY SYSTEM	ASSESSMENT FREQUENCY
Cardiovascular	
Vital signs	Hourly
Skin color and capillary refill	Every 1 to 2 hours
Pulses	Every 4 to 8 hours
Heart sounds	Every 4 to 8 hours
Fluid balance indicators	Every 4 to 8 hours
GI	
Abdominal size and tenderness	Every 4 to 8 hours
Bowel sounds	Every 4 to 8 hours
Neurologic	
Orientation	Every 1 to 2 hours
Ability to move all body parts on command	Every 1 to 2 hours
Cognitive functioning	Every 2 to 4 hours
Pupillary response	Every 4 to 8 hours
Renal	
Urine output	Every 1 to 2 hours
Respiratory	
Oxygenation indicators	Every 1 to 2 hours
Breath sounds	Every 4 to 8 hours
Skin and mucous membranes	
Total body, checking for decreased perfusion	Every 8 hours
Extremities, checking color, capillary refill, and integrity	Every 4 to 8 hours

rationale for these medications and how to avoid adverse reactions. For instance, tell the patient on iron supplements that a high-fiber diet helps prevent constipation and that taking iron with food offsets its unpleasant taste.

• Inform the patient that he'll need periodic CBCs with RBC monitoring even after the crisis ends. Emphasize that these tests help identify such conditions as slow, continuous sickling, nutrition-related anemias, and altered fluid status.

• Teach the patient how to prevent infection during activities of daily living. For example, he should wear gloves when gardening, avoid tight clothing, not go barefoot, get vaccinations as recommended, abstain from smoking, and seek prompt medical attention for respiratory and oropharyngeal infections.

• To help prevent future crises, teach the patient to avoid conditions that may trigger sickle cell crisis—for example, temperature extremes, excessive exercise, dehydration, unpressurized aircrafts, and high altitudes.

4

Respiratory disorders

The respiratory system accomplishes alveolar gas exchange. In this exchange, pulmonary capillary blood takes on oxygen and gives off carbon dioxide. When disease or trauma interferes with the respiratory system's vital work, the patient's ability to sustain life is immediately threatened.

Some respiratory disorders, such as respiratory acidosis or alkalosis, may gradually develop into an acute crisis. Others, such as pulmonary embolism and near drowning, are immediately life-threatening and can quickly lead to death if detection and emergency intervention are delayed. Unfortunately, many acute respiratory disorders provide little or no warning of the impending danger to the patient.

As a primary caregiver, you must be able to detect both subtle and gross changes in your patient's respiratory function. Through your assessment, you can determine the adequacy of the patient's gas exchange as well as evaluate his response to respiratory therapy. In addition, your supportive care—such as administering oxygen and drug therapy properly and protecting the patient from injury that could result from an altered mental status—can do much to prevent residual deficits and help speed the patient's recovery.

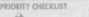

PRIORITY CHECKLIST

Initial respiratory care

Check for:
- ☐ history of chronic respiratory conditions
- ☐ history of acute episodes of breathing difficulties
- ☐ history of medical therapy for underlying respiratory problems, including drug history
- ☐ history of precipitating factors such as allergies or chest trauma
- ☐ history of medical-surgical conditions, especially those associated with acute respiratory disorders
- ☐ patent airway
- ☐ abnormal respiratory rate, rhythm, or depth
- ☐ diminished or abnormal breath sounds
- ☐ changes in skin color
- ☐ altered mental status
- ☐ anxiety or restlessness
- ☐ signs and symptoms of hypoxia
- ☐ changes in organ function
- ☐ abnormal respiratory function test results.

Intervene by:
- ☐ notifying the doctor
- ☐ maintaining a patent airway
- ☐ administering oxygen therapy
- ☐ repositioning the patient to maximize chest expansion
- ☐ starting an I.V. line
- ☐ obtaining arterial blood gas levels
- ☐ monitoring vital signs continuously.

Prepare for:
- ☐ intubation and ventilation
- ☐ emergency drug administration
- ☐ invasive procedures such as a tracheotomy or chest tube insertion
- ☐ noninvasive procedures such as chest X-rays or chest physiotherapy.

UPPER AIRWAY OBSTRUCTION

A medical emergency, upper airway obstruction occurs when an upper airway structure (trachea, larynx, pharynx, nose, or mouth) becomes partially or totally blocked. As a result, the patient's oxygen supply decreases or may be completely cut off. If not treated promptly, upper airway obstruction can lead to hypoxemia and progress quickly (within minutes if obstruction is complete) to severe hypoxia, loss of consciousness, and death.

CAUSES

Numerous conditions can cause an upper airway obstruction—for example, epiglottitis, pharyngitis, airway trauma, and tumors. (To learn the most common causes, see *Reviewing causes of upper airway obstruction.*)

COMPLICATIONS

An upper airway obstruction may lead to tissue hypoxia, metabolic acidosis, and respiratory and cardiac arrest. Furthermore, if a sharp or irregularly shaped object caused the obstruction, the airway may be irritated or damaged, which may lead to edema and worsening obstruction.

ASSESSMENT

The patient's history may reveal a predisposing cause. For example, preexisting pulmonary disease or a history of a tumor predisposes him to an airway obstruction. Likewise, drug or alcohol use or a disease that affects motor coordination or mental function increases the patient's risk for choking.

Inspection will reveal varying signs, depending on the cause, location, and severity of the obstruction. With a partial airway obstruction, the patient may grasp at his throat and gag or choke. However, he will be able to speak. Stridor may be audible during inspiration or throughout the respiratory cycle. You may observe nasal flaring and dyspnea along with intercostal muscle retraction.

If a patient's upper airway is completely obstructed, he'll clutch his throat (the universal sign of distress) and will not be able to talk.

Airflow from his nose and mouth will be absent. You may also see increased salivation, diaphoresis, cyanosis, and lethargy that may quickly progress to unconsciousness.

Auscultation of the lung fields may reveal decreased breath sounds and wheezing with a partial obstruction or absent breath sounds with a total obstruction.

DIAGNOSTIC TESTS

For a patient with a partial obstruction, the following diagnostic tests may help determine the cause and extent of obstruction.
• *Radiographic studies, such as X-rays and computed tomography scan,* reveal the location, shape, and extent of the obstruction.
• *Bronchoscopy and laryngoscopy* define the location, size, and nature of the obstruction.
• *Arterial blood gas (ABG) studies* show a decreased partial pressure of oxygen in arterial blood, an increased partial pressure of carbon dioxide in arterial blood, and both metabolic and respiratory acidosis in a patient with a near-complete obstruction.
• *Pulmonary function studies* may show a normal inspiratory flow but abnormal expiratory flow in a patient with a variable intrathoracic obstruction. A patient with a variable extrathoracic obstruction has abnormal inspiratory flow.
• *Flow-volume loop studies* chart the volume and flow of air during inspiration and expiration. A patient with a variable intrathoracic obstruction shows a plateau in the expiratory flow curve; a flattened inspiratory flow curve occurs with a variable extrathoracic obstruction. A plateau in both the expiratory and inspiratory curves indicates a fixed obstruction.

Because a complete airway obstruction is life-threatening and demands immediate attention, the patient's diagnosis will be based on the presenting signs and symptoms alone.

TREATMENT

In upper airway obstruction, treatment aims to open the airway and restore baseline respirations, thereby reversing hypoxia. With a partial obstruction, you may insert an artificial airway or, if the patient can cough force-

Reviewing causes of upper airway obstruction

CAUSE	DESCRIPTION	SIGNS AND SYMPTOMS
Airway trauma	Injury occurring during intubation or extubation with an artificial airway	Stridor and distress, usually within 1 hour after extubation
Angioedema	Acute, painless, dermal, subcutaneous, or submucosal swelling of short duration; frequently associated with urticaria or anaphylaxis	Generalized edema involving the face, neck, lips, larynx, hands, feet, genitalia, or viscera
Bilateral vocal cord paralysis	Speech loss from vocal cord lesion on both sides of larynx	Stridor, dyspnea
Epiglottitis	Acute inflammation of the epiglottis with edema; may cause complete laryngeal obstruction 2 to 5 hours after onset	Cherry-red epiglottis, high fever, stridor, sore throat, dysphagia, drooling, restlessness, irritability, inspiratory retractions
Ludwig's angina	Indurated cellulitis of the mouth floor after mucosal laceration or dental infection; resultant edema	Edema of the mouth and tongue; abscesses of second and third mandibular molars
Mediastinal tumor	Obstructive lesion of the mediastinum	Chest pain, retrosternal pressure, cough, hoarseness, clubbing, tracheal deviation, mediastinal mass
Palatal paresis	Incomplete paralysis of the palate	Stridor, dyspnea
Pharyngeal abscess	Localized collection of pus in the pharynx	Fever, dysphagia, trismus, drooling, cervical adenopathy, hoarseness, stridor
Pharyngitis	Inflammation or infection of the pharynx	Sore throat
Polychondritis (relapsing)	Progressive inflammation and destruction of cartilage; may cause tracheal or bronchial collapse	Inflammation, floppy ear, saddle nose
Sleep apnea syndrome	Cessation of airflow through nose and mouth for at least 10 seconds during sleep; may accompany obesity	Hypersomnia, snoring, distorted sleep
Thyroid enlargement	Enlarged thyroid with positive thyroid scan; may be related to previous thyroid surgery	Dyspnea, enlarged goiter
Tracheal stricture	Narrowing of the trachea, often occurring several weeks after tracheotomy or prolonged intubation	Stridor, localized wheezing
Tracheal tumor	Obstructive lesion of the trachea	Paroxysmal dyspnea, hoarseness, hemoptysis
Tracheomalacia	Softening of tracheal cartilage, often following extubation	Stridor, ineffective cough, fever, malaise, recurrent infection (due to tracheal injury)

fully, encourage him to expel the foreign body. However, if signs indicate decreasing air exchange, treat the patient as though he has a complete obstruction.

If finger-sweeps, back blows, or abdominal thrusts (also called the Heimlich maneuver) can't remove a complete obstruction, the doctor may attempt to remove the object by bronchoscopy or through the use of forceps or suctioning equipment. Last-resort treatment options include cricothyrotomy and transtracheal catheter ventilation. These measures provide a temporary airway until the patient can be tracheally intubated or taken to the operating room for a tracheotomy.

The patient may require oxygen therapy or even intubation to correct hypoxemia. If the patient's obstruction resulted from inflammation (for example, from diphtheria, allergic reactions, croup, or epiglottitis) or edema (for example, from a thermal injury), humidified oxygen therapy may be given to help decrease swelling and allow the airway to open.

Various medications may also be used as adjunctive therapy in the treatment of an upper airway obstruction. For example, I.V. corticosteroids, such as dexamethasone or methylprednisolone, further decrease edema and swelling; epinephrine reduces swelling from an allergic reaction; and antibiotics treat an underlying infection.

KEY NURSING DIAGNOSES AND PATIENT OUTCOMES

Anxiety related to threat of death caused by upper airway obstruction. Based on this nursing diagnosis, you'll establish these patient outcomes. The patient will:
• use available support systems to lessen anxiety
• demonstrate abated physical symptoms of anxiety.

Impaired gas exchange related to atelectasis or edema distal to the obstruction. Based on this nursing diagnosis, you'll establish these patient outcomes. The patient will:
• regain and maintain ABG values within the normal range
• remain alert and oriented to person, place, and time

• report an ability to breathe easily.

Ineffective airway clearance related to specific cause of obstruction. Based on this nursing diagnosis, you'll establish these patient outcomes. The patient will:
• regain and maintain a patent airway and have adequate air movement in and out of his lungs
• demonstrate a respiratory rate that fluctuates no more than 5 breaths/minute from the baseline.

NURSING INTERVENTIONS
• Attempt to remove the obstruction with finger-sweeps, back blows, or abdominal thrusts, as needed.
• Administer oxygen by face mask or artificial airway to ensure adequate oxygenation of tissues.
• Assist with inserting an artificial airway, as needed.
• If intubation or a tracheotomy is required, be prepared to assist with the procedure and provide appropriate ventilatory care.
• Provide emotional support to the patient to decrease his anxiety.
• Assist with cricothyrotomy or percutaneous transtracheal catheter insertion, as required.
• Administer corticosteroids, epinephrine, or antibiotics as ordered.

Monitoring
• Assess the patient's respiratory status (rate and breath sounds) for signs of increased respiratory distress.
• Watch the cardiac monitor for arrhythmias arising from hypoxemia.
• Monitor ABG values frequently to determine the degree of hypoxemia.
• If the patient is receiving mechanical ventilation, monitor ventilator settings, including tidal volume, flow rate, and percentage of oxygen.

Patient teaching
• If the patient is not acutely ill, briefly teach him about his condition and explain why it is occurring. Tell him how the condition will be treated and explain each new procedure before beginning.

• If the patient is intubated and on a ventilator, explain how the ventilator will help him breathe. Also explain that he won't be able to talk while he's intubated or has a tracheostomy, but that he can communicate through notes.

ACUTE EPIGLOTTITIS

A life-threatening emergency, this acute inflammation of the epiglottis and surrounding area rapidly causes edema and induration. Untreated, the disease results in complete airway obstruction. Epiglottitis proves fatal in 8% to 12% of patients.

CAUSES

Epiglottitis usually results from infection with the bacterium *Haemophilus influenzae* type B and, occasionally, pneumococci or group A streptococci.

COMPLICATIONS

Airway obstruction and death may occur within 2 hours of onset.

ASSESSMENT

The history may reveal an earlier upper respiratory tract infection. Additional complaints include a sore throat, dysphagia, and the sudden onset of a high fever.

On inspection, the patient may be febrile, drooling, pale or cyanotic, restless, apprehensive, and irritable. You may also observe nasal flaring. The patient may sit in a tripod position: upright and leaning forward with the chin thrust out, mouth open, and tongue protruding. This position helps relieve severe respiratory distress. The patient's voice usually sounds thick and muffled.

Because manipulation may trigger sudden airway obstruction, attempt throat inspection only when immediate intubation can be performed if necessary. (See *Airway crisis*.) The patient's throat will appear red and inflamed.

Auscultation of the lung fields may reveal rhonchi and diminished breath sounds, usually transmitted from the upper airway.

Airway crisis

Epiglottitis can progress to complete airway obstruction within minutes. To prepare for this medical emergency, keep the following tips in mind:
• Watch for increasing restlessness, tachycardia, fever, dyspnea, and intercostal and substernal retractions. These are warning signs of total airway obstruction and the need for an emergency tracheotomy.
• Keep the following equipment available at the patient's bedside in case of sudden, complete airway obstruction: a tracheotomy tray, endotracheal tubes, a hand-held resuscitation bag, oxygen equipment, and a laryngoscope with blades of various sizes.
• Remember that using a tongue blade or throat culture swab can initiate sudden, complete airway obstruction.
• Before examining the patient's throat, request trained personnel (such as an anesthesiologist) to stand by if emergency airway insertion should be needed.

DIAGNOSTIC TESTS

• *Lateral neck X-rays* show an enlarged epiglottis and a distended hypopharynx.
• *Direct laryngoscopy* reveals the hallmark of acute epiglottitis: a swollen, beefy-red epiglottis. The throat examination should follow X-ray studies and, in most cases, should *not* be performed if significant obstruction is suspected or if immediate intubation isn't possible.

Additional X-rays of the chest and cervical trachea help to confirm the diagnosis.

TREATMENT

A patient with acute epiglottitis and airway obstruction requires emergency hospitalization. He should be placed in a cool-mist tent with added oxygen. If complete or near-complete airway obstruction occurs, he may also need emergency endotracheal intubation or a tracheotomy. Arterial blood gas (ABG) monitoring or pulse oximetry may be used to assess his progress.

Treatment may also include parenteral fluids to prevent dehydration when the disease interferes with swallowing, and a 10-day course of parenteral antibiotics – usually ampicillin. If the patient is allergic to penicillin or could have ampicillin-resistant endemic *H. influenzae* epiglottitis, chloramphenicol or another antibiotic may be prescribed.

Although controversial, corticosteroids may be prescribed to reduce edema during early treatment. Oxygen therapy may also be used.

KEY NURSING DIAGNOSES AND PATIENT OUTCOMES

High risk for suffocation related to airway closure caused by swelling and edema. Based on this nursing diagnosis, you'll establish these patient outcomes. The patient will:
• have his condition identified quickly and treated promptly
• maintain a patent airway.

Impaired gas exchange related to altered oxygen supply caused by partial airway obstruction. Based on this nursing diagnosis, you'll establish these patient outcomes. The patient will:
• express feelings of comfort in maintaining air exchange
• regain and maintain normal ABG values
• exhibit no signs and symptoms of hypoxia.

Ineffective airway clearance related to swelling and edema in the throat. Based on this nursing diagnosis, you'll establish these patient outcomes. The patient will:
• demonstrate controlled coughing techniques
• exhibit normal breath sounds
• maintain a patent airway.

NURSING INTERVENTIONS

• Place the patient in a sitting position to ease his respiratory difficulty unless he finds another position more comfortable.
• Place the patient in a cool-mist tent. Change the sheets frequently because they quickly become saturated.
• Calm the patient during X-ray studies of his chest and cervical trachea.

• Minimize external stimuli.
• Start an I.V. line for antibiotic therapy and fluid replacement if the patient can't maintain adequate fluid intake. Draw blood for laboratory analysis, as ordered.
• If the patient has a tracheostomy, anticipate his needs because he'll be unable to voice them. Provide emotional support. Reassure him and his family that a tracheostomy is a short-term intervention (usually in place from 4 to 7 days).

Monitoring

• Frequently assess the patient's temperature, vital signs, and respiratory rate and pattern. Also monitor ABG levels (to detect hypoxia and hypercapnia) and pulse oximetry values (to detect decreasing oxygen saturation). Rising temperature, increasing pulse rate, and hypotension are signs of secondary infection. Report any changes.
• Observe the patient continuously for signs of impending airway closure, which may develop at any time.
• Record intake and output precisely to monitor for dehydration.

Patient teaching

• Inform the patient and family that epiglottal swelling usually subsides after 24 hours of antibiotic therapy. The epiglottis usually returns to normal size within 72 hours.
• If the patient's home care regimen includes oral antibiotic therapy, emphasize the need for completing the entire prescription. Explain proper administration. Discuss drug storage, dosage, adverse effects, and whether or not the medication can be taken with food or milk.
• If the patient should require the haemophilus b conjugate vaccine, discuss the rationale for immunization, and help the family obtain the vaccine.

STATUS ASTHMATICUS

A prolonged asthmatic attack, status asthmaticus is a life-threatening complication of asthma that can last for days to weeks. It can be fatal even with optimal therapy.

CAUSES

Status asthmaticus occurs when a prolonged asthmatic attack doesn't respond to conventional asthma therapy with bronchodilators. A variety of stimuli or precipitating factors can cause an asthma attack, including dust, pollen, animal dander, food and cooking odors, perfume or cologne, cleaning products, air pollutants, mold spores, grains, exercise, and cold, dry air.

Medications, such as aspirin, nonsteroidal anti-inflammatory drugs, and beta-adrenergic agents (including eyedrops), can also trigger asthma attacks. Additionally, viral infections, overuse of bronchodilators, an autonomic imbalance, and psychological or emotional upheaval can bring on an attack in an asthmatic patient.

Asthma is a disease of reversible airflow obstruction, characterized by bronchospasm, inflammation and edema of the airway mucosa, and increased sputum production. Because the patient is unresponsive to conventional bronchodilator therapy used to treat an asthma attack, his ventilation becomes increasingly impaired in status asthmaticus as airway resistance and respiratory work increase and expiratory flow decreases. Although he works harder to breathe, he can't improve his oxygen supply, so he becomes hypoxic and eventually hypercapnic. As he tires, his compensatory mechanisms become less and less effective. If this process isn't reversed promptly, the patient will die. (See *How status asthmaticus progresses*.)

COMPLICATIONS

Respiratory alkalosis, respiratory acidosis, hypoxia, and cyanosis may all develop from status asthmaticus. Ultimately, respiratory failure may result.

ASSESSMENT

The patient's history may reveal the precipitating factor for the current asthma attack, such as recent exposure to animal dander, presence of a viral infection, or a recent emotional upheaval. A review of the patient's history may also reveal that, during a previous

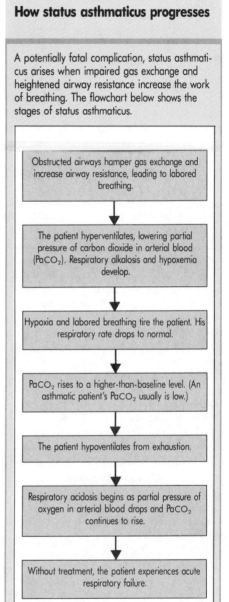

How status asthmaticus progresses

A potentially fatal complication, status asthmaticus arises when impaired gas exchange and heightened airway resistance increase the work of breathing. The flowchart below shows the stages of status asthmaticus.

Obstructed airways hamper gas exchange and increase airway resistance, leading to labored breathing.

↓

The patient hyperventilates, lowering partial pressure of carbon dioxide in arterial blood ($PaCO_2$). Respiratory alkalosis and hypoxemia develop.

↓

Hypoxia and labored breathing tire the patient. His respiratory rate drops to normal.

↓

$PaCO_2$ rises to a higher-than-baseline level. (An asthmatic patient's $PaCO_2$ usually is low.)

↓

The patient hypoventilates from exhaustion.

↓

Respiratory acidosis begins as partial pressure of oxygen in arterial blood drops and $PaCO_2$ continues to rise.

↓

Without treatment, the patient experiences acute respiratory failure.

asthma attack, the patient developed syncope or required mechanical ventilation.

◆ NURSING ALERT. Patients with a history of syncope during asthma attacks or of requiring intubation are at increased risk for a fatal attack. Despite any treatment given, the patient will typically report increasing difficulty breathing.

On inspection, the patient will appear apprehensive, pale, diaphoretic, breathless, and exhausted from fighting for air. In addition, he'll usually be severely dyspneic and have great difficulty talking. Note tachypnea with obvious use of the accessory muscles of respiration; active, prolonged expirations (with an inspiration-expiration ratio of 1:2 to 1:4); and, perhaps, nasal flaring. Coughing may not be evident because the patient may be unable to cough.

The patient may display signs of hypoxemia, such as anxiety, restlessness, and confusion. If he begins to fall asleep or looks cyanotic, he may be developing acute respiratory failure.

Percussion of the chest reveals hyperresonance. Palpation may disclose vocal fremitus. In addition, palpation of peripheral pulses reveals a rapid, thready pulse. You may also discover pulsus paradoxus, a drop of more than 12 mm Hg in systolic blood pressure during inspiration. This phenomenon, which indicates a severe airflow obstruction, is linked to decreased filling of the right atrium, decreased lung compliance, and increased intrathoracic pressure.

Auscultation may disclose inspiratory and expiratory wheezing before you even place a stethoscope on the patient's chest. However, in a severe attack, you may not hear wheezing because the patient lacks sufficient air movement in his chest. Heart sounds will be distant, and heart rate and blood pressure will usually be increased.

DIAGNOSTIC TESTS

• *Pulmonary function tests* reveal signs of airway obstruction (decreased flow rates and forced expiratory volume in 1st second of expiration [FEV_1], low-normal or decreased vital capacity, increased total lung and residual capacity, and decreased peak expiratory flow rate [PEFR].) The patient with status asthmaticus may have difficulty performing these tests. PEFR requires only a forceful breath rather than a full, sustained exhalation; therefore, this test is easier for the patient to perform. FEV_1 and PEFR are monitored over time to determine trends in lung function. Falling FEV_1 and PEFR indicate worsening airway obstruction.

Typically, the patient experiencing an asthmatic attack has decreased partial pressure of carbon dioxide in arterial blood ($PaCO_2$) and decreased partial pressure of oxygen in arterial blood (PaO_2.) However, in status asthmaticus, the $PaCO_2$ may be normal or increased, indicating severe bronchial obstruction, and the FEV_1 will probably be less than 25% of the predicted value. Initiating treatment tends to improve the airflow. However, even when the asthma attack appears controlled, the spirometric values (FEV_1 and forced expiratory flow) remain abnormal. Residual volume remains abnormal for the longest period – up to 3 weeks after the attack.

• *ABG analyses* or *pulse oximetry measurements* are necessary to diagnose status asthmaticus.

• *Chest X-ray* can diagnose or monitor the progress of status asthmaticus. The X-ray may show hyperinflation with areas of focal atelectasis.

• *Laboratory tests* may reveal an increased serum IgE concentration and an increased eosinophil count as the result of an allergic reaction.

TREATMENT

In status asthmaticus, treatment consists of beta-agonist bronchodilators, corticosteroids, oral sympathomimetics, sympathomimetic aerosol therapy (such as metaproterenol and albuterol), epinephrine injected subcutaneously for rapid effect, terbutaline, aminophylline, and theophylline. (See *Identifying epinephrine dosage in status asthmaticus.*) Bronchodilators are given via aerosol therapy at intervals dictated by the severity of the patient's symptoms – as often as hourly or continuously.

Systemic corticosteroids, such as methylprednisolone, given I.V. reduce inflammation and edema of the airway mucosa. The dosage depends on the patient's size, the severity of the attack, and his previous corticosteroid therapy (if any).

ABG analysis and pulse oximetry help assess respiratory status, particularly after ventilator therapy or a change in oxygen concentration. If the patient is hypoxemic, aerosolized oxygen, rather than compressed air, will be administered.

The patient will require antibiotic therapy if he shows any sign of infections. Also, he may need fluid replacement.

KEY NURSING DIAGNOSES AND PATIENT OUTCOMES

Impaired gas exchange related to altered oxygen supply caused by severe bronchoconstriction. Based on this nursing diagnosis, you'll establish these patient outcomes. The patient will:
• regain and maintain normal breath sounds
• have ABG values return to normal
• exhibit no signs and symptoms of hypoxia.

Inability to sustain spontaneous ventilation related to exhaustion caused by prolonged asthmatic attack. Based on this nursing diagnosis, you'll establish these patient outcomes. The patient will:
• have his condition identified quickly and treated promptly with intubation and mechanical ventilation
• breathe spontaneously after the withdrawal of ventilator support.

Ineffective breathing pattern related to fatigue from prolonged asthmatic attack. Based on this nursing diagnosis, you'll establish these patient outcomes. The patient will:
• regain and maintain maximum lung expansion with adequate ventilation
• exhibit a respiratory rate within 5 breaths/minute of baseline
• no longer use accessory respiratory muscles.

NURSING INTERVENTIONS
• Maintain the patient in semi-Fowler's position and encourage diaphragmatic breathing. Stay with him and encourage him to relax.
• As ordered, administer humidified oxygen by nasal cannula at 2 to 4 liters/minute to ease breathing and to increase arterial oxygen saturation. Later, adjust oxygen according to the

---

DOSAGE FINDER

Identifying epinephrine dosage in status asthmaticus

To treat bronchospasm, give an adult 0.1 to 0.25 mg (1 to 2.5 ml of a 1:10,000 dilution) I.V. slowly over 5 to 10 minutes. As ordered, follow this with an infusion of 1 to 4 mcg/minute.

In S.C. administration, give 200 to 500 mcg every 20 minutes to 4 hours up to a maximum of 1 mg.

In oral inhalation, give two to three inhalations of a 2.25% solution. Then, if necessary, give two to three inhalations four to six times a day.

If you're using a nebulizer, give 5 ml of a 0.1% solution for 15 minutes every 3 to 4 hours.

---

patient's vital functions and ABG measurements. If necessary, assist with intubation and provide supportive care for mechanical ventilation.
• Administer drugs as ordered. Continue epinephrine or a sympathomimetic as ordered.
• If aminophylline has not been administered as yet, prepare to administer the drug I.V. as a loading dose followed by a continuous I.V. drip as ordered. Use an I.V. infusion pump to safely control the continuous infusion rate of aminophylline. Because young patients and those who smoke or take barbiturates have increased aminophylline metabolism, expect to administer a larger dose to these patients. Simultaneously, give a loading dose of corticosteroid medication I.V. or I.M., as ordered, if not already done.
• Question sedative and narcotic orders because these drugs can depress the respiratory system.
• Combat dehydration with I.V. fluids until the patient can tolerate oral fluids, which will help loosen secretions.
• Encourage the patient to express his fears and concerns about his illness. Answer his questions honestly. Encourage him to identify and follow care measures and activities that promote relaxation.

Monitoring

• Assess the patient's respiratory function closely, paying close attention to his respiratory rate, pattern, and depth. Alert the doctor immediately to any sudden or dramatic changes as well as to a worsening condition.
• Monitor oxygenation with periodic ABG samples and continuous pulse oximetry. Rising carbon dioxide, falling pH, and increasing respiratory fatigue are signs that call for intubation and mechanical ventilation.
• Obtain frequent vital signs, remaining especially alert for pulsus paradoxus.
• Evaluate the patient's response to drug therapy.

♦ NURSING ALERT. Watch for signs and symptoms of aminophylline toxicity. Elderly patients with hepatic or cardiac insufficiency or those taking erythromycin are predisposed to aminophylline toxicity.
• Assess the patient for dehydration, which may increase the thickness of the secretions and make them harder to remove; this, in turn, may cause airway plugging.
• Monitor for signs and symptoms of complications, such as acute respiratory failure.

Patient teaching

• After the patient's condition stabilizes, focus your patient education on preventing recurring attacks. Teach the patient and family the factors that can trigger asthma and the early warning signs of wheezing and shortness of breath. Teach the patient how to use the metered dose inhaler correctly. Advise him about possible adverse effects associated with his medications, and instruct him to notify his doctor if symptoms occur.
• Urge the patient to drink plenty of fluids (at least 3 qt [3 liters] daily) to maintain hydration and prevent thickening of airway secretions. Show him how to breathe deeply. Instruct him to cough up secretions accumulated overnight and to allow time for medications to work. He can best loosen secretions by coughing correctly—inhaling fully and gently, then bending over with his arms crossed over the abdomen before coughing.

• Teach the patient and his family about diaphragmatic and pursed-lip breathing. Encourage the patient to perform relaxation exercises whenever he feels himself becoming anxious.
• Encourage the patient to eat a well-balanced diet to prevent respiratory infection and fatigue. Help him identify foods that trigger an attack. Teach him and his family to avoid known allergens and irritants, such as aerosol sprays, smoke, and automobile exhausts. Refer the patient to community resources, such as the American Lung Association and the National Allergy and Asthma Network.

ADULT RESPIRATORY DISTRESS SYNDROME

A form of pulmonary edema, adult respiratory distress syndrome (ARDS) can quickly lead to acute respiratory failure. Also known as shock, stiff, white, wet, or Da Nang lung, ARDS may follow direct or indirect lung injury.

Increased permeability of the alveolocapillary membranes allows fluid to accumulate in the lung interstitium, alveolar spaces, and small airways, causing the lung to stiffen. This impairs ventilation, reducing oxygenation of pulmonary capillary blood. Difficult to recognize, the disorder can prove fatal within 48 hours of onset if not promptly diagnosed and treated.

Although this four-stage syndrome can progress to intractable and fatal hypoxemia, patients who recover may have little or no permanent lung damage.

In some patients, the syndrome may coexist with disseminated intravascular coagulation (DIC). Whether ARDS stems from DIC or develops independently remains unclear. Patients with three concurrent ARDS risk factors have an 85% probability of developing ARDS.

CAUSES

Trauma is the most common cause of ARDS, possibly because trauma-related factors, such as fat emboli, sepsis, shock, pulmonary contusions, and multiple transfusions, increase the likelihood that microemboli will develop.

Other common causes of ARDS include anaphylaxis, aspiration of gastric contents, diffuse pneumonia (especially viral), drug overdose (for example, heroin, aspirin, and ethchlorvynol), idiosyncratic drug reaction (to ampicillin and hydrochlorothiazide), inhalation of noxious gases (such as nitrous oxide, ammonia, and chlorine), near drowning, and oxygen toxicity.

Less common causes of ARDS include coronary artery bypass grafting, hemodialysis, leukemia, acute miliary tuberculosis, pancreatitis, thrombotic thrombocytopenic purpura, uremia, and venous air embolism.

COMPLICATIONS

ARDS can lead to metabolic and respiratory acidosis and ensuing cardiac arrest.

ASSESSMENT

As you conduct your assessment, be alert for rapid, shallow breathing, dyspnea, tachycardia, hypoxemia, intercostal and suprasternal retractions, crackles and rhonchi, restlessness, apprehension, mental sluggishness, and motor dysfunction. ARDS is staged from I to IV, and each stage has typical signs. (See *Recognizing ARDS stages.*)

DIAGNOSTIC TESTS

• *Arterial blood gas (ABG) analysis* (with the patient breathing room air) initially shows a reduced partial pressure of oxygen in arterial blood, or PaO_2 (less than 60 mm Hg), and a decreased partial pressure of carbon dioxide in arterial blood, or $PaCO_2$ (less than 35 mm Hg). Hypoxemia, despite increased supplemental oxygen, is the hallmark of ARDS. The resulting blood pH usually reflects respiratory alkalosis. As ARDS worsens, ABG values show respiratory acidosis (increasing $PaCO_2$ [more than 45 mm Hg]) and metabolic acidosis (decreasing bicarbonate levels [less than 22 mEq/liter]) and declining PaO_2, despite oxygen therapy.

• *Pulmonary artery catheterization* helps identify the cause of pulmonary edema by measuring pulmonary artery wedge pressure

Recognizing ARDS stages

Adult respiratory distress syndrome (ARDS) is staged from I to IV as follows.

Stage I
In this first stage, the patient may complain of dyspnea, especially on exertion. Respiratory and pulse rates are normal to high. Auscultation may reveal diminished breath sounds.

Stage II
Respiratory distress becomes more apparent in stage II. The patient may use accessory muscles to breathe and appear pallid, anxious, and restless. He may have a dry cough with thick, frothy sputum and bloody, sticky secretions. Palpation may disclose cool, clammy skin. Tachycardia and tachypnea may accompany elevated blood pressure. Auscultation may detect basilar crackles. (Stage II signs and symptoms may be incorrectly attributed to other causes, such as multiple trauma.)

Stage III
The patient may struggle to breathe if he's in stage III. A vital signs check reveals tachypnea (more than 30 breaths/minute), tachycardia with arrhythmias (usually premature ventricular contractions), and a labile blood pressure. Inspection may reveal a productive cough and pale, cyanotic skin. Auscultation may disclose crackles and rhonchi. The patient will need intubation and ventilation.

Stage IV
At this late stage, the patient has acute respiratory failure with severe hypoxia. His mental status is deteriorating, and he may become comatose. His skin appears pale and cyanotic. Spontaneous respirations are not evident. Bradycardia with arrhythmias accompanies hypotension. Metabolic and respiratory acidosis develop. When ARDS reaches this stage, the patient is at high risk for fibrosis. Pulmonary damage becomes life-threatening.

(PAWP). This procedure also allows collection of samples of pulmonary artery and mixed venous blood that show decreased oxygen saturation, reflecting tissue hypoxia. PAWP values in ARDS are 12 mm Hg or less.

• *Serial chest X-rays* in early stages show bilateral infiltrates. In later stages, findings demonstrate lung fields with a ground-glass appearance and, eventually (with irreversible hypoxemia), "whiteouts" of both lung fields.

Differential diagnosis must rule out cardiogenic pulmonary edema, pulmonary vasculitis, and diffuse pulmonary hemorrhage. Etiologic tests may involve sputum analyses (including Gram stain and culture and sensitivity), blood cultures (to identify infectious organisms), toxicology tests (to screen for drug ingestion), and various serum amylase tests (to rule out pancreatitis).

TREATMENT

Therapy focuses on correcting the cause of the syndrome if possible and preventing progression of life-threatening hypoxemia and respiratory acidosis. Supportive care consists of administering humidified oxygen by a tight-fitting mask, which facilitates the use of continuous positive airway pressure (CPAP). However, this therapy alone seldom fulfills the ARDS patient's ventilatory requirements. If the patient's hypoxemia doesn't subside with this treatment, he may require intubation, mechanical ventilation, and positive end-expiratory pressure (PEEP). Other supportive measures include fluid restriction, diuretic therapy, and correction of electrolyte and acid-base imbalances.

When a patient with ARDS needs mechanical ventilation, sedatives, narcotics, or neuromuscular blocking agents (such as vecuronium) may be ordered to minimize restlessness (and thereby oxygen consumption and carbon dioxide production) and to facilitate ventilation.

When ARDS results from fat emboli or a chemical injury, a short course of high-dose corticosteroids may help if given early. Treatment with sodium bicarbonate may be necessary to reverse severe metabolic acidosis. Fluids and vasopressors may be needed to maintain blood pressure. Nonviral infections require treatment with antimicrobial drugs.

KEY NURSING DIAGNOSES AND PATIENT OUTCOMES

Anxiety related to potential threat of death because of ARDS. Based on this nursing diagnosis, you'll establish these patient outcomes. The patient will:

• state or write down feelings of anxiety about his condition and death
• use support systems to assist with coping
• demonstrate diminished physical symptoms of anxiety.

Impaired gas exchange related to direct or indirect lung injury. Based on this nursing diagnosis, you'll establish these patient outcomes. The patient will:

• demonstrate adequate gas exchange with therapy, evidenced by ABG values that return to normal and restoration of normal respiratory function
• recover from ARDS with no residual lung damage.

Inability to sustain spontaneous ventilation related to pulmonary edema and fibrosis. Based on this nursing diagnosis, you'll establish these patient outcomes. The patient will:

• recover from lung tissue damage
• resume spontaneous ventilation with treatment
• regain and maintain normal ABG values.

NURSING INTERVENTIONS

• Maintain a patent airway by suctioning. Use sterile, nontraumatic technique. Ensure adequate humidification to help liquefy tenacious secretions.
• If the patient is on mechanical ventilation, drain any condensate from the tubing promptly to ensure maximum oxygen delivery.
• Provide alternative means of communication for the patient on mechanical ventilation.
• Be prepared to administer CPAP to the patient with severe hypoxemia.
• To maintain PEEP, suction only as needed. High-frequency jet ventilation may also be required.
• Give sedatives, as ordered, to reduce restlessness.

• If the patient has a pulmonary artery catheter in place, change dressings according to hospital guidelines, using strict aseptic technique.

• Reposition the patient often.

• Note and record any changes in respiratory status or temperature or hypotension that may indicate a deteriorating condition. Notify the doctor.

• Record caloric intake. Administer tube feedings and parenteral nutrition as ordered. Plan patient care to allow periods of uninterrupted sleep. To promote health and prevent fatigue, arrange for alternate periods of rest and activity.

• Maintain joint mobility by performing passive range-of-motion exercises. If possible, help the patient perform active exercises.

• Provide meticulous skin care. To prevent skin breakdown, reposition the endotracheal tube from side to side every 24 hours.

• Provide emotional support. Answer the patient's and family's questions as fully as possible to allay their fears and concerns.

Monitoring

• Frequently assess the patient's respiratory status. Be alert for inspiratory retractions. Note respiratory rate, rhythm, and depth. Watch for dyspnea and accessory muscle use. Listen for adventitious or diminished breath sounds. Check for clear, frothy sputum (indicating pulmonary edema).

• Monitor the patient's level of consciousness, noting confusion or mental sluggishness.

• Be alert for signs of treatment-induced complications, including arrhythmias, DIC, GI bleeding, infection, malnutrition, paralytic ileus, pneumothorax, pulmonary fibrosis, renal failure, thrombocytopenia, and tracheal stenosis.

• Closely monitor the patient's heart rate and blood pressure. Watch for arrhythmias that may result from hypoxemia, acid-base disturbances, or electrolyte imbalance.

• With pulmonary artery catheterization, know the desired PAWP level; check readings often, and watch for decreasing mixed venous oxygen saturation.

• Frequently evaluate the patient's serum electrolyte levels. Measure intake and output. Weigh the patient daily.

• Check ventilator settings frequently. Monitor ABG levels.

• Monitor and record the patient's response to medication.

• Because PEEP may lower cardiac output, check for hypotension, tachycardia, and decreased urine output.

• Evaluate the patient's nutritional intake.

• If the patient has injuries that affect the lungs, watch for adverse respiratory changes, especially in the first few days after the injury, when his condition may appear to be improving.

Patient teaching

• Explain the disorder to the patient and his family. Tell them what signs and symptoms may occur, and review the treatment that may be required.

• Orient the patient and his family to the unit and hospital surroundings. Provide them with simple explanations and demonstrations of treatments.

• Tell the recuperating patient that recovery will take some time and that he'll feel weak for a while. Urge him to share his concerns with the staff.

ACUTE RESPIRATORY FAILURE

When the lungs can't adequately maintain arterial oxygenation or eliminate carbon dioxide, acute respiratory failure results. Left untreated, the condition leads to tissue hypoxia. In patients with essentially normal lung tissue, acute respiratory failure usually produces a partial pressure of carbon dioxide in arterial blood ($Paco_2$) greater than 50 mm Hg and a partial pressure of oxygen in arterial blood (Pao_2) below 50 mm Hg.

These limits, however, don't apply to patients with chronic obstructive pulmonary disease (COPD). These patients consistently have a high $Paco_2$ (hypercapnia) and a low Pao_2 (hypoxemia) level. So for them, only acute deterioration in arterial blood gas (ABG) values – and corresponding clinical deterioration – signals acute respiratory failure.

CAUSES

Acute respiratory failure may develop from any condition that increases the work of breathing and decreases the respiratory drive. These conditions may result from respiratory tract infection (such as bronchitis or pneumonia), bronchospasm, or accumulated secretions secondary to cough suppression. Other common causes are related to ventilatory failure, in which the brain fails to direct respiration, and gas exchange failure, in which respiratory structures fail to function properly. (See *Mechanics of acute respiratory failure.*)

COMPLICATIONS

Tissue hypoxia, metabolic acidosis, and respiratory and cardiac arrest are among possible complications.

ASSESSMENT

Because acute respiratory failure is life-threatening, you probably won't have time to conduct an in-depth patient interview. Instead, you'll rely on family members or the patient's medical records to discover the precipitating incident.

On inspection, you'll note cyanosis of the oral mucosa, lips, and nail beds; nasal flaring; and ashen skin. You may observe the patient yawning and using accessory muscles to breathe. He may appear restless, anxious, depressed, lethargic, agitated, or confused. Additionally, he usually exhibits tachypnea, which signals impending respiratory failure.

Palpation may reveal cold, clammy skin and asymmetrical chest movement, which suggests pneumothorax. If tactile fremitus is present, you'll notice that it decreases over an obstructed bronchus or pleural effusion but increases over consolidated lung tissue.

Percussion—especially in patients with COPD—reveals hyperresonance. If acute respiratory failure results from atelectasis or pneumonia, percussion usually produces a dull or flat sound.

Auscultation typically discloses diminished breath sounds. In patients with pneumothorax, breath sounds may be absent. In other cases of respiratory failure, you may hear such adventitious breath sounds as wheezes (in asthma) and rhonchi (in bronchitis). If you hear crackles, suspect pulmonary edema as the cause of respiratory failure.

DIAGNOSTIC TESTS

• *ABG analysis* is the key to diagnosis (and subsequent treatment) of acute respiratory failure. Progressively deteriorating ABG values and pH—compared with the patient's "normal" values—strongly suggest acute respiratory failure. In patients with essentially normal lung tissue, a pH below 7.35 usually indicates acute respiratory failure. In patients with COPD, the pH is even lower.

• *Chest X-rays* identify underlying pulmonary diseases or conditions, such as emphysema, atelectasis, lesions, pneumothorax, infiltrates, and effusions.

• *Electrocardiography (ECG)* can demonstrate arrhythmias. Common ECG patterns point to cor pulmonale and myocardial hypoxia.

• *Pulse oximetry* reveals decreasing arterial oxygen saturation.

• *Blood tests,* such as a white blood cell count, detect underlying causes. Abnormally low hematocrit and hemoglobin levels signal blood loss, which indicates decreased oxygen-carrying capacity.

• *Serum electrolyte findings* vary. Hypokalemia may result from compensatory hyperventilation, the body's attempt to correct alkalosis; hypochloremia usually occurs in metabolic alkalosis.

• *Pulmonary artery catheterization* helps to distinguish between pulmonary and cardiovascular causes of acute respiratory failure and monitors hemodynamic pressures.

Additional tests, such as a blood culture, Gram stain, and sputum culture, may identify the pathogen.

TREATMENT

Acute respiratory failure constitutes an emergency. The patient will need cautious use of oxygen therapy (nasal prongs or a Venturi mask) to raise his Pao_2. If significant respiratory acidosis persists, mechanical ventilation with an endotracheal, nasotracheal, or a tra-

Mechanics of acute respiratory failure

Three major malfunctions account for impaired gas exchange and subsequent acute respiratory failure. They include alveolar hypoventilation, ventilation-perfusion mismatch, and intrapulmonary (right-to-left) shunting.

Alveolar hypoventilation

Decreased oxygen saturation may result when chronic airway obstruction reduces alveolar minute ventilation. In such cases, partial pressure of oxygen in arterial blood (PaO_2) falls and partial pressure of carbon dioxide in arterial blood rises. Hypoxia results.

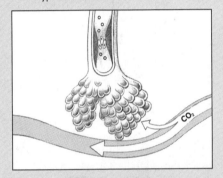

Ventilation-perfusion mismatch

The most common cause of hypoxemia, imbalances in ventilation and perfusion occur when conditions such as pulmonary embolism or adult respiratory distress syndrome interrupt normal gas exchange in a specific lung region. Either too little ventilation with normal blood flow or too little blood flow with normal ventilation may cause the imbalance. Whichever happens, the result is the same: PaO_2 falls.

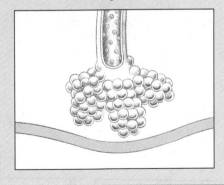

Right-to-left shunting

Untreated ventilation or perfusion imbalances can lead to right-to-left shunting in which blood passes from the heart's right side to its left without being oxygenated.

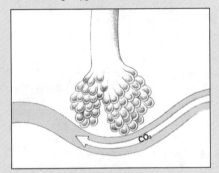

Implications

The hypoxemia and hypercapnia characteristic of respiratory failure stimulate strong compensatory responses by all body systems, including the respiratory, cardiovascular, and central nervous systems.

In response to hypoxemia, for example, the sympathetic nervous system triggers vasoconstriction, increases peripheral resistance, and boosts the heart rate.

The body responds to hypercapnia with cerebral depression, hypotension, circulatory failure, and an increased heart rate and cardiac output. Both hypoxemia and hypercapnia cause the brain's respiratory control center to first increase respiratory depth (tidal volume) and then increase the respiratory rate. As respiratory failure worsens, intercostal, supraclavicular, and suprasternal retractions may also occur.

High-frequency jet ventilation

This technique was developed for use when high peak airway pressures or large intrapleural air leaks preclude conventional mechanical ventilation. The high-frequency jet ventilation (HFJV) system employs a narrow injector cannula to deliver short, rapid bursts of oxygen to the airways under low pressure.

Advantages
This combination of high respiratory rate, low tidal volumes, and low pressure enhances alveolar gas exchange without elevating peak inspiratory pressures and compromising cardiac output—the major drawback of conventional high-volume, high-pressure mechanical ventilation. Thus, HFJV is valuable for patients with hemodynamic instability and those at high risk for pulmonary barotrauma, such as young children. It's also useful for ventilating patients during bronchoscopy, laryngoscopy, and laryngeal surgery because its narrow cannula doesn't obstruct the operating field.

A potential new use of HFJV is in emergency respiratory situations. Because the cannula can be inserted directly into the trachea through a cricothyrotomy, HFJV may be used when upper airway trauma or obstruction precludes intubation. Use of HFJV in cardiopulmonary resuscitation allows continuous ventilation during chest compression. And its use in patients with chest trauma decreases chest wall movement and improves stability, enhancing ventilation.

cheostomy tube may be necessary. High-frequency jet ventilation may be initiated if the patient's condition doesn't improve with conventional mechanical ventilation. (See *High-frequency jet ventilation* and *Responding to mechanical ventilator alarms.*)

Treatment routinely includes antibiotics (for infection), bronchodilators and, possibly, corticosteroids.

If the patient also has cor pulmonale and decreased cardiac output, fluid restriction and administration of positive inotropic agents, vasopressors, and diuretics may be ordered.

KEY NURSING DIAGNOSES AND PATIENT OUTCOMES

Impaired gas exchange related to altered oxygen supply caused by the underlying pulmonary condition. Based on this nursing diagnosis, you'll establish these patient outcomes. The patient will:
• exhibit PaO_2 and breath sounds that return to baseline
• experience no dyspnea
• cough and deep-breathe adequately to keep airways clear, which enhances oxygenation.

Ineffective airway clearance related to decreased energy, fatigue, or presence of tracheobronchial secretions. Based on this nursing diagnosis, you'll establish these patient outcomes. The patient will:
• cough and deep-breathe adequately to expectorate secretions
• demonstrate skill in conserving energy while attempting to clear airway
• maintain a patent airway.

Ineffective breathing pattern related to decreased energy or fatigue caused by underlying pulmonary condition or metabolic acidosis. Based on this nursing diagnosis, you'll establish these patient outcomes. The patient will:
• achieve maximum lung expansion with adequate ventilation
• demonstrate skill in conserving energy while carrying out activities of daily living
• exhibit a respiratory rate and pattern and ABG values that return to baseline and remain within this normal range.

NURSING INTERVENTIONS
• Orient the patient to the treatment unit. Most patients with acute respiratory failure receive intensive care. Acquainting the patient with procedures, sounds, and sights helps to minimize his anxiety.
• To reverse hypoxemia, administer oxygen at appropriate concentrations to maintain a PaO_2 of at least 60 mm Hg. The patient with COPD usually requires only small amounts of supplemental oxygen.
• Maintain a patent airway. If your patient retains carbon dioxide, encourage him to cough

Responding to mechanical ventilator alarms

Mechanical ventilators have preset alarms triggered by changes in the patient's respiratory rate, which signal changes (some potentially fatal) in the patient's condition. Use this chart to identify the potential causes of these alarms and the actions you must take to resolve them.

ALARM	POSSIBLE CAUSE	ACTIONS
High pressure The pressure required to ventilate the patient exceeds the preset pressure, usually set at 10 to 15 cm H_2O above normal peak airway pressure.	• Pneumothorax, decreased lung compliance • Excessive secretions, coughing, airway plugging • Changes in patient position • Kinked ventilator tubing	• Assess breath sounds and chest wall expansion, percuss for hyperresonance, and verify endotracheal (ET) tube placement. • Provide suctioning. • Reposition patient. • Unkink tubing; check ventilator circuit.
Low pressure The resistance to the inspiratory flow is less than the preset amount, usually set at 10 cm H_2O below peak airway pressure.	• Patient disconnected from ventilator • Break in ventilator circuit	• Check for disconnected ventilator tubing; reconnect patient. • Check ventilator for loose connections; notify respiratory therapist if break isn't obvious or can't be corrected quickly. • Use manual resuscitator to support patient if problem can't be solved quickly.
Apnea The period of apnea exceeds preset time; ventilator defaults to assist-control mode (not available on all ventilators).	• Patient fatigue • Decreased level of consciousness (LOC)	• Assess patient for fatigue and changes in LOC. • Notify doctor if patient's condition has changed. • Alert respiratory therapist to ventilator changes.
Respiratory rate The respiratory rate falls below or exceeds the preset rate.	• Patient anxiety • Hypoxia	• Reassure patient; use relaxation techniques; give medication as ordered. • Evaluate for signs and symptoms of hypoxia, such as decreased LOC, confusion, cyanosis, tachycardia, and arrhythmias; assess need for arterial blood gas analysis or pulse oximetry reading.
Low exhaled tidal volume The exhaled tidal volume falls below preset alarm volume.	• Leak in ET or tracheal tube cuff • Airway secretions, increasing airway resistance, decreased lung compliance • Increased respiratory rate • Leak in ventilator system	• Assess ET or tracheal tube cuff for patency; add air if needed and if cuff pressure doesn't exceed 18 mm Hg (22 cm H_2O). • Suction airway secretions, assess peak airway pressure, and assess breath sounds and chest wall expansion. • Assess patient's respiratory rate. • Assess ventilator circuit for leaks; notify respiratory therapist if you detect one.

and breathe deeply with pursed lips. If he's alert, have him use an incentive spirometer. If he's intubated and lethargic, reposition him every 1 to 2 hours. Use postural drainage and chest physiotherapy to help clear secretions.
• Perform oral hygiene measures frequently.
• Apply soft wrist restraints for the confused patient if needed. This will prevent him from disconnecting the oxygen setup. However, remember that these restraints can increase anxiety, fear, and agitation.
• Position the patient for comfort and optimal gas exchange. Place the call button within the patient's reach.
• Maintain the patient in a normothermic state to reduce his body's demand for oxygen.
• Pace patient care activities to maximize the patient's energy level and provide needed rest.
• If the patient requires mechanical ventilation, check ventilator settings, cuff pressures, and ABG values often to ensure correct fraction of inspired oxygen (FIO_2) settings, which are determined by ABG levels. Draw blood samples for ABG analysis 20 to 30 minutes after every change in the FIO_2 setting.
• Check mechanical ventilator alarms frequently to ensure that they are on and functioning. Respond to any alarm immediately and take corrective action quickly.
• Suction the trachea as needed after oxygenation. Provide humidification to liquefy secretions.
• Prevent infection by using sterile technique while suctioning and by changing ventilator tubing every 24 hours.
• Prevent tracheal erosion, which can result from an overinflated artificial airway cuff compressing the tracheal wall's vasculature. Use the minimal-leak technique and a cuffed tube with high residual volume (low-pressure cuff), a foam cuff, or a pressure-regulating valve on the cuff. Measure cuff pressure every 8 hours.
• Implement measures to prevent nasal tissue necrosis. Position and maintain the nasotracheal tube midline within the nostrils, and provide meticulous care. Periodically, loosen the tape securing the tube to prevent skin breakdown. Avoid excessive movement of any

tubes, and make sure that the ventilator tubing has adequate support.
• If the patient is receiving corticosteroids, administer antacids or histamine-receptor antagonists, as ordered.
• Help the patient communicate without words. Offer him a pen and tablet, a word chart, or an alphabet board.

Monitoring

• Monitor the patient for a positive response to oxygen therapy, such as improved breathing, color, and ABG values.
• Observe the patient closely for respiratory arrest. Auscultate for breath sounds. Report any changes in ABG values immediately. Notify the doctor of any deterioration in oxygen saturation levels as detected by pulse oximetry.
• Watch for treatment complications, especially oxygen toxicity and adult respiratory distress syndrome.
• Frequently assess vital signs. Note and report an increasing pulse rate, rising or falling respiratory rate, declining blood pressure, or fever.
• Monitor and record serum electrolyte levels carefully. Take steps to correct imbalances. Monitor fluid balance by recording the patient's intake and output and daily weight.
• Check the cardiac monitor for arrhythmias.
• If the patient requires mechanical ventilation, monitor changes in ABG values after each change in the FIO_2 setting.
• When suctioning the patient, check for any changes in sputum quality, consistency, or color.
• Watch for complications of mechanical ventilation, such as reduced cardiac output, pneumothorax or other barotrauma, increased pulmonary vascular resistance, diminished urine output, increased intracranial pressure, and GI bleeding.
• Routinely assess endotracheal tube position and patency. Make sure the tube is placed properly and taped securely. Immediately after intubation, check for accidental intubation of the esophagus or the mainstem bronchus, which may have occurred during tube insertion. Also be alert for transtracheal or la-

ryngeal perforation, aspiration, broken teeth, nosebleeds, vagal reflexes (such as bradycardia), arrhythmias, and hypertension.
• After tube placement, watch for complications, such as tube displacement, herniation of the tube's cuff, respiratory infection, and tracheal malacia and stenosis.
• Monitor for signs of stress ulcers, which are common in intubated patients, especially those in the intensive care unit. Inspect gastric secretions for blood, especially if the patient has a nasogastric tube or reports epigastric tenderness, nausea, or vomiting. Also monitor hemoglobin and hematocrit levels, and check all stools for blood.

Patient teaching

• Describe all tests and procedures to the patient and his family. Discuss the reasons for suctioning, chest physiotherapy, blood tests and, if used, soft wrist restraints.
• If the patient is intubated or has a tracheostomy, explain why he can't speak. Suggest alternative means of communication.
• Identify reportable signs of respiratory infection.
• If applicable, teach the patient about the effects of smoking. Provide resources to help him stop smoking.

ACUTE PULMONARY EDEMA

Marked by an accumulation of fluid in extravascular spaces of the lung, pulmonary edema is a common complication of cardiac disorders. The disorder may occur as a chronic condition, or it may develop quickly and lead rapidly to death, as in the case of acute pulmonary edema. (See *Nursing care in acute pulmonary edema*, pages 70 and 71.)

CAUSES

Pulmonary edema usually results from left ventricular failure caused by arteriosclerotic, cardiomyopathic, hypertensive, or valvular heart disease. The disorder stems from either of two mechanisms: increased pulmonary capillary hydrostatic pressure or decreased colloid osmotic pressure. Normally, the two

pressures are in balance. When this balance changes, pulmonary edema results.

If pulmonary capillary hydrostatic pressure increases, the compromised left ventricle requires increased filling pressures to maintain adequate output; these pressures are transmitted to the left atrium, pulmonary veins, and pulmonary capillary bed. This forces fluids and solutes from the intravascular compartment into the interstitium of the lungs. As the interstitium overloads with fluid, fluid floods the peripheral alveoli and impairs gas exchange.

If colloid osmotic pressure decreases, the natural pulling force that contains intravascular fluids is lost—nothing opposes the hydrostatic force. Thus, fluid flows freely into the interstitium and alveoli, resulting in pulmonary edema.

Other factors that may predispose the patient to pulmonary edema include:
• barbiturate or opiate poisoning
• congestive heart failure
• infusion of excessive volumes of I.V. fluids or an overly rapid infusion
• impaired pulmonary lymphatic drainage (from Hodgkin's disease or obliterative lymphangitis after radiation)
• inhalation of irritating gases
• mitral stenosis and left atrial myxoma (which impair left atrial emptying)
• pneumonia
• pulmonary veno-occlusive disease.

COMPLICATIONS

Acute pulmonary edema may progress to respiratory and metabolic acidosis, with subsequent cardiac or respiratory arrest.

ASSESSMENT

The history may include a predisposing factor for pulmonary edema. The patient typically complains of a persistent cough. He may report getting a cold and being dyspneic on exertion. He may experience paroxysmal nocturnal dyspnea and orthopnea.

On inspection, you may note restlessness and anxiety. With severe pulmonary edema, the patient's breathing may be visibly labored and rapid. His cough may sound intense and pro-

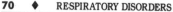

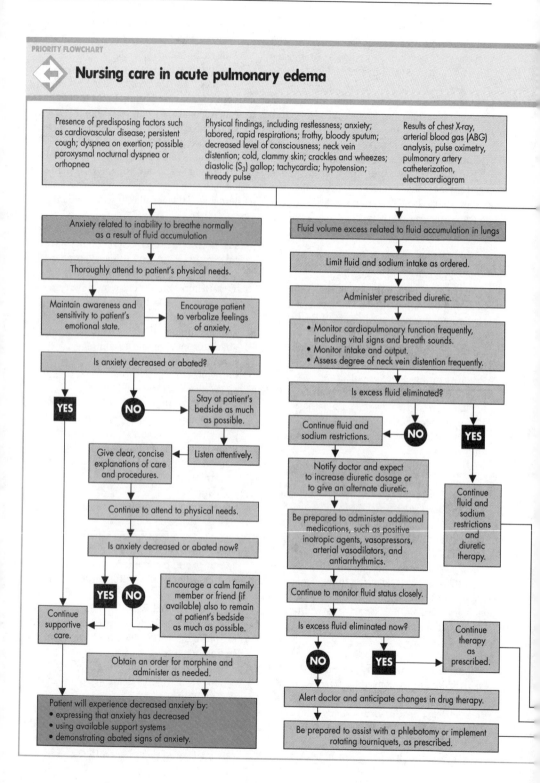

PRIORITY FLOWCHART

Nursing care in acute pulmonary edema

Presence of predisposing factors such as cardiovascular disease; persistent cough; dyspnea on exertion; possible paroxysmal nocturnal dyspnea or orthopnea

Physical findings, including restlessness; anxiety; labored, rapid respirations; frothy, bloody sputum; decreased level of consciousness; neck vein distention; cold, clammy skin; crackles and wheezes; diastolic (S_3) gallop; tachycardia; hypotension; thready pulse

Results of chest X-ray, arterial blood gas (ABG) analysis, pulse oximetry, pulmonary artery catheterization, electrocardiogram

---

Anxiety related to inability to breathe normally as a result of fluid accumulation

Thoroughly attend to patient's physical needs.

Maintain awareness and sensitivity to patient's emotional state.

Encourage patient to verbalize feelings of anxiety.

Is anxiety decreased or abated?

YES

NO → Stay at patient's bedside as much as possible.

↓

Listen attentively.

Give clear, concise explanations of care and procedures.

Continue to attend to physical needs.

Is anxiety decreased or abated now?

YES **NO**

Encourage a calm family member or friend (if available) also to remain at patient's bedside as much as possible.

Continue supportive care.

Obtain an order for morphine and administer as needed.

Patient will experience decreased anxiety by:
• expressing that anxiety has decreased
• using available support systems
• demonstrating abated signs of anxiety.

Fluid volume excess related to fluid accumulation in lungs

Limit fluid and sodium intake as ordered.

Administer prescribed diuretic.

• Monitor cardiopulmonary function frequently, including vital signs and breath sounds.
• Monitor intake and output.
• Assess degree of neck vein distention frequently.

Is excess fluid eliminated?

Continue fluid and sodium restrictions. ← **NO**   **YES**

Notify doctor and expect to increase diuretic dosage or to give an alternate diuretic.

Be prepared to administer additional medications, such as positive inotropic agents, vasopressors, arterial vasodilators, and antiarrhythmics.

Continue fluid and sodium restrictions and diuretic therapy.

Continue to monitor fluid status closely.

Is excess fluid eliminated now?

NO   **YES** →

Continue therapy as prescribed.

Alert doctor and anticipate changes in drug therapy.

Be prepared to assist with a phlebotomy or implement rotating tourniquets, as prescribed.

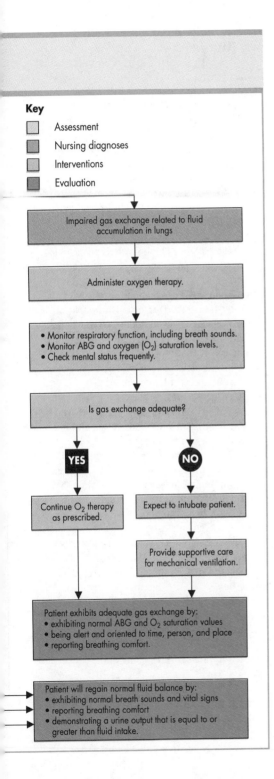

Key

☐ Assessment
☐ Nursing diagnoses
☐ Interventions
■ Evaluation

Impaired gas exchange related to fluid accumulation in lungs

Administer oxygen therapy.

• Monitor respiratory function, including breath sounds.
• Monitor ABG and oxygen (O_2) saturation levels.
• Check mental status frequently.

Is gas exchange adequate?

YES / **NO**

Continue O_2 therapy as prescribed.

Expect to intubate patient.

Provide supportive care for mechanical ventilation.

Patient exhibits adequate gas exchange by:
• exhibiting normal ABG and O_2 saturation values
• being alert and oriented to time, person, and place
• reporting breathing comfort.

Patient will regain normal fluid balance by:
• exhibiting normal breath sounds and vital signs
• reporting breathing comfort
• demonstrating a urine output that is equal to or greater than fluid intake.

duce frothy, bloody sputum. In advanced stages, the patient's level of consciousness decreases.

Typical palpation findings include neck vein distention. In acute pulmonary edema, the skin feels sweaty, cold, and clammy. Auscultation may reveal crepitant crackles and a diastolic (S_3) gallop. In severe pulmonary edema, the crackles become more diffuse, and you may hear wheezing as the alveoli and bronchioles fill with fluid.

Additional findings include worsening tachycardia, falling blood pressure, thready pulse, and decreased cardiac output. In advanced pulmonary edema, breath sounds diminish.

DIAGNOSTIC TESTS

Clinical features of pulmonary edema permit a working diagnosis. Diagnostic tests provide the following information.

• *Arterial blood gas (ABG) analysis* usually shows hypoxia with variable partial pressure of carbon dioxide in arterial blood, depending on the patient's degree of fatigue. ABG results may also identify metabolic acidosis.

• *Chest X-rays* show diffuse haziness of the lung fields and, usually, cardiomegaly and pleural effusion.

• *Pulse oximetry* may reveal decreasing arterial oxygen saturation levels.

• *Pulmonary artery catheterization* identifies left ventricular failure (indicated by elevated pulmonary artery wedge pressure). This finding helps to rule out adult respiratory distress syndrome, in which wedge pressure usually remains normal.

• *Electrocardiography* may disclose evidence of previous or current myocardial infarction.

TREATMENT

In pulmonary edema, treatment aims to reduce extravascular fluid, to improve gas exchange and myocardial function and, if possible, to correct underlying disease. High concentrations of oxygen can be administered by nasal cannula or mask. (Typically, the patient with pulmonary edema doesn't tolerate a mask.) If the patient's arterial oxygen levels remain too low, assisted ventilation can improve oxygen delivery to the tissues and usually improves his acid-base balance. A bronchodilator, such as aminophylline, may decrease bronchospasm and enhance myocardial contractility. Appropriate diuretics, such as furosemide, ethacrynic acid, and bumetanide, increase urination, which helps to mobilize extravascular fluid.

Treatment of myocardial dysfunction includes positive inotropic agents, such as digitalis glycosides and amrinone, to enhance contractility. Pressor agents may be given to enhance contractility and to promote vasoconstriction in peripheral vessels.

Antiarrhythmics may also be given, particularly in arrhythmias related to decreased cardiac output. Occasionally, arterial vasodilators, such as nitroprusside, can decrease peripheral vascular resistance, preload, and afterload.

Morphine may reduce anxiety and dyspnea and dilate the systemic venous bed, promoting blood flow from pulmonary circulation to the periphery.

Other treatments include rotating tourniquets and phlebotomy (both reduce preload). Phlebotomy will also remove hemoglobin, which may worsen the patient's hypoxemia.

KEY NURSING DIAGNOSES AND PATIENT OUTCOMES

Anxiety related to inability to breathe normally as a result of fluid accumulation. Based on this nursing diagnosis, you'll establish these patient outcomes. The patient will:
• express feelings of anxiety
• use support systems to assist with coping
• demonstrate abated physical symptoms of anxiety.

Fluid volume excess related to fluid accumulation in lungs. Based on this nursing diagnosis, you'll establish these patient outcomes. The patient will:
• eliminate excess fluid safely with treatment
• develop no complications, such as respiratory or metabolic acidosis
• regain and maintain a normal fluid balance.

Impaired gas exchange related to fluid accumulation in lungs. Based on this nursing di-

agnosis, you'll establish these patient outcomes. The patient will:
• demonstrate no severe signs or symptoms of tissue hypoxia
• regain and maintain normal ABG levels
• regain normal gas exchange with alleviation of pulmonary edema.

NURSING INTERVENTIONS

• Help the patient relax to promote oxygenation, control bronchospasm, and enhance myocardial contractility.
• Reassure the patient, who will be frightened by his inability to breathe normally. Provide emotional support to his family as well.
• Place the patient in high Fowler's position to enhance lung expansion.
• Administer oxygen as ordered.
• Administer nitroprusside in dextrose 5% in water by I.V. drip. During administration, protect the solution from light by wrapping the bottle or bag with aluminum foil. Discard the unused solution after 4 hours.
• Carefully record the time morphine is given and the amount administered.

Monitoring

• Assess the patient's condition frequently, and document his response to treatment. Monitor ABG and pulse oximetry values, oral and I.V. fluid intake, urine output and, in the patient with a pulmonary artery catheter, pulmonary end-diastolic and pulmonary artery wedge pressures. Check the cardiac monitor often. Report changes immediately.
• Watch for complications of treatment, such as electrolyte depletion. Also watch for complications of oxygen therapy and mechanical ventilation.
• Monitor vital signs every 15 to 30 minutes while administering nitroprusside. Watch for arrhythmias in patients receiving digitalis glycosides and for marked respiratory depression in those receiving morphine.

Patient teaching

• Urge the patient to comply with the prescribed medication regimen to avoid future episodes of pulmonary edema.

• Review all prescribed medications with the patient. If he takes digoxin, show him how to monitor his own pulse rate, and warn him to report signs of toxicity. Encourage consumption of potassium-rich foods to lower the risk of toxicity and cardiac arrhythmias. If he takes a vasodilator, teach him the signs of hypotension, and emphasize the need to avoid alcohol.
• Explain all procedures to the patient and his family.
• Emphasize the importance of reporting early signs of fluid overload.
• Explain the reasons for sodium restrictions. List high-sodium foods and drugs.
• Discuss ways to conserve physical energy.

PULMONARY EMBOLISM

An obstruction of the pulmonary arterial bed, pulmonary embolism occurs when a mass — such as a dislodged thrombus — lodges in a pulmonary artery branch, partially or completely obstructing it. This causes a ventilation-perfusion mismatch, resulting in hypoxemia, as well as intrapulmonary shunting.

Pulmonary embolism strikes approximately 500,000 adults each year in the United States, causing 50,000 deaths. The prognosis varies. Although the pulmonary infarction that results from embolism may be so mild as to be asymptomatic, massive embolism (more than 50% obstruction of pulmonary arterial circulation) and infarction can cause rapid death.

CAUSES

In most patients, pulmonary embolism results from a dislodged thrombus that originates in the leg veins. More than half of such thrombi arise in the deep veins of the legs; usually, multiple thrombi arise. Other, less common sources of thrombi include the right side of the heart, the upper extremities, and the pelvic, renal, and hepatic veins.

Such thrombus formation results from vascular wall damage, venous stasis, or hypercoagulability of the blood. Trauma, clot dissolution, sudden muscle spasm, intravascular pressure changes, or a change in peripheral blood flow can cause the thrombus to loosen or fragment. Then the thrombus — now called an embolus — floats to the heart's right side and enters the lung through the pulmonary artery. There, the embolus may dissolve, continue to fragment, or grow.

By occluding the pulmonary artery, the embolus prevents alveoli from producing enough surfactant to maintain alveolar integrity. As a result, alveoli collapse and atelectasis develops. If the embolus enlarges, it may clog most or all pulmonary vessels and cause death.

Rarely, pulmonary embolism results from other sources, including bone, air, fat, amniotic fluid, tumor cells, or a foreign object such as a needle, catheter part, or talc (from drugs intended for oral administration that are injected I.V. by addicts).

The risk increases with long-term immobility, certain predisposing disorders, venous injury, and increased blood coagulability. (See *Risk factors in pulmonary embolism,* page 74.)

COMPLICATIONS

If the embolus totally obstructs the arterial blood supply, pulmonary infarction (lung tissue death) occurs, a complication that affects about 10% of pulmonary embolism patients. It's more likely to occur if the patient has chronic cardiac or pulmonary disease.

Other complications include embolus extension, which blocks vessels beyond the occlusion; hepatic congestion and necrosis; pulmonary abscess; shock and adult respiratory distress syndrome; massive atelectasis; venous overload; ventilation-perfusion mismatch; and massive embolism, resulting in death.

ASSESSMENT

The patient's history may reveal a predisposing condition. He may also complain of shortness of breath for no apparent reason as well as pleuritic or anginal pain. The severity of these symptoms depends on the extent of damage. The signs and symptoms produced by small or fragmented emboli depend on the emboli's size, number, and location. If the embolus totally occludes the main pulmonary ar-

Risk factors in pulmonary embolism

Many disorders and treatments heighten the risk of pulmonary embolism. At particular risk are surgical patients. For example, the anesthetic used during surgery can injure lung vessels, and surgery itself or prolonged bed rest can promote venous stasis, which compounds the risk.

Predisposing disorders
• Lung disorders, especially chronic types
• Cardiac disorders
• Infection
• Diabetes mellitus
• History of thromboembolism, thrombophlebitis, or vascular insufficiency
• Sickle cell disease
• Autoimmune hemolytic anemia
• Polycythemia
• Osteomyelitis
• Long-bone fracture
• Manipulation or disconnection of central lines
• Cancer

Venous stasis
• Prolonged bed rest or immobilization
• Obesity
• Age over 40
• Burns
• Recent childbirth
• Orthopedic casts

Venous injury
• Surgery, particularly of the legs, pelvis, abdomen, or thorax
• Leg or pelvic fractures or injuries
• I.V. drug abuse
• I.V. therapy

Increased blood coagulability
• Use of high-estrogen oral contraceptives

On inspection, you may note a productive cough, possibly producing blood-tinged sputum. Less commonly, you may observe chest splinting, massive hemoptysis, leg edema and, with a large embolus, cyanosis, syncope, and distended neck veins. If you observe restlessness – a sign of hypoxia – the patient may have circulatory collapse.

Palpation may reveal a warm, tender area in the extremities, a possible area of thrombosis. On auscultation, you may hear transient pleural friction rub and crackles at the embolus site. You may also note an S_3 and S_4 gallop, with increased intensity of the pulmonic component of S_2.

In pleural infarction, the patient's history may include heart disease and left ventricular failure. The patient may complain of sudden, sharp pleuritic chest pain accompanied by progressive dyspnea. On inspection, you may note that he has a fever and is coughing up blood-tinged sputum. Auscultation may reveal a pleural friction rub.

DIAGNOSTIC TESTS
• *Lung perfusion scan (lung scintiscan)* can show a pulmonary embolus.
• *Ventilation scan*, usually performed with a lung perfusion scan, confirms the diagnosis.
• *Pulmonary angiography* may show a pulmonary vessel filling defect or an abrupt vessel ending, both of which indicate pulmonary embolism. Although the most definitive test, it's used only if the diagnosis can't be confirmed any other way and anticoagulant therapy would put the patient at significant risk.
• *Electrocardiography (ECG)* helps distinguish pulmonary embolism from myocardial infarction. If the patient has an extensive embolism, the ECG shows right axis deviation; right bundle-branch block; tall, peaked P waves; depressed ST segments; T-wave inversions (a sign of right ventricular heart strain); and supraventricular tachyarrhythmias.
• *Chest X-ray* helps rule out other pulmonary diseases, although it's inconclusive in the 1 to 2 hours after embolism. It may also show areas of atelectasis, an elevated diaphragm, pleural effusion, a prominent pulmonary artery and,

tery, the patient will have severe signs and symptoms.

When you begin your assessment, you may find that the patient is tachycardic. He may also have a low-grade fever. If circulatory collapse has occurred, he'll have a weak, rapid pulse rate and hypotension.

occasionally, the characteristic wedge-shaped infiltrate that suggests pulmonary infarction.
• *Arterial blood gas (ABG) analysis* sometimes reveals decreased partial pressure of oxygen in arterial blood and decreased partial pressure of carbon dioxide in arterial blood from tachypnea.
• *Thoracentesis* may rule out empyema, a sign of pneumonia, if the patient has pleural effusion.
• *Magnetic resonance imaging* can identify blood flow changes that point to an embolus or can identify the embolus itself.

TREATMENT

The goal of treatment is to maintain adequate cardiovascular and pulmonary function until the obstruction resolves and to prevent any recurrence. (Most emboli resolve within 10 to 14 days.)

Treatment for an embolism caused by a thrombus generally consists of oxygen therapy, as needed, and anticoagulation with heparin to inhibit new thrombus formation. The patient on heparin therapy needs daily coagulation studies (partial thromboplastin time [PTT]). The patient may also receive warfarin for 3 to 6 months, depending on his risk factors; if so, his prothrombin time (PT) will be monitored daily and then biweekly.

If the patient has a massive pulmonary embolism and shock, he may need fibrinolytic therapy with urokinase, streptokinase, or alteplase. Initially, these thrombolytic agents dissolve clots within 12 to 24 hours. Seven days later, these drugs lyse clots to the same degree as heparin therapy alone.

If the embolus causes hypotension, the patient may need a vasopressor. A septic embolus requires antibiotic therapy, not anticoagulants, and evaluation for the infection's source (most likely endocarditis).

If the patient can't take anticoagulants or develops recurrent emboli during anticoagulant therapy, he'll need surgery. Surgery consists of vena caval ligation, plication, or insertion of a device (umbrella filter) to filter blood returning to the heart and lungs. Angiographic demonstration of pulmonary embolism should take place before surgery.

To prevent postoperative venous thromboembolism, the patient may require rotating tourniquets applied to his legs. Or he can receive a combination of heparin and dihydroergotamine, which is more effective than heparin alone.

If the patient has a fat embolus, he'll need oxygen therapy. He may also need mechanical ventilation, corticosteroids and, if pulmonary edema arises, diuretics.

KEY NURSING DIAGNOSES AND PATIENT OUTCOMES

Altered cardiopulmonary tissue perfusion related to obstruction of pulmonary artery. Based on this nursing diagnosis, you'll establish these patient outcomes. The patient will:
• regain and maintain adequate cardiopulmonary tissue perfusion and cellular oxygenation
• show no signs or symptoms of pulmonary infarction or emboli extension
• eliminate risk factors when possible to prevent recurrence.

Anxiety related to situational crisis. Based on this nursing diagnosis, you'll establish these patient outcomes. The patient will:
• express feelings of anxiety
• cope with his condition without showing signs of severe anxiety.

Impaired gas exchange related to collapsed alveoli. Based on this nursing diagnosis, you'll establish these patient outcomes. The patient will:
• regain and maintain adequate ventilation
• regain and maintain normal ABG levels
• show no signs and symptoms of severe hypoxia.

NURSING INTERVENTIONS
• As ordered, give oxygen by nasal cannula or mask. If breathing is severely compromised, provide endotracheal intubation with assisted ventilation, as ordered.
• Administer heparin, as ordered, by I.V. push or by continuous drip. Don't administer I.M. injections.
• If the patient has pleuritic chest pain, administer the ordered analgesic.

• After the patient's condition stabilizes, encourage him to move about and assist him with isometric and range-of-motion exercises.

◆ NURSING ALERT. *Never* vigorously massage the patient's legs; doing so could cause thrombi to dislodge.

• Prepare the patient for surgery as indicated. After surgery, make sure he ambulates as soon as possible to prevent venous stasis.

• Provide the patient with adequate nutrition and fluids to promote healing.

• If needed, provide incentive spirometry to help the patient with deep breathing. Provide tissues and a bag for easy disposal of tissues.

• Offer the patient diversional activities to promote relaxation and relieve restlessness.

Monitoring

• Assess the patient's respiratory status closely. If he has worsening dyspnea, check his ABG levels.

• Monitor coagulation studies daily. Effective heparin therapy raises PTT to about 2 to 2½ times normal values. During heparin therapy, watch closely for epistaxis, petechiae, and other signs of abnormal bleeding. Also check the patient's stools for occult blood.

• Watch for possible complications of anticoagulant treatment, including gastric bleeding, cerebrovascular accident, and hemorrhage.

• Check the patient's temperature and the color of his feet to detect venous stasis.

Patient teaching

• Explain all procedures and treatments to the patient and his family.

• Teach the patient and his family the signs and symptoms of thrombophlebitis and pulmonary embolism.

• Teach the patient on anticoagulant therapy the signs of bleeding to watch for (bloody stools, blood in urine, large bruises).

• Instruct the patient that he can help prevent bleeding by shaving with an electric razor and by brushing his teeth with a soft toothbrush.

• Emphasize the importance of taking medication exactly as ordered. Tell the patient not to take any other medications, especially aspirin, without asking the doctor.

• Instruct the patient taking warfarin not to significantly vary the amount of vitamin K he consumes daily. Doing so could interfere with anticoagulant therapy.

• Stress the importance of follow-up laboratory tests, such as PT, to monitor anticoagulant therapy.

• Tell the patient that he must inform all his health care providers—including dentists—that he's receiving anticoagulant therapy.

• To prevent pulmonary emboli in a high-risk patient, encourage him to walk and exercise his legs and to wear support or antiembolism stockings. Also, tell him not to cross or massage his legs.

FAT EMBOLI SYNDROME

A life-threatening disorder, fat emboli syndrome occurs when fat cells or globules enter venous circulation. This typically happens following a long-bone fracture, although other types of fractures—such as pelvic fractures, and crush injuries—as well as multiple fractures may also cause fat emboli.

In 90% of patients, fat emboli syndrome occurs within 24 to 48 hours after the injury, although it may occur as much as 10 days later. If not treated quickly, this disorder can lead to acute respiratory distress and death. Overall, this syndrome carries a high mortality.

Fat emboli syndrome can occur in either sex and at any age. However, it most commonly occurs in men between ages 20 and 40 and in elderly patients between ages 70 and 80.

CAUSES

Conditions other than long-bone fractures that may trigger fat emboli include pancreatitis, diabetic coma, osteomyelitis, and sickle cell anemia. Patients at risk for developing fat emboli syndrome include those with hyperglycemia, hypercholesterolemia, increased capillary fragility, or an inability to cope with physiologic stress.

After fat globules enter the venous circulation, they eventually block capillaries in major organs, especially the lungs. The pathophysiology of fat emboli syndrome isn't well understood; however, experts have suggested a mechanical and a biochemical theory. (See *What happens in fat emboli syndrome,* page 78.)

COMPLICATIONS

Fat globule and free fatty acid deposits may lead to acute respiratory distress and major organ dysfunction, especially in the brain, heart, liver, and spleen.

ASSESSMENT

The patient's history may reveal a long-bone fracture within the previous 3 days or a disorder known to be associated with fat emboli syndrome, such as hyperglycemia, hypercholesterolemia, or capillary fragility. The patient may complain of chest pain on inspiration.

Upon inspection during the early stages of fat emboli syndrome, you may notice a mental status change, such as confusion, which may progress to delirium or coma. During the first 4 to 6 hours after onset of fat emboli syndrome, petechiae may appear over the patient's torso, axillary folds, conjunctival sacs and retina, and soft palate mucosa. The patient may also have tachypnea.

Palpation may reveal localized muscle weakness, spasticity, and rigidity from muscle irritation. Upon auscultation, you may notice tachycardia and an irregular heartbeat along with crackles and wheezing.

The patient may also have a fever due to brain center irritation as well as signs and symptoms of cardiovascular collapse.

DIAGNOSTIC TESTS

The diagnosis of fat emboli syndrome is based on clinical findings from the patient's history and physical examination as well as the following diagnostic studies.
• *Serial urine examinations* for fat initially reveal fat globules, but within 3 days after the onset of symptoms, the fat globules disappear in about 50% of patients.
• *Serum lipase content* is typically elevated. As the amount of fat in the urine decreases, about 50% of the patients show an increased serum lipase content.

• *Arterial blood gas (ABG) measurements* typically reveal a partial pressure of oxygen in arterial blood less than 60 mm Hg.
• *Electrocardiography (ECG)* may show tachycardia, prominent S waves, T-wave inversions, multiple arrhythmias, and right bundle-branch block, all due to chemical irritation.
• *Platelet count* falls below 150,000/mm^3.
• *Hemoglobin level* falls during the early stages of fat emboli syndrome for unknown reasons.

TREATMENT

In fat emboli syndrome, treatment is mainly supportive. Fluids may be administered I.V. to prevent shock and to dilute free fatty acids. Although usually ineffective, various drug therapies may be tried to prevent death. These include corticosteroids (to counteract the inflammatory response to free fatty acids), heparin (for its lipolytic action in breaking down fat globules), ethanol (for its vasodilating action and its ability to inhibit lung lipase activity), and dextran (to improve tissue perfusion and expand plasma volume).

KEY NURSING DIAGNOSES AND PATIENT OUTCOMES

Decreased cardiac output related to deposit of fat globules and free fatty acids in cardiac muscle. Based on this nursing diagnosis, you'll establish these patient outcomes. The patient will:
• remain free of chest pain
• demonstrates no cardiac arrhythmias on the ECG
• maintain adequate cardiac output as exhibited by a normal pulse, blood pressure, and mental status.

Impaired gas exchange related to obstruction of the pulmonary vascular bed by fat globules. Based on this nursing diagnosis, you'll establish these patient outcomes. The patient will:
• regain and maintain ABG values within the normal range
• demonstrate a respiratory rate that fluctuates no more than 5 breaths/minute from the baseline

What happens in fat emboli syndrome

Although the pathophysiology of fat emboli syndrome isn't well understood, its effects are. A fracture initiates the pathophysiologic process that leads to pneumonitis from lipase release; this may eventually cause death.

Two theories, which are explained below, have been formulated to explain the pathophysiology of fat emboli syndrome.

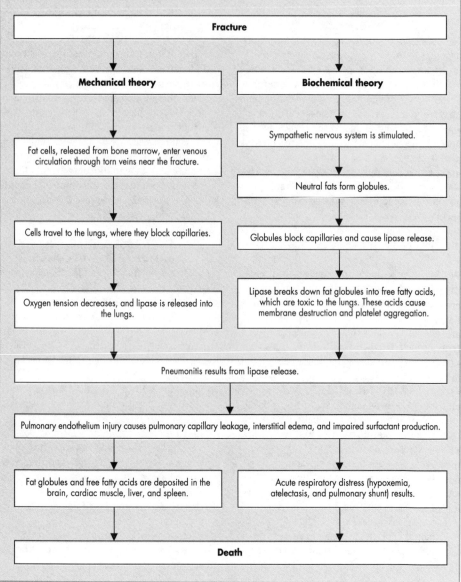

• remain alert and oriented to person, place, and time.

High risk for injury related to change in level of consciousness (LOC). Based on this nursing diagnosis, you'll establish these patient outcomes. The patient will:
• remain safe and protected in his environment
• sustain no injuries
• regain normal LOC as exhibited by being alert and oriented to person, place, and time.

NURSING INTERVENTIONS

• Transfer the patient to the intensive care unit if he isn't already there.
• Provide supportive care as prescribed.
• Give fluids to prevent shock and to dilute free fatty acids.
• Administer oxygen, as ordered, to ensure adequate oxygenation of tissues. If necessary, assist with intubation and provide appropriate ventilatory care.
• Administer medications as prescribed.
• Prepare the patient and family for a potentially fatal outcome and help them find effective coping strategies.

Monitoring

• Check for signs of increasing respiratory distress, such as tachycardia, wheezing, crackles, and a change in LOC.
• Monitor ABG values, complete blood count, and blood chemistry values for abnormalities.
• Observe the patient's ECG, and remain alert for any changes.
• Monitor the patient's temperature and other vital signs for changes.

Patient teaching

• Explain why the patient needs to be cared for in the intensive care unit. Also explain each new procedure before beginning.
• Stress the importance of alerting the nurse if symptoms worsen.

PULMONARY CONTUSION

When trauma to the chest bruises delicate lung tissue, a pulmonary contusion may result. The contusion may even occur on the lung on the opposite side of the impact. This is known as a contrecoup pulmonary contusion. Because signs and symptoms may not appear for several hours, the disorder cannot be immediately ruled out following a chest injury, even if the patient is free of symptoms.

Pulmonary contusions are classified as mild, moderate, or severe. A mild pulmonary contusion is one in which damage is limited to one segment of the lung or less; in a moderate pulmonary contusion, damage may extend from one segment to an entire lobe; and, in a severe pulmonary contusion, damage may extend to more than one lobe. The more severe the contusion, the greater the mortality risk.

CAUSES

Pulmonary contusion results from any type of blunt or penetrating chest trauma. It also often accompanies a flail chest.

The disorder develops when the trauma damages the lung parenchyma, causing hemorrhage and edema in the affected area. The leakage of blood and colloids into the alveoli compromises gas exchange and impairs ventilation. This leads to systemic hypoxia and, possibly, respiratory arrest.

COMPLICATIONS

Atelectasis, shock, infection (especially pneumonia), adult respiratory distress syndrome, and respiratory arrest may all result from a pulmonary contusion.

ASSESSMENT

The patient's history should reveal some type of chest trauma. The patient may complain of dyspnea and chest pain.

Upon inspection, you may observe hemoptysis, pallor or cyanosis, dyspnea, nasal flaring, accessory muscle use, extreme anxiety, or other signs and symptoms of respiratory distress. You may also notice bruising and disfigurement in the chest area.

Auscultation may reveal decreased breath sounds with crackles in the area of the contusion because of fluid leakage into the alveoli. In addition, an increased heart or respiratory rate may be an early sign of respiratory difficulty; decreased blood pressure may indicate impending shock.

An elevated temperature may indicate infection.

DIAGNOSTIC TESTS

• *Chest X-rays* identify the location and extent of the pulmonary contusion. They also reveal any underlying pulmonary diseases or conditions, such as emphysema, atelectasis, pneumothorax, infiltrates, and effusion, that would affect the type of respiratory care required.
• *Arterial blood gas (ABG) measurements* detect the degree of hypoxemia. Although ABG values may be normal initially, progressively deteriorating ABG values strongly suggest the development of acute respiratory failure.
• *Complete blood count (CBC)* detects problems arising from a pulmonary contusion. For example, an elevated white blood cell (WBC) count signals infection. Also, abnormally low hematocrit and hemoglobin levels signal blood loss and decreased oxygen-carrying capacity.

TREATMENT

Appropriate treatment aims to keep the patient adequately oxygenated. If the patient has no signs or symptoms of marked respiratory distress, oxygen may be administered by nasal cannula or mask. However, if he is experiencing respiratory distress, he'll require intubation and mechanical ventilation, possibly with positive end-expiratory pressure.

Diuretics are indicated if the patient shows signs of increased lung fluid, such as a productive cough, frothy sputum, tachycardia, or increased crackles. Prophylactic antibiotic therapy is routinely administered to minimize the risk of infection. Although controversial, corticosteroids may also be administered.

If the pulmonary contusion is severe and the patient exhibits signs of shock (decreased blood pressure, pallor, diaphoresis, and increased pulse or respiratory rate), he may need

colloids to replace volume and maintain oncotic pressure. In addition, an emergency thoracotomy may be necessary to remove the contused area.

KEY NURSING DIAGNOSES AND PATIENT OUTCOMES

High risk for infection related to depressed respiratory function. Based on this nursing diagnosis, you'll establish these patient outcomes. The patient will:
• maintain a normal temperature
• maintain a WBC count within the normal range
• produce a normal quantity and quality of sputum.

Impaired gas exchange related to hemorrhage and fluid leakage into alveoli caused by pulmonary contusion. Based on this nursing diagnosis, you'll establish these patient outcomes. The patient will:
• maintain ABG values within the normal range
• demonstrate effective coughing and deep-breathing exercises every 2 to 4 hours
• exhibit a normal respiratory rate.

Pain related to bruising of lung tissue as a result of pulmonary contusion. Based on this nursing diagnosis, you'll establish these patient outcomes. The patient will:
• describe the factors that intensify pain and modify his behavior accordingly
• state and then carry out appropriate interventions for pain relief
• express a feeling of comfort and relief from pain.

NURSING INTERVENTIONS

• Administer oxygen therapy as needed. If necessary, assist the doctor with intubation and provide appropriate ventilatory care.
• Provide pulmonary hygiene and intermittent positive-pressure breathing or mini-nebulizer treatments to decrease bronchospasm and to increase secretion mobilization as prescribed.
• Administer prophylactic antibiotics, as prescribed, to minimize the risk of infection.
• Expect to administer diuretics, as prescribed, to relieve lung congestion, if present.

• Maintain adequate hydration. Infuse I.V. fluids at the rate prescribed to maintain fluid balance.

• Position the patient for comfort and optimal gas exchange. Place the call button within the patient's reach.

• Assist the patient with activities to minimize pain and administer analgesics as prescribed.

Monitoring

• Assess the patient's respiratory rate and breath sounds for signs of respiratory distress (tachypnea, increased crackles, or changes in level of consciousness).

• If the patient is intubated, monitor ventilator settings, including tidal volume, peak airway pressure, minute ventilation, flow rate, and percentage of oxygen.

• Monitor ABG values often to ensure adequate oxygenation.

• Observe the patient for signs and symptoms of shock (pallor, decreased blood pressure, diaphoresis, and increased pulse or respiratory rate). Measure the patient's intake and output.

• Watch for arrhythmias.

• Monitor CBC values, being alert for an increased WBC count (signaling infection) or decreased hemoglobin levels and hematocrit (signaling blood loss).

• Watch for temperature elevations, which could suggest infection.

• Check chest X-rays to determine the progress of healing.

Patient teaching

• Reinforce the doctor's explanation of the patient's condition and treatment plan. Make sure the patient and his family understand the care required.

• Teach the patient about the type of respiratory therapy he needs (such as incentive spirometry and oxygen therapy). Also, teach him how to cough and deep-breathe to remove secretions, to prevent atelectasis, and to maintain good pulmonary hygiene.

• Stress the importance of alerting the nurse if respiratory symptoms worsen.

• If the patient is intubated, explain how the ventilator will help him breathe. Reassure him that, although he can't talk while intubated, he can communicate through notes or letter blocks.

HEMOTHORAX

This potentially life-threatening disorder occurs when blood enters the pleural cavity from damaged intercostal, pleural, or mediastinal vessels (or occasionally from the lung's parenchymal vessels). Depending on the amount of blood and the underlying cause of bleeding, hemothorax can cause varying degrees of lung collapse. About 25% of patients with chest trauma (blunt or penetrating) experience hemothorax. Pneumothorax (air in the pleural cavity) commonly accompanies hemothorax.

CAUSES

Hemothorax usually results from either blunt or penetrating chest trauma. Less often, it occurs because of thoracic surgery, pulmonary infarction, neoplasm, dissecting thoracic aneurysm, or anticoagulant therapy.

COMPLICATIONS

Hemothorax may result in mediastinal shift, ventilatory compromise, lung collapse and, without successful intervention, cardiac and respiratory arrest.

ASSESSMENT

The patient history typically reflects recent trauma. In addition, the patient may complain of chest pain and sudden difficulty breathing, which may be mild to severe, depending on the amount of blood in the pleural cavity.

Inspection typically discloses a patient with tachypnea, dusky skin color, diaphoresis, and hemoptysis (bloody, frothy sputum). If hemothorax progresses to respiratory failure, the patient may show restlessness, anxiety, cyanosis, and stupor. As the chest rises and falls, you may notice that the affected side expands and stiffens; the unaffected side may rise with the patient's gasping respirations.

Percussion may disclose dullness over the affected side of the chest; auscultation may

How hemothorax size affects signs and symptoms

A common method of classifying hemothorax is by size — small, moderate, or massive. Hemothorax size determines which signs and symptoms your patient will develop and how much blood is lost. Consequently, you can usually estimate the seriousness of your patient's injury if you know how large the hemothorax is. Use the chart below to compare signs and symptoms and diagnostic findings for each size.

SIZE	SIGNS AND SYMPTOMS	DIAGNOSTIC FINDINGS
Small hemothorax Less than 400-ml blood loss	Usually none	• With less than 250 ml of accumulated fluid, no recognizable chest X-ray changes. With 250 to 400 ml of fluid, chest X-ray shows blunting of costophrenic angle.
Moderate hemothorax 500- to 2,000-ml blood loss	• Indications of internal hemorrhage (such as pallor, restlessness, anxiety, tachycardia, and decreased blood pressure) • Dyspnea • Chest tightening • Asymmetrical chest movement • Ecchymosis over the affected lung • Bloody sputum	• Dullness over the affected side heard during percussion • Decreased or absent breath sounds over the affected side heard during auscultation; exaggerated bronchovesicular breath sounds above fluid level (less common) • Decreased tactile fremitus over the affected side during palpation • Decreased hemoglobin level (less common) • Blood or serosanguineous fluid obtained from thoracentesis • Fluid occupying one-third of the involved lung, as shown on chest X-ray
Massive hemothorax More than 2,000-ml blood loss	• Dyspnea • Tachypnea • Hypotension • Hypoxia • Cyanosis • Hypovolemic shock	Same as those for moderate hemothorax, plus the following: • fluid occupying half of the involved lung, as shown on chest X-ray • decreased hemoglobin levels • absent breath sounds and dullness noted during auscultation and percussion

detect decreased or absent breath sounds over the affected side, tachycardia, and hypotension. (For further information, see *How hemothorax size affects signs and symptoms.*)

DIAGNOSTIC TESTS

• *Thoracentesis* performed for diagnosis and therapy may yield blood or serosanguineous fluid. Fluid specimens may be sent to the laboratory for analysis.
• *Chest X-rays* display pleural fluid and detect mediastinal shift.
• *Arterial blood gas (ABG) analysis* documents respiratory failure.

• *Hemoglobin levels* may be decreased, depending on blood loss.

TREATMENT

In hemothorax, treatment aims to stabilize the patient's condition, stop the bleeding, evacuate blood from the pleural cavity, and reexpand the affected lung. Mild hemothorax usually clears in 10 to 14 days, requiring only observation for further bleeding. In severe hemothorax, treatment includes thoracentesis to remove blood and other fluids from the pleural cavity and then insertion of a chest tube into the sixth intercostal space at the posterior axillary line. Typically, a large-diameter chest tube is used to prevent clotting. Suction may also be used. If the chest tube doesn't improve the patient's condition, the surgeon may need to perform a thoracotomy to evacuate blood and clots and control bleeding.

Autotransfusion may be used if the patient's blood loss approaches or exceeds 1,000 ml. (See *Understanding autotransfusion*, page 84.)

Other treatment measures include oxygen therapy, I.V. therapy to restore fluid volume, and administration of analgesics.

KEY NURSING DIAGNOSES AND PATIENT OUTCOMES

Altered cerebral tissue perfusion related to hypotension. Based on this nursing diagnosis, you'll establish these patient outcomes. The patient will:
• avoid permanent neurologic deficit caused by altered cerebral tissue perfusion
• remain awake, alert, and oriented to time, person, and place
• regain and maintain normal blood pressure.

Anxiety related to situational crisis. Based on this nursing diagnosis, you'll establish these patient outcomes. The patient will:
• identify sources of his anxiety and express his feelings of anxiety
• use available support systems to help cope with his anxiety
• report fewer physical symptoms related to anxiety.

Impaired gas exchange related to lung dysfunction. Based on this nursing diagnosis, you'll establish these patient outcomes. The patient will:
• quickly regain normal lung function with emergency treatment
• maintain adequate gas exchange after treatment, as shown by normal ABG values and absence of signs and symptoms of hypoxia
• exhibit nonlabored respirations, as shown by equal rise and fall of the chest wall with inspiration and expiration.

NURSING INTERVENTIONS

• Listen to the patient's fears and concerns. Offer reassurance as appropriate. Remain with him during periods of stress and anxiety. En-

courage him to identify actions and care measures that promote comfort and relaxation. Be sure to perform these measures and encourage the patient and his family to do so as well. Include the patient and his family in care-related decisions whenever possible.
• As ordered, give oxygen by face mask or nasal cannula.
• Administer blood transfusions, as ordered, using a large-bore needle. Assist with autotransfusion, as indicated.
• To correct shock, give I.V. fluids and blood transfusions, as ordered. Use a central venous pressure line to monitor treatment progress.
• Give pain medication, as ordered, and record its effectiveness.
• Assist with thoracentesis, as indicated.
• Assist with chest tube insertion and provide appropriate care of the tube.
• Prepare the patient for surgery, as indicated.

Monitoring

• Check the patient's ABG values often. Also monitor hemoglobin levels and hematocrit, white blood cell count, and coagulation studies to determine blood replacement needs.
• Watch for complications signaled by pallor and gasping respirations.
• Monitor the patient's vital signs diligently. Watch for increasing pulse and respiratory rates and falling blood pressure, which may indicate shock or massive bleeding.
• Monitor chest tube drainage. Immediately report a chest tube that's warm and full of blood and a rapidly rising, bloody fluid level in the drainage collection chamber. The patient may need emergency surgery.

Patient teaching

• Explain all procedures to the patient and his family. Encourage the patient to ask questions.
• If appropriate, provide preoperative and postoperative teaching. Explain and prepare the patient and his family for mechanical ventilation if necessary.
• Encourage the patient to perform deep-breathing exercises every hour whenever he's awake to promote gas exchange.

Understanding autotransfusion

Used most often in patients with chest wounds—especially those that involve hemothorax—autotransfusion is a procedure in which the patient's own blood is collected, filtered, and then reinfused. It may also be used when two or three units of pooled blood can be recovered—for example, in cardiac or orthopedic surgery.

Autotransfusion eliminates the patient's risk of transfusion reaction or contracting a blood-borne disease, such as cytomegalovirus, hepatitis, and human immunodeficiency virus. It's contraindicated in sepsis or cancer.

How autotransfusion works

A large-bore chest tube connected to a closed drainage system is used to collect the patient's blood from a wound or chest cavity. This blood passes through a filter, which catches most potential thrombi, including clumps of fibrin and damaged red blood cells (RBCs). The filtered blood passes into a collection bag. From the bag, the blood is usually reinfused immediately. Or it may be processed in a commercial cell washer that reduces anticoagulated whole blood to washed RBCs for later infusion.

Assisting with autotransfusion

• Set up the blood collection system as you would any closed chest drainage system. Attach the collection bag according to the manufacturer's instructions.
• If ordered, inject an anticoagulant, such as heparin or acid-citrate-dextrose solution, into the self-sealing port on the connector of the patient's drainage tubing.
• During reinfusion, monitor the patient for complications, such as blood clotting, hemolysis, coagulopathies, thrombocytopenia, particulate and air emboli, sepsis, and citrate toxicity (from the acid-citrate-dextrose solution).

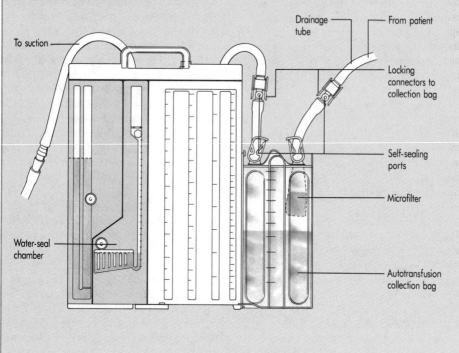

• Instruct the patient not to cough during thoracentesis.
• Discuss the rationale for chest tube therapy with the patient and his family.

PNEUMOTHORAX

An accumulation of air or gas between the parietal and visceral pleurae characterizes pneumothorax. The amount of air or gas trapped in the intrapleural space determines the degree of lung collapse. Common types of pneumothorax are open, closed, and tension. (See *Nursing care in pneumothorax,* pages 86 and 87.)

CAUSES

Open pneumothorax—also called an open or sucking chest wound—results when atmospheric air (positive pressure) flows directly into the pleural cavity (negative pressure). As the air pressure in the pleural cavity becomes positive, the lung collapses on the affected side, resulting in substantially decreased total lung capacity, vital capacity, and lung compliance. The resulting ventilation-perfusion imbalances lead to hypoxia. Types of open pneumothorax include penetrating pneumothorax and traumatic pneumothorax.

Closed pneumothorax occurs when air enters the pleural space from within the lung, causing increased pleural pressure and preventing lung expansion during normal inspiration. Closed pneumothorax may be called traumatic pneumothorax when blunt chest trauma causes lung tissue to rupture, which results in air leakage.

Spontaneous pneumothorax, another type of closed pneumothorax, is more common in men than in women. It's common in older patients with chronic pulmonary disease, but it may occur in healthy, tall, young adults. Both types of closed pneumothorax can result in a collapsed lung with hypoxia and decreased total lung capacity, vital capacity, and lung compliance. The total amount of lung collapse can range from 5% to 95%.

In tension pneumothorax, air in the pleural space is under higher pressure than air in adjacent lung and vascular structures. The accumulating pressure causes the lung to collapse. As air accumulates and intrapleural pressures rise, the mediastinum shifts away from the affected side and decreases venous return. This forces the heart, trachea, esophagus, and great vessels to the unaffected side, compressing the heart and the contralateral lung. Without immediate treatment, this emergency can become rapidly fatal.

COMPLICATIONS

Extensive pneumothorax can lead to fatal pulmonary and circulatory impairment.

ASSESSMENT

The patient history reveals sudden, sharp, pleuritic pain, which is exacerbated by chest movement, breathing, and coughing. The patient may also report shortness of breath.

Inspection typically reveals asymmetrical chest wall movement with overexpansion and rigidity on the affected side. The patient may appear cyanotic. In tension pneumothorax, he may have distended neck veins and pallor and may exhibit anxiety. (Test results may confirm increased central venous pressure.)

Palpation may reveal crackling beneath the skin, indicating subcutaneous emphysema (air in tissues) and decreased vocal fremitus. In tension pneumothorax, palpation may disclose tracheal deviation away from the affected side and a weak, rapid pulse. Percussion may demonstrate hyperresonance on the affected side, and auscultation may disclose decreased or absent breath sounds over the collapsed lung. The patient may be hypotensive with tension pneumothorax. Spontaneous pneumothorax that releases only a small amount of air into the pleural space may cause no signs and symptoms.

DIAGNOSTIC TESTS

• *Chest X-rays* reveal air in the pleural space and, possibly, a mediastinal shift, which confirms the diagnosis.

PRIORITY FLOWCHART

Nursing care in pneumothorax

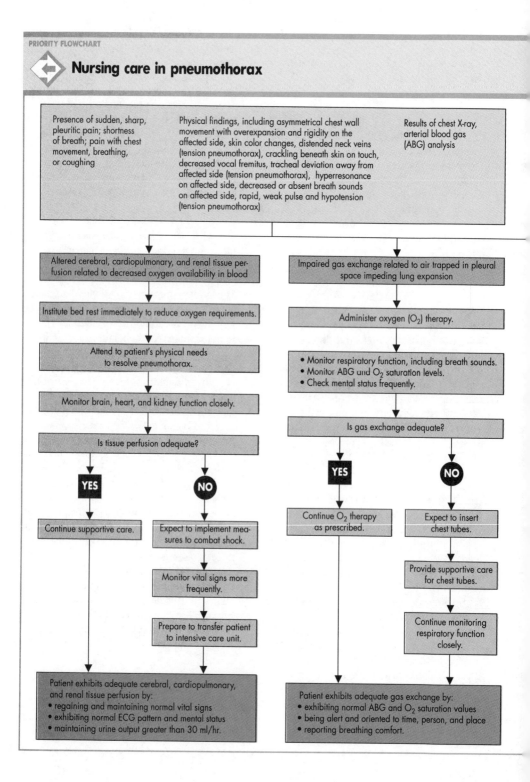

Presence of sudden, sharp, pleuritic pain; shortness of breath; pain with chest movement, breathing, or coughing

Physical findings, including asymmetrical chest wall movement with overexpansion and rigidity on the affected side, skin color changes, distended neck veins (tension pneumothorax), crackling beneath skin on touch, decreased vocal fremitus, tracheal deviation away from affected side (tension pneumothorax), hyperresonance on affected side, decreased or absent breath sounds on affected side, rapid, weak pulse and hypotension (tension pneumothorax)

Results of chest X-ray, arterial blood gas (ABG) analysis

Altered cerebral, cardiopulmonary, and renal tissue perfusion related to decreased oxygen availability in blood

Institute bed rest immediately to reduce oxygen requirements.

Attend to patient's physical needs to resolve pneumothorax.

Monitor brain, heart, and kidney function closely.

Is tissue perfusion adequate?

YES

NO

Continue supportive care.

Expect to implement measures to combat shock.

Monitor vital signs more frequently.

Prepare to transfer patient to intensive care unit.

Patient exhibits adequate cerebral, cardiopulmonary, and renal tissue perfusion by:
• regaining and maintaining normal vital signs
• exhibiting normal ECG pattern and mental status
• maintaining urine output greater than 30 ml/hr.

Impaired gas exchange related to air trapped in pleural space impeding lung expansion

Administer oxygen (O_2) therapy.

• Monitor respiratory function, including breath sounds.
• Monitor ABG and O_2 saturation levels.
• Check mental status frequently.

Is gas exchange adequate?

YES

NO

Continue O_2 therapy as prescribed.

Expect to insert chest tubes.

Provide supportive care for chest tubes.

Continue monitoring respiratory function closely.

Patient exhibits adequate gas exchange by:
• exhibiting normal ABG and O_2 saturation values
• being alert and oriented to time, person, and place
• reporting breathing comfort.

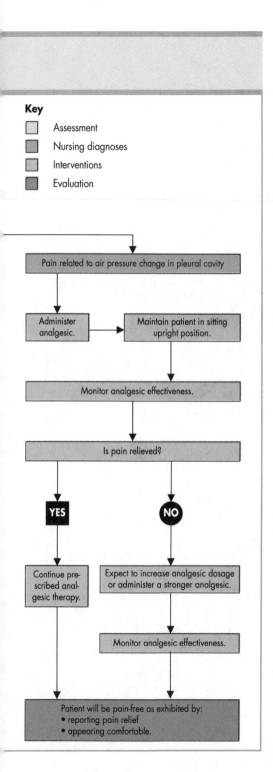

Key

Assessment

Nursing diagnoses

Interventions

Evaluation

Pain related to air pressure change in pleural cavity

Administer analgesic.

Maintain patient in sitting upright position.

Monitor analgesic effectiveness.

Is pain relieved?

YES

NO

Continue prescribed analgesic therapy.

Expect to increase analgesic dosage or administer a stronger analgesic.

Monitor analgesic effectiveness.

Patient will be pain-free as exhibited by:
• reporting pain relief
• appearing comfortable.

• *Arterial blood gas (ABG) studies* may show hypoxemia, possibly accompanied by respiratory acidosis and hypercapnia. Arterial oxygen saturation levels may fall initially but typically return to normal within 24 hours.

TREATMENT

Typically, treatment is conservative for spontaneous pneumothorax with no signs of increased pleural pressure (indicating tension pneumothorax), with lung collapse less than 30%, and with no dyspnea or other indications of physiologic compromise. Such treatment consists of bed rest, careful monitoring (of blood pressure and pulse and respiratory rates), oxygen administration and, possibly, aspiration of air with a large-bore needle attached to a syringe.

If more than 30% of the lung collapses, treatment to reexpand the lung includes placing a thoracostomy tube in the second or third intercostal space at the midclavicular line. The thoracostomy tube then connects to an underwater seal or to low-pressure suction. (See *Managing chest drainage problems*, page 88.)

Recurring spontaneous pneumothorax requires thoracotomy and pleurectomy. These procedures prevent recurrence by causing the lung to adhere to the parietal pleura. Traumatic and tension pneumothorax require chest tube drainage; traumatic pneumothorax may also require surgical repair. Analgesics may be prescribed.

KEY NURSING DIAGNOSES AND PATIENT OUTCOMES

Altered cardiopulmonary, cerebral, or renal tissue perfusion related to decreased oxygen availability in blood. Based on this nursing diagnosis, you'll establish these patient outcomes. The patient will:
• restrict his activities to reduce tissue oxygen needs until pneumothorax is resolved
• exhibit no signs or symptoms of tissue hypoxia.

Impaired gas exchange related to air trapped in pleural space impeding lung expansion. Based on this nursing diagnosis, you'll establish these patient outcomes. The patient will:

Managing chest drainage problems

PROBLEM	INTERVENTIONS
Patient positioned improperly	• Keep the collection chamber below chest level. • Place the patient in semi-Fowler's position when in bed to promote drainage. • Avoid dependent loops in the tubing; coil the tubing flat on the bed and then let it fall in a straight line to the drainage unit.
Absent tidaling (rise and fall of solution in the rod submerged in the water seal)	• Check for twisted tubing and untwist it. • Inspect the connections for clots.
Air leak	• Apply pressure to the skin around the chest tube insertion site. Observe if the bubbling stops; if so, the leak may be in the patient end of the tube, and additional sutures will be needed at the insertion site. • Briefly clamp the chest tube close to the patient. If the leak persists, it is in the tubing. Continue to briefly clamp the tubing at intervals to determine where the leak is. • Keep connections taped securely and the chest dressing occlusive.
Accidental disconnection of the chest tube from the chest drainage system	• If the patient doesn't have an air leak, the tube can be briefly clamped or pinched shut until the tube is reconnected to the drainage system. • Reestablish the system quickly.
Accidental removal of the chest tube	• Apply direct pressure to the chest tube site. • Cover the area with a sterile dressing and call the doctor immediately.

• regain and maintain adequate ventilation with prompt treatment
• regain and maintain normal ABG levels
• show resolution of pneumothorax on chest X-ray with treatment.

Pain related to air pressure change in pleural cavity. Based on this nursing diagnosis, you'll establish these patient outcomes. The patient will:
• express feelings of chest comfort following analgesic administration
• sit upright to increase comfort
• become pain-free with resolution of pneumothorax.

NURSING INTERVENTIONS

• Listen to the patient's fears and concerns. Offer reassurance as appropriate. Include the patient and his family in care-related decisions whenever possible.
• Keep the patient as comfortable as possible, and administer analgesics as necessary. The patient with pneumothorax usually feels most comfortable sitting upright.
• Administer oxygen therapy, as prescribed.
• Prepare the patient for chest tube insertion or thoracotomy, as indicated.
• If a chest tube is in place, change the dressing around the chest tube insertion site at least every 24 hours. Be careful not to create tension pneumothorax with a dressing that's too tight. Keep the site clean.

◆ NURSING ALERT. Don't dislodge or reposition the tube. If it becomes dislodged, immediately place a petroleum gauze dressing over the opening and call the doctor.
• Give analgesics as needed.

Monitoring

• Assess the patient regularly, noting the rate, depth, and ease of his breathing. Monitor ABG levels regularly, as ordered.
• Watch for complications, signaled by pallor, gasping respirations, and sudden chest pain.

Carefully monitor vital signs at least every hour for indications of shock, increasing respiratory distress, or mediastinal shift. Listen for breath sounds over both lungs.
• Watch for signs of tension pneumothorax (especially if the patient has chest tubes inserted). These include falling blood pressure and rising pulse and respiratory rates, which could be fatal without prompt treatment. Also palpate the tissue around any chest tube insertion site for subcutaneous air, and auscultate for changes in breath sounds that indicate improving or worsening respiration. Watch for signs of drainage, infection, and air leakage (bubbling in the water-seal chamber), which can result from a hole or tear in the lung.
• Assess the effectiveness of administered analgesics, and monitor the patient for adverse reactions.

Patient teaching

• Reassure the patient. Explain what pneumothorax is, what causes it, and all diagnostic tests and procedures. If the patient is having surgery or chest tubes inserted, explain why he needs these procedures. Reassure him that the chest tubes will make him more comfortable.
• Encourage the patient to perform deep-breathing exercises every hour when awake.
• Discuss the potential for recurrent spontaneous pneumothorax, and review its signs and symptoms. Emphasize the need for immediate medical intervention if these should occur.

PENETRATING CHEST WOUNDS

Depending on its size, a penetrating chest wound may cause varying degrees of damage to bones, soft tissue, blood vessels, and nerves.

The risk of death and disease from a chest wound depends on the size and severity of the wound. Gunshot wounds usually are more serious than stab wounds because they cause more severe lacerations and rapid blood loss and because ricochet often damages large areas and multiple organs. With prompt, aggressive treatment, up to 90% of patients with penetrating chest wounds recover.

CAUSES

Stab wounds from a knife or an ice pick and gunshot wounds are the most common penetrating chest wounds. Wartime explosions or firearms fired at close range are the usual causes of large, gaping wounds.

COMPLICATIONS

Penetrating chest wounds may lead to arrhythmias, cardiac tamponade, mediastinitis, subcutaneous emphysema, and bronchopleural fistula.

ASSESSMENT

The patient's history reveals the cause of the chest wound. The patient may groan and cry with pain. The chest wound may be obvious, possibly accompanied by a sucking sound as the diaphragm contracts and air enters the chest cavity through the opening in the chest wall.

The patient's level of consciousness depends on the extent of the injury. If he's awake and alert, he may be in severe pain. This will cause him to splint his respirations, reducing his vital capacity.

Inspection reveals the location and type of chest wound. (If you observe the wound in the lower thoracic area, consider it a thoracoabdominal injury until proven otherwise.) If hemopneumothorax is present, the patient will appear dyspneic, tachypneic, anxious, and cyanotic. He may try to sit up to catch his breath. You may note tracheal deviation, depending on the severity of the injury.

On palpation, you may note a weak, thready pulse, which may result from massive blood loss and hypovolemic shock. Percussion reveals dullness over areas of blood collection in the pleural or pericardial sac. Auscultation detects decreased blood pressure and tachycardia from anxiety and blood loss. It also reveals diminished breath sounds over the area of lung collapse in hemopneumothorax. (See *How severe is the wound?* page 90.)

How severe is the wound?

Examining the wound site helps you to determine the severity of a penetrating wound. To help assess the severity of a stab wound, you'll also need to determine the type and size of the weapon used to inflict the wound and the location and angle of entry. For a gunshot wound, you'll need to determine the following:
• weapon and missile type
• missile velocity
• victim's distance from weapon
• location of entrance and exit wounds.

DIAGNOSTIC TESTS

• *Chest X-rays* allow evaluation of the injury and confirm chest tube placement.
• *Arterial blood gas (ABG) analysis* helps evaluate the patient's respiratory status.
• *A complete blood count* may show low hemoglobin and hematocrit levels, reflecting severe blood loss.

TREATMENT

In a penetrating chest wound, treatment involves maintaining a patent airway and providing ventilatory support as needed. Chest tube insertion allows the reestablishment of intrathoracic pressure and drainage of blood from a hemothorax. (See *Positioning for chest tube insertion.*)

The patient's wound may need surgical repair. The patient also may need analgesics, antibiotics, and tetanus prophylaxis as well as infusion of blood products and I.V. fluids.

KEY NURSING DIAGNOSES AND PATIENT OUTCOMES

Decreased cardiac output related to blood loss. Based on this nursing diagnosis, you'll establish these patient outcomes. The patient will:
• maintain hemodynamic stability exhibited by stable vital signs and orientation to time, person, and place
• exhibit no significant complications such as chest pain, syncope, or arrhythmias

• regain and maintain adequate cardiac output with effective treatment of penetrating chest wound.

Impaired gas exchange related to lung dysfunction. Based on this nursing diagnosis, you'll establish these patient outcomes. The patient will:
• quickly regain normal lung function with emergency treatment
• maintain adequate gas exchange after treatment, as shown by normal ABG values and absence of signs and symptoms of hypoxia.

Ineffective breathing pattern related to pain and lung dysfunction. Based on this nursing diagnosis, you'll establish these patient outcomes. The patient will:
• regain and maintain nonlabored respirations, as shown by equal rise and fall of the chest wall with inspiration and expiration
• report breathing comfort after analgesic administration
• exhibit normal chest expansion visible on X-ray.

NURSING INTERVENTIONS

• Immediately evaluate the patient's ABCs – airway, breathing, and circulation. Establish a patent airway, and provide ventilatory support as needed.
• Apply wound dressings, as necessary, always using sterile technique.
• Place an occlusive dressing (for example, petroleum gauze) over a sucking wound. If signs of a tension pneumothorax develop, temporarily remove the occlusive dressing to create a simple pneumothorax.
• Assist with insertion of central lines for monitoring and fluid replacement, if indicated.
• Ensure adequate I.V. access with at least two large-bore peripheral catheters.
• Obtain blood samples for typing and cross-matching.
• Use appropriate measures to control bleeding, as indicated. Replace blood and fluids as necessary.
• If warranted, obtain and set up equipment for autotransfusion, particularly when blood loss is massive.

Positioning for chest tube insertion

When preparing a patient for chest tube insertion, position him so that the doctor has easy access to the insertion site.

If your patient has a *pneumothorax,* place him in high Fowler's, semi-Fowler's, or the supine position or have him lie on his unaffected side with his arms overhead. The doctor will insert the tube in the anterior chest at the midclavicular line in the second or third intercostal space.

If your patient has a *hemothorax,* have him lean over the overbed table, straddle a chair with his arms leaning over the back, or lie on his unaffected side with his arms overhead. The doctor will insert the tube in the fourth to sixth intercostal space at the midaxillary line.

If the patient has had a *thoracotomy,* the doctor usually will insert the chest tube during surgery. The patient will lie on his unaffected side with his arms elevated. This patient may receive two chest tubes: basilar and apical.

Semi-Fowler's position

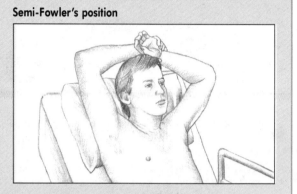

Leaning forward

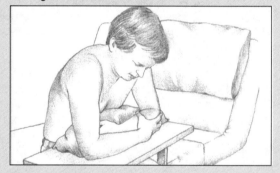

Lying on side

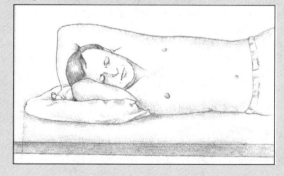

• Assist with chest X-ray and placement of chest tubes (using water-seal drainage) to re-establish intrathoracic pressure and to drain blood in a hemothorax. A second X-ray will evaluate the position of tubes and their function.
• Provide ordered analgesics to relieve pain.

Monitoring

• Monitor the patient's cardiopulmonary status continuously. Check his pulses and breath sounds frequently for rate and quality.
• Estimate the patient's blood loss.

  ◆ NURSING ALERT. Always remember to look for bleeding under the patient when estimating blood loss.
• Throughout treatment, monitor central venous pressure and vital signs to detect hypovolemia and hemorrhagic shock.
• After chest tubes are in place, watch for bleeding and substantial air leakage through chest tubes, a sign of lung lacerations. Also watch for a blood loss of more than 100 ml/hour through chest tubes, the result of arterial lacerations. Report such findings at once.

Patient teaching

• Reassure the patient, especially if he's the victim of a violent crime. Report the incident to the police in accordance with local laws. Help contact the patient's family, and offer them reassurance.
• Reinforce the doctor's explanation of the patient's condition and treatment plan. Make sure the patient and his family understand the care required.
• Teach the patient about the type of respiratory therapy he needs. Also teach him breathing exercises to maintain effective pulmonary function. Explain the need for turning, coughing, and deep breathing.
• Discuss the medications prescribed for pain, including their adverse effects.
• Teach splinting techniques for turning, deep breathing, and ambulation.
• Encourage the patient not to smoke. Explain that smoking increases tracheobronchial secretions and decreases arterial oxygen saturation.

• Advise the patient to notify the doctor if pain worsens or is accompanied by fever, a productive cough, and shortness of breath. These signs may indicate infection.
• Warn the patient to avoid contact sports until the pain disappears and the doctor permits him to resume such activities.

RESPIRATORY ACIDOSIS

This acid-base disturbance is characterized by reduced alveolar ventilation and hypercapnia (partial pressure of carbon dioxide in arterial blood [$Paco_2$] greater than 45 mm Hg). Respiratory acidosis can be acute and life-threatening (resulting from sudden failure in ventilation) or chronic (resulting from long-term pulmonary disease).

The prognosis depends on the severity of the underlying disturbance and the patient's general clinical condition.

CAUSES

Factors that predispose a patient to respiratory acidosis include:
• *drugs* that depress the respiratory control center's sensitivity, such as narcotics, anesthetics, hypnotics, and sedatives
• *central nervous system (CNS) trauma*, such as medullary injury, which may impair ventilatory drive
• *chronic metabolic alkalosis*, which may occur when respiratory compensatory mechanisms attempt to normalize pH by decreasing alveolar ventilation
• *neuromuscular diseases*, such as Guillain-Barré syndrome, myasthenia gravis, and poliomyelitis, in which respiratory muscles fail to respond properly to respiratory drive, reducing alveolar ventilation.

In addition, respiratory acidosis can result from an airway obstruction or parenchymal lung disease that interferes with alveolar ventilation or from chronic obstructive pulmonary disease (COPD), asthma, severe adult respiratory distress syndrome, chronic bronchitis, large pneumothorax, extensive pneumonia, and pulmonary edema.

Interpreting ABG values

Arterial blood gas (ABG) values provide crucial information about the efficiency of your patient's gas exchange and acid-base balance. You can also use ABG values to monitor the effects of respiratory interventions.

Although ABG measurement requires blood sampling, an invasive procedure that sometimes causes pain (especially for patients without an arterial line), the information it provides allows more thorough assessment of gas exchange. Normal ABG values are:
• blood pH: 7.35 to 7.45
• partial pressure of oxygen in arterial blood (PaO_2): 80 to 100 mm Hg (decreases with age)
• partial pressure of carbon dioxide in arterial blood ($PaCO_2$): 35 to 45 mm Hg
• bicarbonate (HCO_3^-): 22 to 26 mEq/liter
• arterial oxygen saturation (SaO_2): 95% to 100%.

Evaluating acid-base balance
To interpret ABG results, start by evaluating acid-base balance. Suspect *alkalosis* as the primary or initiating disorder if the pH exceeds 7.45. Suspect *acidosis* if the pH is below 7.35. With a normal pH, other ABG values may be normal if the patient has compensated for his problem. For example, the kidneys can compensate by retaining HCO_3^- if the lungs can't eliminate enough carbon dioxide.

To determine the specific type of alkalosis or acidosis, analyze the $PaCO_2$ and HCO_3^- values. If the former is abnormal but the latter normal, suspect acute respiratory alkalosis or acidosis without metabolic compensation by the kidneys. If the HCO_3^- value is abnormal but the $PaCO_2$ value is normal, suspect metabolic alkalosis or acidosis.

A borderline normal high or low pH combined with an abnormal $PaCO_2$ or HCO_3^- value indicates whether or not the acid-base disorder is compensated. With compensated respiratory acidosis, pH is borderline low, $PaCO_2$ is high, and HCO_3^- is high.

Assessing oxygenation
To assess your patient's oxygenation, check the PaO_2 and SaO_2. Note the fraction of inspired oxygen he was receiving when the blood sample was drawn. Decreased PaO_2 and SaO_2 values may indicate hypoxemia.

Be sure to track serial ABG measurements, noting whether any significant changes followed medical or nursing interventions.

COMPLICATIONS
Acute or chronic respiratory acidosis can produce shock and cardiac arrest.

ASSESSMENT
The patient may initially complain of headache and dyspnea. He may also have a predisposing condition for respiratory acidosis. On inspection, you may see that he's dyspneic and diaphoretic. He may report nausea and vomiting.

Palpation may detect bounding pulses. Auscultation may reveal rapid and shallow respirations, tachycardia and, possibly, hypotension.

Ophthalmoscopic examination may uncover papilledema. And neurologic examination may disclose a decreased level of consciousness (LOC) ranging from restlessness, confusion, and apprehension to somnolence, with a fine or flapping tremor (asterixis) and depressed reflexes.

DIAGNOSTIC TESTS
• *Arterial blood gas (ABG) analysis* confirms respiratory acidosis. $PaCO_2$ rises above the normal 45 mm Hg; pH typically falls below the normal range of 7.35 to 7.45; and bicarbonate (HCO_3^-) levels are normal in acute respiratory acidosis but elevated in chronic respiratory acidosis. (See *Interpreting ABG values.*)

TREATMENT

Effective treatment aims to correct the source of alveolar hypoventilation. If alveolar ventilation is significantly reduced, the patient may need mechanical ventilation until the underlying condition can be treated. Treatment includes bronchodilators, oxygen, and antibiotics in COPD; drug therapy for conditions such as myasthenia gravis; removal of foreign bodies from the airway in cases of obstruction; antibiotics for pneumonia; dialysis to eliminate toxic drugs; and correction of metabolic alkalosis.

Dangerously low pH levels (less than 7.15) can produce profound CNS and cardiovascular deterioration and may require administration of I.V. sodium bicarbonate. In chronic lung disease, elevated $Paco_2$ levels may persist despite treatment.

KEY NURSING DIAGNOSES AND PATIENT OUTCOMES

Fear related to threat of death. Based on this nursing diagnosis, you'll establish these patient outcomes. The patient will:
• identify and express his fear
• use available support systems to help him cope with fear
• show no physical signs or symptoms of fear.

Impaired gas exchange related to alveolar hypoventilation. Based on this nursing diagnosis, you'll establish these patient outcomes. The patient will:
• regain and maintain normal ABG values
• exhibit no signs and symptoms of profound CNS or cardiovascular deterioration
• demonstrate compliance with the prescribed treatment for the underlying cause of respiratory acidosis.

Ineffective breathing pattern related to rapid, shallow respirations. Based on this nursing diagnosis, you'll establish these patient outcomes. The patient will:
• reestablish his respiratory rate within normal limits
• express a feeling of comfort with his breathing pattern
• have normal breath sounds on auscultation.

NURSING INTERVENTIONS

• Be prepared to treat or remove the underlying cause, such as an airway obstruction.
• Maintain adequate hydration by administering I.V. fluids.
• Give oxygen (only at low concentrations in patients with COPD) if the partial pressure of oxygen in arterial blood drops.
• Give aerosolized or I.V. bronchodilators as prescribed.
• Start mechanical ventilation if hypoventilation cannot be corrected immediately. Maintain a patent airway and provide adequate humidification if acidosis requires mechanical ventilation.
• Perform tracheal suctioning regularly and chest physiotherapy, if ordered.
• Reassure the patient as much as possible, depending on his LOC. Allay the fears and concerns of family members by keeping them informed about the patient's status.

Monitoring

• To detect developing respiratory acidosis, closely monitor patients with COPD and chronic carbon dioxide retention for signs of acidosis. Also closely monitor all patients who receive narcotics and sedatives.
• Be alert for critical changes in the patient's respiratory, CNS, and cardiovascular functions. Report such changes immediately. Also monitor and report variations in ABG levels and electrolyte status.
• Monitor and record the patient's response to administered aerosolized or I.V. bronchodilators.
• Continuously monitor ventilator settings if the patient requires intubation.

Patient teaching

• Instruct the patient who's recovering from a general anesthetic to turn, cough, and perform deep-breathing and coughing exercises frequently to prevent respiratory acidosis.
• If the patient receives home oxygen therapy for COPD, stress the importance of maintaining the ordered concentration and flow rate.
• Explain the reasons for ABG analysis. Discuss the blood-drawing technique and tell the

patient that he may feel slight discomfort from the needle stick.
• Alert the patient to possible adverse effects of prescribed medications. Tell him to call the doctor if any occur.

RESPIRATORY ALKALOSIS

Marked by a decrease in the partial pressure of carbon dioxide in arterial blood ($Paco_2$) to less than 35 mm Hg and a rise in blood pH above 7.45, respiratory alkalosis results from alveolar hyperventilation. Uncomplicated respiratory alkalosis leads to reduced hydrogen ion concentration, which raises the blood pH. Hypocapnia occurs when the lungs eliminate more carbon dioxide than the body produces at the cellular level. In the acute stage, respiratory alkalosis is also called hyperventilation syndrome and can be life-threatening.

CAUSES
Predisposing factors include:
• congestive heart failure
• injury to the respiratory control center of the central nervous system (CNS)
• extreme anxiety
• fever
• overventilation during mechanical ventilation
• pulmonary embolism
• salicylate intoxication (early).

COMPLICATIONS
In severe respiratory alkalosis, related cardiac arrhythmias may fail to respond to conventional treatment. Seizures may also occur.

ASSESSMENT
The patient history may reveal a predisposing factor associated with respiratory alkalosis. The patient may complain of light-headedness or paresthesia.

On inspection, the patient may seem anxious, with visibly rapid breathing. In severe respiratory alkalosis, tetany may be apparent, with visible twitching and flexion of the wrists and ankles.

Auscultation may reveal tachycardia and deep, rapid breathing.

DIAGNOSTIC TESTS
• *Arterial blood gas (ABG) analysis* confirms respiratory alkalosis and rules out compensation for metabolic acidosis. $Paco_2$ falls below 35 mm Hg; blood pH rises in proportion to the fall in $Paco_2$ in the acute stage but drops toward normal in the chronic stage. The bicarbonate (HCO_3^-) level is normal in the acute stage but below normal in the chronic stage. (For further information, see *Interpreting ABG values,* page 93.)
• *Serum electrolyte studies* detect metabolic acid-base disorders.

TREATMENT
In respiratory alkalosis, treatment attempts to eradicate the underlying condition—for example, by removing ingested toxins or by treating fever, sepsis, or a CNS injury. In severe respiratory alkalosis, the patient may need to breathe into a paper bag, which helps relieve acute anxiety and increase carbon dioxide levels. If respiratory alkalosis results from anxiety, sedatives and tranquilizers may help the patient.

Prevention of hyperventilation in patients receiving mechanical ventilation requires monitoring ABG levels and adjusting dead space or minute volume.

KEY NURSING DIAGNOSES AND PATIENT OUTCOMES
Anxiety related to threat of death. Based on this nursing diagnosis, you'll establish these patient outcomes. The patient will:
• express feelings of anxiety
• employ stress-reduction techniques to prevent or minimize anxiety
• exhibit a decrease in anxiety symptoms when respiratory alkalosis resolves.

Impaired gas exchange related to alveolar hyperventilation. Based on this nursing diagnosis, you'll establish these patient outcomes. The patient will:
• regain and maintain normal ABG values

• show no signs or symptoms of severe respiratory alkalosis, such as cardiac arrhythmias and seizures
• comply with prescribed treatment to correct the cause of respiratory alkalosis.

Ineffective breathing pattern related to deep, rapid breathing. Based on this nursing diagnosis, you'll establish these patient outcomes. The patient will:
• regain a normal respiratory rate and pattern
• express a feeling of comfort with his breathing pattern
• have normal breath sounds on auscultation.

NURSING INTERVENTIONS
• Provide supportive care for the underlying cause of respiratory alkalosis, as ordered.
• Stay with the patient during periods of extreme stress and anxiety. Offer reassurance and maintain a calm, quiet environment.
• If the patient is coping with anxiety-induced respiratory alkalosis, help him identify factors that precipitate anxiety. Also help him find coping mechanisms and activities that promote relaxation.

Monitoring
• Watch for and report changes in neurologic, neuromuscular, and cardiovascular functioning.
• Remember that twitching and cardiac arrhythmias may be associated with alkalemia and electrolyte imbalances. Monitor ABG and serum electrolyte levels closely. Report any variations immediately.

Patient teaching
• Explain all care procedures to the patient. Allow ample time to answer his questions.
• Instruct the patient in anxiety-reducing techniques, such as guided imagery, meditation, or yoga. Teach him how to counter hyperventilation with a controlled-breathing pattern.

NEAR DROWNING

In near drowning, the victim has survived (at least temporarily) the physiologic effects of submersion in fluid. Hypoxemia and acidosis constitute his primary clinical problems.

Near drowning occurs in three forms. In "dry" near drowning, the victim doesn't aspirate fluid but suffers respiratory obstruction or asphyxia (10% to 15% of patients). In "wet" near drowning, the victim aspirates fluid and suffers from asphyxia or secondary changes from fluid aspiration (about 85% of patients). And in secondary near drowning, the victim suffers recurrence of respiratory distress (usually aspiration pneumonia or pulmonary edema) within minutes or 1 to 2 days after the near-drowning episode.

CAUSES
Near drowning typically results from an inability to swim. In swimmers, it can result from panic, a boating accident, sudden acute illness (such as a seizure or myocardial infarction), a blow to the head while in the water, venomous stings from aquatic animals, heavy drinking before swimming, a suicide attempt, or decompression sickness from deep-water diving.

COMPLICATIONS
Near drowning may result in neurologic impairment, seizure disorders, and pulmonary or cardiac disease.

ASSESSMENT
The patient's history (obtained from a family member, a friend, or emergency personnel, if necessary) reveals the cause of the near-drowning episode. The patient may display a host of signs and symptoms. If he's conscious, he may complain of a headache or substernal chest pain.

Your initial assessment of the patient's vital signs may detect fever; rapid, slow, or absent pulse; and shallow, gasping, or absent respirations. If the patient was exposed to cold temperatures, he may be hypothermic.

On initial observation, the patient may be unconscious, semiconscious, or awake. If he's awake, he usually appears apprehensive, irritable, restless, or lethargic, and he may vomit. Inspection may reveal cyanosis or pink, frothy sputum (indicating pulmonary edema). Palpation of the abdomen may disclose distention.

Auscultation of the lungs may reveal crackles, rhonchi, wheezing, or apnea. You may note tachycardia, arrhythmias, or cardiac arrest when you auscultate the heart. The patient also may be hypotensive.

DIAGNOSTIC TESTS

• *Arterial blood gas (ABG) analysis* shows the degree of hypoxia, intrapulmonary shunt, and acid-base balance.
• *Serum electrolyte levels* monitor electrolyte balance.
• *Complete blood count* determines hemolysis.
• *Blood urea nitrogen* and *serum creatinine levels* and *urinalysis* evaluate renal function.
• *Cervical spine X-ray* rules out fracture.
• *Serial chest X-rays* evaluate pulmonary changes.
• *Electrocardiography (ECG)* detects myocardial ischemia.

TREATMENT

Prehospital care includes measures to protect the spinal cord, cardiopulmonary resuscitation (CPR), as needed, and supplemental oxygen.

After the patient reaches the hospital, CPR continues. His oxygenation and circulation are maintained. X-rays confirm cervical spine integrity, and his blood pH and electrolyte imbalances are corrected. If he's hypothermic, steps are taken to rewarm him.

ABG results help guide pulmonary therapy and determine the need for sodium bicarbonate to treat metabolic acidosis. If the patient can't maintain an open airway, has abnormal ABG levels and pH, or can't breathe spontaneously, he may need endotracheal intubation and mechanical ventilation. If he develops bronchospasm, he may need bronchodilators. Central venous pressure or pulmonary artery wedge pressure determines the need for fluid replacement and cardiac drugs. The patient also may require treatment for pulmonary edema. Nasogastric (NG) tube drainage prevents vomiting, and an indwelling urinary catheter allows monitoring of urine output.

KEY NURSING DIAGNOSES AND PATIENT OUTCOMES

High risk for aspiration related to submersion in water during near-drowning episode. Based on this nursing diagnosis, you'll establish these patient outcomes. The patient will:
• have his condition detected and treated immediately
• recover normal lung function.

Hypothermia related to prolonged exposure to cold water. Based on this nursing diagnosis, you'll establish these patient outcomes. The patient will:
• regain and maintain normal body temperature
• exhibit no complications associated with hypothermia, such as residual neurologic deficits or hypovolemic shock if warmed too quickly.

Inability to sustain spontaneous ventilation related to lung dysfunction caused by near drowning. Based on this nursing diagnosis, you'll establish these patient outcomes. The patient will:
• maintain adequate ventilation through mechanical means until spontaneous ventilation returns
• maintain normal ABG and oxygen saturation values
• regain normal breathing pattern.

NURSING INTERVENTIONS

• Continue CPR as indicated. Assist with intubation and mechanical ventilation if patient can't maintain spontaneous ventilations.
• If the patient is hypothermic, start rewarming procedures during CPR. Don't stop CPR until the patient's body temperature ranges between 86° and 90.5° F (30° and 32.5° C).
• Protect the cervical spine until fracture is ruled out.
• Ensure peripheral I.V. access and administer I.V. fluids as necessary.
• If ordered, insert an NG tube to remove swallowed water and reduce the risk of vomiting and aspiration.

• Insert an indwelling urinary catheter to monitor urine output. Metabolic acidosis may develop to compensate for impaired renal function.

• Administer bronchodilators as ordered.

Monitoring

• Assess ABG levels and obtain an ECG. The patient will probably need continuous cardiac monitoring.

• Continually monitor the patient's vital signs and neurologic status. He may suffer central nervous system damage despite adequate treatment for hypoxia and shock.

• Obtain baseline serum electrolyte levels; continue monitoring these levels.

• If a central line is in place, monitor hemodynamic parameters: cardiac output, central venous pressure, pulmonary artery wedge pressure, heart rate, and arterial blood pressure.

• If the patient has been submerged in cold water, use a rectal probe to determine the degree of hypothermia.

Patient teaching

• To prevent near drowning, advise the patient to avoid use of alcohol or drugs before swimming, to observe water safety measures (such as the "buddy system"), and to take a water safety course given by the American Red Cross, YMCA, or YWCA.

5

Cardiovascular disorders

Despite new knowledge and new procedures for detecting and treating disorders of the heart and blood vessels, cardiovascular disease remains the leading cause of death in North America. As a result, no matter where you practice nursing, you're likely to encounter patients with potentially life-threatening cardiovascular disorders.

In this section, you'll find definitive nursing information on a range of acute cardiovascular disorders. These range from arrhythmias and cardiogenic shock to myocardial contusions. This section also covers coronary artery disease and myocardial infarction—the most prevalent forms of heart disease—along with hypertensive crisis, heart failure, dissecting aortic aneurysm, and acute arterial occlusion.

Because a cardiovascular crisis often occurs suddenly and may rapidly become fatal, your prompt assessment and interventions could prove lifesaving. Besides interpreting electrocardiograms and cardiac enzyme studies, you'll need to be prepared to give emergency drugs, insert a peripheral I.V. line, and provide other rapid interventions. You may also need to perform life-support measures to avert brain damage or death.

Initial cardiovascular care

Check for:
- [ ] history of cardiovascular disease, especially hypertension, arterial occlusive disease, arrhythmias, or ischemic heart disease
- [ ] history of chest pain, palpitations, shortness of breath, edema, or fatigue
- [ ] medication history, especially antihypertensive, anginal, or antiarrhythmic drugs, diuretics, digitalis glycosides, or anticoagulants
- [ ] history of smoking and alcohol intake
- [ ] recent history of chest trauma
- [ ] exercise and activity intolerance
- [ ] respiratory dysfunction, abnormal vital signs, or chest pain
- [ ] electrocardiogram (ECG) abnormalities or changes from previous ECGs
- [ ] abnormal heart or breath sounds or both
- [ ] presence and quality of peripheral pulses
- [ ] skin color and temperature changes
- [ ] evidence of fluid retention
- [ ] abnormal neurologic function.

Intervene by:
- [ ] notifying doctor immediately of acute change in patient's cardiovascular status
- [ ] initiating cardiopulmonary resuscitation, as indicated
- [ ] inserting an I.V. line and obtaining an ECG
- [ ] administering oxygen and enforcing bed rest
- [ ] monitoring vital signs closely.

Prepare for:
- [ ] emergency drug therapy
- [ ] invasive and noninvasive diagnostic tests
- [ ] immediate surgery, if indicated
- [ ] defibrillation or temporary pacemaker insertion
- [ ] hemodynamic monitoring.

CORONARY ARTERY DISEASE

The dominant effect of coronary artery disease (CAD), the loss of oxygen and nutrients to myocardial tissue, results from diminished coronary blood flow. Fatty fibrous plaques, calcium-plaque deposits, or combinations of both narrow the lumens of coronary arteries, reducing the volume of blood that can flow through them.

A major cause of death, this disease is nearly epidemic in the Western world. CAD is more prevalent in men, whites, and middle-aged and older people than in women or in people of other races and ages. More than 50% of men ages 60 or older show signs of CAD on autopsy.

CAUSES

Atherosclerosis, the most common cause of CAD, has been linked to many risk factors. Some risk factors, such as the following, can't be controlled:

• *Age.* Atherosclerosis usually occurs after age 40.
• *Sex.* Men are eight times more susceptible than premenopausal women to atherosclerosis.
• *Heredity.* A positive family history of CAD increases the risk.
• *Race.* White men are more susceptible than nonwhite men to atherosclerosis; nonwhite women are more susceptible than white women.

However, the patient can modify other risk factors, such as the following, with good medical care and appropriate lifestyle changes:

• *Blood pressure.* Systolic pressure that exceeds 160 mm Hg or diastolic pressure that exceeds 95 mm Hg increases the risk.
• *Serum cholesterol levels.* Increased low-density lipoprotein and decreased high-density lipoprotein levels substantially heighten the risk.
• *Smoking.* Cigarette smokers are twice as likely to have a myocardial infarction (MI) and four times as likely to experience sudden death as nonsmokers. The risk dramatically drops within 1 year after smoking ceases.

• *Obesity.* Added weight augments the risk for diabetes mellitus, hypertension, and elevated serum cholesterol levels.
• *Physical activity.* Regular exercise reduces the risk.
• *Stress.* Added stress or type A personality increases the risk.
• *Diabetes mellitus.* This disorder raises the risk, especially in women.
• *Other modifiable factors.* Increased levels of serum fibrinogen and uric acid, elevated hematocrit, reduced vital capacity, high resting heart rate, thyrotoxicosis, and use of oral contraceptives heighten the risk.

Uncommon causes of reduced coronary artery blood flow include dissecting aneurysms, infectious vasculitis, syphilis, and congenital defects in the coronary vascular system. Coronary artery spasms may also impede blood flow. (See *Understanding coronary artery spasm.*)

COMPLICATIONS

When a coronary artery goes into spasm or is occluded by plaques, blood flow to the part of the myocardium that's supplied by that vessel decreases, causing angina pectoris. Failure to remedy the occlusion causes ischemia and, eventually, myocardial tissue infarction.

ASSESSMENT

The classic symptom of CAD is angina, the direct result of inadequate flow of oxygen to the myocardium. The patient usually describes it as a burning, squeezing, or crushing tightness in the substernal or precordial chest that may radiate to the left arm, neck, jaw, or shoulder blade. Typically, the patient clenches his fist over his chest or rubs his left arm when describing the pain. Nausea, vomiting, fainting, sweating, and cool extremities may accompany the tightness.

Angina commonly occurs after physical exertion but may also follow emotional excitement, exposure to cold, or a large meal. Angina can also develop during sleep and may awaken the patient.

The patient's history will suggest any pattern to the type and onset of pain. If the pain is predictable and relieved by rest or nitrates, it's called stable angina. If it increases in fre-

Understanding coronary artery spasm

Characterized by spontaneous, sustained contraction of one or more coronary arteries, coronary artery spasm can cause ischemia and dysfunction of the heart muscle. This disorder may also trigger Prinzmetal's angina and even myocardial infarction (MI) in patients with unoccluded coronary arteries.

Causes
The direct cause of coronary artery spasm is unknown, but possible contributing factors include:
• altered influx of calcium across the cell membrane
• intimal hemorrhage into the medial layer of the blood vessel
• hyperventilation
• elevated catecholamine levels
• fatty buildup in the lumen.

Signs and symptoms
The major symptom of coronary artery spasm is angina. But unlike classic angina, this pain commonly occurs spontaneously and may be unrelated to physical exertion or emotional stress; it may, however, follow cocaine use. It is usually more severe than classic angina, lasts longer, and may be cyclic — recurring every day at the same time. Ischemic episodes may cause arrhythmias, altered heart rate, lower blood pressure and, occasionally, fainting caused by decreased cardiac output. Spasm in the left coronary artery may result in mitral valve prolapse, producing a loud systolic murmur and, possibly, pulmonary edema, with dyspnea, crackles, and hemoptysis. MI and sudden death may occur.

Treatment
After diagnosis by coronary angiography and 12-lead electrocardiography, the patient may receive calcium channel blockers (verapamil, nifedipine, or diltiazem) to reduce coronary artery spasm and to decrease vascular resistance, and nitrates (nitroglycerin or isosorbide dinitrate) to relieve chest pain. During cardiac catheterization, the patient with clean arteries may receive ergotamine to induce the spasm and aid in the diagnosis.

Nursing interventions
When caring for a patient with coronary artery spasm, explain all necessary procedures and teach him how to take his medications safely. If he's receiving nifedipine or other calcium channel blocker, monitor his blood pressure, pulse rate, and ECG to detect arrhythmias. Because nifedipine may cause peripheral and periorbital edema, watch for fluid retention.

If the patient is also receiving a digitalis glycoside, monitor its levels and check for signs of digitalis toxicity.

Because coronary artery spasm is sometimes associated with atherosclerotic disease, advise the patient to stop smoking, avoid overeating, use alcohol sparingly, and maintain a balance between exercise and rest.

---

quency and duration and is more easily induced, it's referred to as unstable or unpredictable angina. Unstable angina generally indicates extensive or worsening disease and, untreated, may progress to MI. An effort-induced pain that occurs with increasing frequency and with decreasing provocation is referred to as crescendo angina. If severe pain occurs at rest without provocation, it's called variant or Prinzmetal's angina.

Inspection may reveal evidence of atherosclerotic disease, such as xanthelasma and xanthoma. Ophthalmoscopic inspection may show increased light reflexes and arteriovenous nicking, suggesting hypertension, an important risk factor for CAD.

Palpation can uncover thickened or absent peripheral arteries, signs of cardiac enlargement, and abnormal contraction of the cardiac impulse, such as left ventricular akinesia or dyskinesia.

Auscultation may detect bruits, an S_3, an S_4, or a late systolic murmur (if mitral insufficiency is present).

Identifying nitroglycerin dosage in CAD

To treat angina pectoris, give an adult a 150- to 600-mcg sublingual or buccal tablet. Or administer one or two metered-dose sprays (400 or 800 mcg) onto or under the tongue. Give one dose every 5 minutes. If relief doesn't occur after the third dose, notify the doctor.

DIAGNOSTIC TESTS

• *Electrocardiography (ECG)* during angina shows ischemia, as demonstrated by T-wave inversion or ST-segment depression and, possibly, arrhythmias, such as premature ventricular contractions. ECG results may or may not be normal during pain-free periods. Arrhythmias may occur without infarction, secondary to ischemia.
• *Treadmill* or *bicycle exercise test* may provoke chest pain and ECG signs of myocardial ischemia in response to physical exertion. Monitoring of electrical rhythm may demonstrate T-wave inversion or ST-segment depression in the ischemic areas.
• *Coronary angiography* reveals coronary artery stenosis or obstruction, collateral circulation, and the arteries' condition beyond the narrowing.
• *Myocardial perfusion imaging* with thallium-201 during treadmill exercise detects ischemic areas of the myocardium, visualized as "cold spots."

TREATMENT

In patients with angina, treatment aims to reduce myocardial oxygen demand or increase the oxygen supply and reduce pain. Activity restrictions may be required to prevent onset of pain. Rather than eliminating activities, performing them more slowly often averts pain. Stress-reduction techniques are also essential, especially if known stressors precipitate pain.

Drug therapy consists primarily of nitrates, such as nitroglycerin and isosorbide dinitrate, calcium channel blockers, or beta-adrenergic blockers. (See *Identifying nitroglycerin dosage in CAD.*)

Obstructive lesions may necessitate atherectomy or coronary artery bypass graft surgery, using vein grafts. Percutaneous transluminal coronary angioplasty (PTCA) may be performed during cardiac catheterization to compress fatty deposits and relieve occlusion.

Laser angioplasty corrects occlusion by vaporizing fatty deposits with the excimer or hot-tip laser device. (See *Relieving occlusion with PTCA and laser angioplasty,* pages 104 and 105.) Rotational ablation (or rotational atherectomy) removes atheromatous plaque with a high-speed, rotating burr covered with diamond crystals.

Because CAD is so widespread, prevention is important. Dietary restrictions aimed at reducing intake of calories (in obesity) and of salt, fats, and cholesterol minimize the risk, especially when supplemented with regular exercise. Abstention from smoking and reduction of stress are also essential.

Other preventive actions include control of hypertension (with diuretics or beta blockers), control of elevated serum cholesterol or triglyceride levels (with antilipemics, such as clofibrate), and measures to minimize platelet aggregation and the danger of blood clots (with aspirin, for example).

KEY NURSING DIAGNOSES AND PATIENT OUTCOMES

Altered cardiopulmonary tissue perfusion related to reduced blood flow to the myocardium caused by coronary artery spasm or occlusion. Based on this nursing diagnosis, you'll establish these patient outcomes. The patient will:
• maintain adequate myocardial tissue perfusion, as exhibited by a normal heart rate and rhythm and the absence of ischemic ECG changes
• verbalize an understanding of the prescribed medical regimen and relate the importance of seeking follow-up care for the rest of his life.

Decreased cardiac output related to adverse effect of CAD on myocardial function.

Based on this nursing diagnosis, you'll establish these patient outcomes. The patient will:
• maintain hemodynamic stability
• regain and maintain normal vital signs and mental alertness
• regain and maintain normal cardiac output.

Pain related to inadequate oxygen flow to the myocardium as a result of reduced myocardial blood flow. Based on this nursing diagnosis, you'll establish these patient outcomes. The patient will:
• experience a reduced severity and frequency of anginal pain episodes by complying with medical or surgical therapy
• identify the factors that trigger anginal pain
• verbalize an understanding of what he needs to do when anginal pain occurs.

NURSING INTERVENTIONS
• Keep nitroglycerin available for immediate use. Instruct the patient to call immediately whenever he feels chest, arm, or neck pain and before taking nitroglycerin.
• After a cardiac catheterization, review the expected course of treatment with the patient and his family. Also, to encourage safe elimination of the contrast medium, increase the I.V. flow rate and make sure the patient drinks plenty of fluids. Add potassium to the I.V. fluid, as ordered.
• Prepare the patient for PTCA or bypass surgery, as indicated.

Monitoring
• During anginal episodes, monitor the patient's blood pressure and heart rate. Take a 12-lead ECG during anginal episodes before administering nitroglycerin or other nitrates. Record the duration of pain, the amount of medication required to relieve it, and any accompanying symptoms.
• Ask the patient to grade the severity of his pain on a scale of 1 to 10. This allows him to give his individual assessment of pain as well as of the effectiveness of pain-relieving medications.
• Following a cardiac catheterization, monitor the patient's catheter site for bleeding and evaluate his distal pulses. Also, periodically check the patient's serum potassium level.

• After rotational ablation, assess the patient for chest pain, hypotension, coronary artery spasm, and bleeding from the catheter site. Provide heparin and antibiotics for 24 to 48 hours, as ordered.

Patient teaching
• Before cardiac catheterization, explain the procedure to the patient.
• Make sure the patient knows why cardiac catheterization is necessary, understands the risks, and realizes that he may need such therapies as PTCA, bypass surgery, atherectomy, and laser angioplasty.
• If the patient is scheduled for surgery, explain the procedure. Provide a tour of the intensive care unit, introduce him to the staff, and discuss the care he can expect after surgery.
• Help the patient determine which activities precipitate episodes of pain so that he can avoid them if possible.
• Help the patient identify and select more effective coping mechanisms to deal with stress. Occupational change may be needed to prevent symptoms, but many patients reject this alternative.
• Stress the need to follow the prescribed drug regimen.
• Explain that recurrent angina symptoms after PTCA or rotational ablation may signal recurring obstruction.
• Encourage the patient to maintain the prescribed low-sodium diet and, if he is also obese, to start a low-calorie diet.
• Encourage regular, moderate exercise. Refer the patient to a cardiac rehabilitation center or cardiovascular fitness program near his home or workplace. The staff can set up a program of exercise that best meets the patient's needs and limitations.
• Suggest that family members or a friend join the patient in his commitment to enhance his exercise program.
• Reassure the patient that he can resume sexual activity and that modifications can allow for sexual fulfillment without fear of overexertion, pain, or reocclusion.
• If necessary, refer the patient to a program to stop smoking. Acknowledge that this will be

Relieving occlusion with PTCA and laser angioplasty

Two forms of angioplasty used to correct coronary artery occlusion include percutaneous transluminal coronary angioplasty (PTCA) and laser angioplasty.

PTCA

This procedure offers some patients with localized disease a nonsurgical alternative to coronary artery bypass graft surgery. In PTCA, a tiny balloon catheter is used to dilate a coronary artery that has been narrowed by an atherosclerotic plaque.

The procedure for PTCA resembles that for cardiac catheterization. A guiding catheter is threaded through a femoral or brachial artery, then backward into the ascending aorta and into the ostium of the right or left coronary artery.

The guide wire is then advanced from the balloon catheter through the coronary artery until its tip is beyond the portion narrowed by plaque formation.

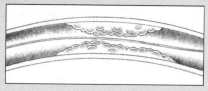

Then the balloon catheter is advanced over the guide wire until the balloon is wedged into the narrowing.

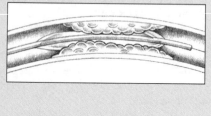

Once in position, the balloon is inflated with a mixture of contrast material and 0.9% sodium chloride solution. The inflated balloon opens the narrowed artery by splitting and compressing the plaque and slightly stretching the artery wall.

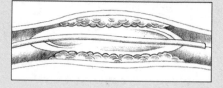

After the balloon reaches 3 to 6.5 atmospheres of pressure, it's deflated. The balloon is then repeatedly inflated until distal perfusion pressure falls about 30%. The catheter and balloon are then removed from the artery.

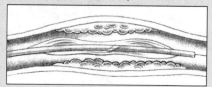

PTCA has widened the narrow part of the artery, improving blood flow to the heart.

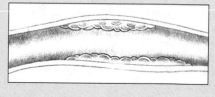

difficult, but tell him that he should make every attempt to stop smoking immediately and never restart.

MYOCARDIAL INFARCTION

A leading cause of death in North America and western Europe, myocardial infarction (MI) results from reduced blood flow through one of the coronary arteries, which causes myo-

Laser angioplasty

Although they're still unperfected, several methods of laser angioplasty effectively relieve stenosis and correct occlusions that balloon angioplasty alone has failed to correct. The hot-tipped laser creates a channel wide enough to admit a balloon catheter, which widens the channel even further. Then the direct-energy laser beam vaporizes or perforates any plaque obstructing the vessel.

A hot-tipped laser moves through a stenotic region.

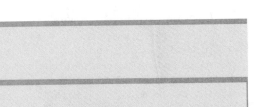

A direct-energy laser beam ablates the plaque.

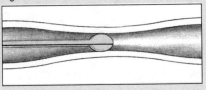

When the channel is opened, the balloon is positioned and then inflated.

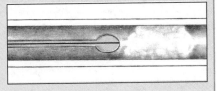

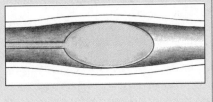

cardial ischemia and necrosis. The infarction site depends on the vessels involved. For instance, occlusion of the circumflex coronary artery causes a lateral wall infarction; occlusion of the left anterior coronary artery causes an anterior wall infarction. Posterior and inferior wall infarctions result from occlusion of the right coronary artery or one of its branches. Right ventricular infarctions can also result from right coronary artery occlusion, can accompany inferior infarctions, and may cause right ventricular failure. In transmural (Q wave) MI, tissue damage extends through all myocardial layers; in subendocardial (non–Q wave) MI, usually only the innermost layer is damaged.

Men are more susceptible to MI than premenopausal women, although incidence is rising among women who smoke or take oral contraceptives. The incidence in postmenopausal women is similar to that in men.

Mortality following MI is about 25% and usually results from cardiac damage or complications. More than 50% of sudden deaths occur within 1 hour after onset of signs and symptoms, before the patient reaches the hospital. Of those who recover, up to 10% die within the first year.

CAUSES

MI results from occlusion of one of the coronary arteries. Such occlusion can stem from atherosclerosis, thrombosis, platelet aggregation, or coronary artery stenosis or spasm. Predisposing factors include:
• aging
• diabetes mellitus
• elevated serum triglyceride, low-density lipoprotein, and cholesterol levels and decreased serum high-density lipoprotein levels
• excessive intake of saturated fats, carbohydrates, or salt
• hypertension
• obesity
• family history of coronary artery disease (CAD)
• sedentary lifestyle
• smoking
• stress or a type A personality (aggressive, competitive, addicted to work, chronically impatient).

In addition, use of drugs such as amphetamines or cocaine can cause an MI.

COMPLICATIONS

Cardiac complications of acute MI include arrhythmias, cardiogenic shock, heart failure causing pulmonary edema, and pericarditis.

Other complications include rupture of the atrial or ventricular septum, ventricular wall, or valves; ventricular aneurysms; mural thrombi causing cerebral or pulmonary emboli; and extensions of the original infarction. Dressler's syndrome (post-MI pericarditis) can occur days to weeks after an MI and cause residual pain, malaise, and fever. (See *Assessing and managing complications of MI.*)

Typically, older patients are more prone to complications and death. Psychological problems can also occur, either from the patient's fear of another MI or from an organic brain disorder caused by tissue hypoxia. Occasionally, a patient may have a personality change.

ASSESSMENT

Typically, the patient reports the cardinal symptom of MI – persistent, crushing substernal pain that may radiate to the left arm, jaw, neck, and shoulder blades. He commonly describes the pain as heavy, squeezing, or crushing, and it may persist for 12 or more hours. However, in some patients – particularly older patients or those with diabetes – pain may not occur; in others, it may be mild and may be confused with indigestion.

Patients with CAD may report increasing frequency, severity, or duration of anginal episodes (especially when not precipitated by exertion, a heavy meal, or cold and wind). The patient may also report a feeling of impending doom, fatigue, nausea, vomiting, and shortness of breath. Sudden death, however, may be the first and only indication of MI.

Inspection may reveal an extremely anxious and restless patient with dyspnea and diaphoresis. If right ventricular failure is present, you may note jugular vein distention. Within the first hour after an anterior MI, about 25% of patients exhibit sympathetic nervous system hyperactivity, such as tachycardia and hypertension. Up to 50% of patients with an inferior MI exhibit parasympathetic nervous system hyperactivity, such as bradycardia and hypotension.

In patients who develop ventricular dysfunction, auscultation may disclose decreased heart sounds, an S_4, an S_3, and paradoxical splitting of S_2. A systolic murmur of mitral insufficiency may be heard with papillary muscle dysfunction secondary to infarction. A pericardial friction rub may also be heard, especially in patients who have a transmural MI or have developed pericarditis.

Fever is unusual at the onset of an MI. However, a low-grade fever may develop during the next few days.

DIAGNOSTIC TESTS

To help diagnose an MI, the patient will undergo a 12-lead electrocardiogram (ECG) as well as serum studies. Expect the following results:

• *Serial 12-lead ECG* will reveal serial ST-segment depression in subendocardial MI and ST-segment elevation and Q waves (representing scarring and necrosis) in transmural MI. However, be aware that during the first few hours after an MI, the ECG may be normal or inconclusive.

• *Total serum creatine kinase (CK) level* will exceed 175 U/liter for men and 140 U/liter for women. (Different measurement methods give different ranges. Check the normal range used by the laboratory at your hospital.)

• *Cardiac muscle isoenzyme CK-MB* will start to rise within 4 hours of an acute MI, peak in 12 to 48 hours, and usually return to normal in 24 to 48 hours. Persistent elevations or increasing levels indicate ongoing myocardial damage.

• *Lactate dehydrogenase isoenzyme ratio (LD_1-LD_2)* will exceed 1.

Other characteristic diagnostic results include the following:

• *Echocardiography* shows ventricular wall dyskinesia with a transmural MI and helps evaluate the ejection fraction.

• *Scans,* using I.V. technetium-99, can identify acutely damaged muscle by picking up accumulation of radioactive nucleotide, which appears as a "hot spot" on the film. Myocardial perfusion imaging with thallium-201 reveals a "cold spot" in most patients during the first few hours after a transmural MI.

Assessing and managing complications of MI

COMPLICATION	ASSESSMENT	TREATMENT
Arrhythmias	Electrocardiogram (ECG) shows premature ventricular contractions, ventricular tachycardia, or ventricular fibrillation; in inferior wall myocardial infarction (MI), bradycardia and junctional rhythms or atrioventricular (AV) block; in anterior wall MI, tachycardia or heart block.	Antiarrhythmics, atropine, cardioversion, defibrillation, and pacemaker
Cardiogenic shock	Catheterization shows decreased cardiac output, increased pulmonary artery systolic and diastolic pressures, decreased cardiac index, increased systemic vascular resistance (SVR), and increased pulmonary artery wedge pressure (PAWP). Signs are hypotension, tachycardia, decreased level of consciousness, decreased urine output, neck vein distention, S_3 and S_4, and cool, pale skin.	I.V. fluids, vasodilators, cardiotonics, digitalis glycosides, intra-aortic balloon pump (IABP), vasopressors, and beta-adrenergic stimulants
Cerebral or pulmonary embolism	Dyspnea, chest pain, or neurologic changes may occur. Nuclear scan shows ventilation-perfusion mismatch in pulmonary embolism. Angiography shows arterial blockage.	Oxygen and heparin and cardiopulmonary resuscitation (CPR); epinephrine; or cardiac pacing
Heart failure	In left ventricular failure, chest X-rays show venous congestion and cardiomegaly. Catheterization shows increases in pulmonary artery systolic and diastolic pressures, PAWP, central venous pressure, and SVR.	Diuretics, vasodilators, inotropics, and digitalis glycosides
Mitral insufficiency	Auscultation reveals apical holosystolic murmur. Dyspnea is prominent. Catheterization shows increased pulmonary artery pressure (PAP) and PAWP. Echocardiogram shows valve dysfunction.	Nitroglycerin, nitroprusside, IABP, and surgical replacement of the mitral valve; possibly concomitant myocardial revascularization with significant coronary artery disease
Pericarditis (Dressler's syndrome)	Auscultation reveals a pericardial friction rub. Chest pain is relieved in sitting position. Sharp pain is unlike previous anginal pain.	Anti-inflammatory agents, such as aspirin or other nonsteroidal anti-inflammatory drugs or corticosteroids
Ventricular aneurysm	Chest X-rays may show cardiomegaly. ECG may show arrhythmias and persistent ST-segment elevation. Left ventriculography shows altered or paradoxical left ventricular motion.	Cardioversion, defibrillation (if ventricular tachycardia or fibrillation occurs), antiarrhythmics, vasodilators, anticoagulants, digitalis glycosides, diuretics and, possibly, surgery
Ventricular rupture	Cardiac tamponade occurs. Arrhythmias, such as ventricular tachycardia and ventricular fibrillation, or sudden death results.	Resuscitation for advanced cardiac life support measures and possible emergency surgical repair if CPR is successful
Ventricular septal rupture	In left-to-right shunt, auscultation reveals a harsh holosystolic murmur and thrill. Catheterization shows increased PAP and PAWP. Increased oxygen saturation of right ventricle and pulmonary artery confirms the diagnosis.	Surgical correction (may be postponed, but usually performed immediately or up to 7 days after septal rupture), IABP, nitroglycerin, nitroprusside, low-dose inotropics (dopamine), and cardiac pacing when high-grade AV blocks occur

DOSAGE FINDER

Identifying morphine dosage in MI

To treat pain associated with myocardial infarction (MI), give an adult 8 to 15 mg I.V., followed by smaller doses every 3 to 4 hours as needed.

TREATMENT

The goals of treatment are to relieve chest pain, to stabilize heart rhythm, and to reduce cardiac workload. Treatment includes revascularization to preserve myocardial tissue. Arrhythmias, the most common problem during the first 48 hours after MI, may require antiarrhythmics, possibly a pacemaker and, rarely, cardioversion.

Drug therapy usually includes:
• lidocaine for ventricular arrhythmias; if lidocaine is ineffective, procainamide, quinidine sulfate, bretylium, or disopyramide
• atropine I.V.
• nitroglycerin (sublingual, topical, transdermal, or I.V.); calcium channel blockers, such as nifedipine, verapamil, and diltiazem (sublingual, oral, or I.V.); or isosorbide dinitrate (sublingual, oral, or I.V.) to relieve pain by redistributing blood to the ischemic area of the myocardium, increasing cardiac output, and reducing myocardial workload
• morphine I.V., the drug of choice for pain and sedation, and possibly meperidine or hydromorphone (See *Identifying morphine dosage in MI.*)
• drugs that increase contractility or blood pressure
• inotropic drugs, such as dobutamine and amrinone, to treat reduced myocardial contractility
• beta-adrenergic blockers, such as propranolol and timolol, after acute MI to help prevent reinfarction.

These other therapies may also be used:
• Oxygen is usually administered (by face mask or nasal cannula) at a modest flow rate for 24 to 48 hours; a lower concentration is necessary if the patient has chronic obstructive pulmonary disease.
• Bed rest with bedside commode is enforced to decrease cardiac workload.
• Pulmonary artery catheterization may be performed to detect left or right ventricular failure and to monitor response to treatment, but it's not routinely done.
• Intra-aortic balloon pump may be used for cardiogenic shock.
• Revascularization therapy can be used if the patient is younger than age 70 and doesn't have a history of cerebrovascular accident, bleeding, GI ulcers, marked hypertension, recent surgery, or chest pain lasting longer than 6 hours. Thrombolytic therapy must be started up to 6 hours after infarction, using intracoronary or systemic streptokinase (I.V.) or tissue plasminogen activator. The best response occurs when treatment begins within the first hour after the onset of symptoms.
• Cardiac catheterization, percutaneous transluminal coronary angioplasty (PTCA), and coronary artery bypass grafting may also be performed.

KEY NURSING DIAGNOSES AND PATIENT OUTCOMES

Altered cardiopulmonary tissue perfusion related to narrowing or closure of one or more coronary arteries. Based on this nursing diagnosis, you'll establish these patient outcomes. The patient will:
• seek emergency intervention immediately to minimize myocardial damage
• exhibit no arrhythmias on ECG
• regain adequate cardiac tissue perfusion.

High risk for injury related to complications of MI. Based on this nursing diagnosis, you'll establish these patient outcomes. The patient will:
• seek immediate medical treatment if complications arise
• avoid permanent deficits caused by complications of MI.

Pain related to myocardial tissue ischemia. Based on this nursing diagnosis, you'll establish these patient outcomes. The patient will:

• express relief of chest discomfort after treatment
• avoid new episodes of chest pain and exhibit no ischemic changes on ECG
• comply with the prescribed treatment regimen to prevent further tissue ischemia.

NURSING INTERVENTIONS

• Administer analgesics, as ordered. Avoid giving I.M. injections because absorption from muscles is unpredictable and I.V. administration provides more rapid symptomatic relief.
• Organize patient care and activities to allow periods of uninterrupted rest.
• Ask the dietary department to provide a clear-liquid diet until nausea subsides. A low-cholesterol, low-sodium diet without caffeine-containing beverages may be ordered.
• Provide a stool softener to prevent straining during defecation, which causes vagal stimulation and may slow the heart rate. Allow the patient to use a bedside commode, and provide as much privacy as possible.
• Assist with range-of-motion exercises. If the patient is immobilized by a severe MI, turn him often. Antiembolism stockings help prevent venostasis and thrombophlebitis.
• Provide emotional support, and help reduce stress and anxiety; administer tranquilizers as needed.
• Prepare the patient for PTCA and thrombolytic therapy, as indicated.

Monitoring

• On admission to the intensive care unit (ICU), monitor and record the patient's ECG, blood pressure, temperature, and heart and breath sounds.
• Assess the patient's degree of pain. Record the severity, location, type, and duration of pain.
• Check the patient's blood pressure after administering nitroglycerin, especially the first dose.
• Frequently monitor ECG rhythm strips to detect heart rate changes and arrhythmias. Analyze rhythm strips and place a representative strip in the patient's chart if you assess any new arrhythmias, if chest pain occurs, or

at least once each shift or according to hospital policy.
• During episodes of chest pain, monitor the patient's ECG, blood pressure, and pulmonary artery pressure measurements (if applicable) to determine changes.
• Watch for crackles, cough, tachypnea, and edema, which may indicate impending left ventricular failure. Carefully monitor daily weight, intake and output, respiratory rate, serum enzyme levels, ECG waveforms, and blood pressure. Auscultate for adventitious breath sounds periodically. (A patient on bed rest commonly has atelectatic crackles, which may disappear after coughing.) Also auscultate for S_3 or S_4 gallops.

Patient teaching

• Explain procedures and answer questions for both the patient and his family. Explain the ICU environment and routine. Remember that you may need to repeat explanations once the emergency situation has resolved.
• To promote compliance with the prescribed medication regimen and other treatment measures, thoroughly explain dosages and therapy. Inform the patient of the drug's adverse effects and advise him to watch for and report signs of toxicity (for example, anorexia, nausea, vomiting, mental depression, vertigo, blurred vision, and yellow vision, if the patient is receiving a digitalis glycoside).
• Review dietary restrictions with the patient. If he must follow a low-sodium or low-fat and low-cholesterol diet, provide a list of foods to avoid. Ask the dietitian to speak to the patient and his family.
• Encourage the patient to participate in a cardiac rehabilitation exercise program. The doctor and the exercise physiologist should determine the level of exercise and then discuss it with the patient and secure his agreement to a stepped-care program.
• Counsel the patient to resume sexual activity progressively. He may need to take nitroglycerin before sexual intercourse to prevent chest pain from the increased activity.
• Advise the patient about appropriate responses to new or recurrent symptoms.

• Advise the patient to report typical or atypical chest pain. Post-MI syndrome may develop, producing chest pain that must be differentiated from recurrent MI, pulmonary infarction, and heart failure.

• Emphasize the need for the patient to stop smoking. If necessary, refer him to a support group.

HEART FAILURE

When the myocardium can't pump effectively enough to meet the body's metabolic needs, heart failure occurs. Usually pump failure occurs from primary or secondary damage to the left ventricle (left ventricular failure). However, left and right ventricular failure usually develop simultaneously. Heart failure is classified as high-output or low-output, acute or chronic, left-sided or right-sided, and forward or backward. (See *Categorizing heart failure*.)

For many patients, the symptoms of heart failure restrict the ability to perform activities of daily living, severely affecting quality of life. Although advances in diagnostic and therapeutic techniques have greatly improved the outlook for these patients, this disorder remains life-threatening, with the prognosis depending on the underlying cause and its response to treatment.

CAUSES

Heart failure frequently results from a primary abnormality of the heart muscle (such as an infarction) that impairs ventricular function to the point that the heart can no longer pump sufficient blood. Heart failure can also result from causes not related to myocardial function. These include:

• insufficient ventricular blood volume caused by mechanical dysfunction during diastole. This occurs in mitral stenosis secondary to rheumatic heart disease or constrictive pericarditis and in atrial fibrillation.

• systolic hemodynamic disturbances – such as excessive cardiac workload caused by volume or pressure overload – that limit the heart's pumping ability. These disturbances can result from mitral or aortic insufficiency, which causes volume overload, and from aortic stenosis or systemic hypertension, which results in increased resistance to ventricular emptying.

In addition, certain conditions can predispose the patient to heart failure, particularly if he has some form of underlying heart disease. These include:

• arrhythmias – such as tachyarrhythmias, which can reduce ventricular filling time; bradycardia, which can reduce cardiac output; and arrhythmias that disrupt the normal atrial and ventricular filling synchrony

• pregnancy and thyrotoxicosis, because of the increased demand for cardiac output

• pulmonary embolism, because it elevates pulmonary artery pressures that can cause right ventricular failure

• infections, because increased metabolic demands further burden the heart

• anemia, because to meet the oxygen needs of the tissues, cardiac output must increase

• increased physical activity, emotional stress, increased sodium or water intake, or failure to comply with the prescribed treatment regimen for the underlying heart disease.

COMPLICATIONS

Pulmonary congestion can lead to pulmonary edema, a life-threatening condition. Decreased perfusion to major organs, especially the brain and kidneys, can cause these organs to fail. Myocardial infarction can occur because the oxygen demands of the overworked heart can't be sufficiently met.

ASSESSMENT

The patient's history reveals a disorder or condition that can precipitate heart failure. The patient often complains of shortness of breath, which, in early stages, occurs during activity, and, in late stages, also at rest. He may report that dyspnea worsens at night when he lies down. He may use two or three pillows to elevate his head to sleep or may have to sleep sitting up in a chair. He may relate that his shortness of breath wakes him up soon after he falls asleep, causing him to sit bolt upright to catch his breath. Often he may remain dyspneic, coughing and wheezing even when he

Categorizing heart failure

Although heart failure is usually classified by the site of failure (left ventricle, right ventricle, or both), it may also be classified by level of cardiac output, stage, and direction (high-output or low-output, acute or chronic, or forward or backward). These classifications represent different clinical aspects of heart failure, not distinct diseases.

Left ventricular failure
Failure of the left ventricle to pump blood to the vital organs and periphery is usually caused by myocardial infarction (MI). Decreased left ventricular output causes fluid to accumulate in the lungs, precipitating dyspnea, orthopnea, and paroxysmal nocturnal dyspnea.

Right ventricular failure
Resulting from failure of the right ventricle to pump sufficient blood to the lungs, this type usually is caused by disorders that increase pulmonary vascular resistance, such as pulmonary embolism, pulmonic stenosis, and pulmonary hypertension. Right ventricular failure produces congestive hepatomegaly, ascites, and edema.

High-output failure
Failure with an elevated cardiac output occurs when tissue demands for oxygenated blood exceed the heart's ability to supply it. High-output failure occurs in arteriovenous fistula, hyperthyroidism, anemia, sickle cell anemia, beriberi, Paget's disease of the bone, and thyrotoxicosis.

Low-output failure
Failure with decreased cardiac output is caused by decreased pumping ability of the myocardium. Low-output failure occurs in coronary artery disease, hypertension, primary myocardial disease, and valvular disease.

Acute failure
This failure occurs suddenly, as in MI or a ruptured heart valve. The sudden reduction in cardiac output results in systemic hypotension without peripheral edema. Acute failure may occur in a chronic condition—for example, when a patient with chronic heart failure experiences an MI. It may also occur in any condition that increases stress on an already diseased heart.

Chronic failure
This type of heart failure occurs gradually and is sustained for long periods. The arterial blood pressure doesn't drop, but peripheral edema is present. Chronic failure may occur in cardiomyopathy, in multivalvular disease, or in a healed, extensive MI.

Forward failure
In forward failure, the heart fails to expel enough blood into the arterial system. Sodium and water retention result from decreased renal perfusion and excessive proximal or distal tubular reabsorption, caused by activation of the renin-angiotensin-aldosterone system.

Backward failure
When backward failure occurs, one ventricle fails to empty its contents normally, and end-diastolic ventricular pressures rise. This, in turn, increases pressure and volume in the atrium and venous system behind the failing ventricle. Elevated systemic venous and capillary pressures cause sodium and water retention and eventual transudation of fluid into the interstitial place.

sits up. This is referred to as paroxysmal nocturnal dyspnea.

The patient may report that his shoes or rings have become too tight, a result of peripheral edema. He may also report increasing fatigue, weakness, insomnia, anorexia, nausea, and a sense of abdominal fullness (particularly in right ventricular failure).

Inspection may reveal a dyspneic, anxious patient in respiratory distress. In mild cases, dyspnea may occur while the patient is lying down or active; in severe cases, it's not related to position. The patient may have a cough that produces pink, frothy sputum. You may note cyanosis of the lips and nail beds, pale skin, diaphoresis, dependent peripheral and sacral edema, and jugular vein distention. Ascites may also be present, especially in patients with right ventricular failure. If heart failure is chronic, the patient may appear cachectic.

When palpating the pulse, you may note that the skin feels cool and clammy. The pulse rate will be rapid, and pulsus alternans may be present. Hepatomegaly and, possibly, splenomegaly also may be present.

Percussion reveals dullness over lung bases that are fluid-filled.

Auscultation of the blood pressure may detect decreased pulse pressure, reflecting reduced stroke volume. Heart auscultation may disclose an S_3 and S_4. Lung auscultation reveals moist, bibasilar crackles. If pulmonary edema is present, you'll hear crackles throughout the lung, accompanied by rhonchi and expiratory wheezing.

DIAGNOSTIC TESTS

• *Electrocardiography* reflects heart strain or enlargement, or ischemia. It may also reveal atrial enlargement, tachycardia, and extrasystoles.
• *Chest X-rays* show increased pulmonary vascular markings, interstitial edema, or pleural effusion and cardiomegaly.
• *Pulmonary artery pressure monitoring* typically demonstrates elevated pulmonary artery and pulmonary artery wedge pressures, elevated left ventricular end-diastolic pressure in left ventricular failure, and elevated right atrial or central venous pressure in right ventricular failure.

TREATMENT

The aim of therapy is to improve pump function by reversing the compensatory mechanisms producing the clinical effects. Treatment may consist of:
• diuresis (with diuretics, such as furosemide, hydrochlorothiazide, spironolactone, ethacrynic acid, bumetanide, or triamterene) to reduce total blood volume and circulatory congestion
• potassium supplements if the patient is receiving a potassium-wasting diuretic such as furosemide
• prolonged bed rest
• oxygen administration to increase oxygen delivery to the myocardium and other vital organ tissues
• inotropic drugs, such as the sympathomimetics dopamine and dobutamine, to strengthen myocardial contractility; or digitalis glycosides, such as digoxin, to enhance cardiac output and decrease heart rate if the patient suffers from congestive heart failure (CHF)
• vasodilators, such as amrinone, or angiotensin-converting enzyme inhibitors, such as captopril, to decrease afterload (See *Identifying drug dosages in heart failure.*)
• antiembolism stockings to prevent venostasis and thromboembolism formation.

After recovery, the patient with CHF usually must continue taking digitalis glycosides, diuretics, and potassium supplements and must remain under medical supervision. If the patient with valve dysfunction has recurrent acute heart failure, surgical replacement may be necessary. If high-output failure is resolved through treatment, recovery is usually complete.

KEY NURSING DIAGNOSES AND PATIENT OUTCOMES

Decreased cardiac output related to reduced stroke volume caused by mechanical, structural, or electrophysiologic heart problems. Based on this nursing diagnosis, you'll establish these patient outcomes. The patient will:
• maintain a normal pulse rate and blood pressure
• avoid dizziness, syncope, arrhythmias, and chest pain
• regain normal cardiac output without residual deficits caused by decreased tissue perfusion.

Fluid volume excess related to blood pooling in the pulmonary system or the systemic circulation caused by myocardial damage. Based on this nursing diagnosis, you'll establish these patient outcomes. The patient will:
• tolerate restricted fluid intake, as ordered, so that it doesn't exceed urine output
• regain and maintain baseline weight

• regain and maintain central venous and pulmonary artery pressures within normal limits (if possible).

Ineffective breathing pattern related to fatigue caused by pulmonary congestion. Based on this nursing diagnosis, you'll establish these patient outcomes. The patient will:
• regain his baseline respiratory rate and maintain stable respirations
• regain and maintain arterial blood gas values within normal limits.

NURSING INTERVENTIONS
• Place the patient in Fowler's position and give supplemental oxygen, as ordered, to ease his breathing.
• Organize all activities to provide maximum rest periods.
• To prevent deep vein thrombosis resulting from vascular congestion, assist the patient with range-of-motion exercises. Enforce bed rest and apply antiembolism stockings.
• Report changes in the patient's condition immediately.

Monitoring
• Weigh the patient daily to help detect fluid retention and observe for peripheral edema. Monitor I.V. intake and urine output (especially if the patient is receiving diuretics).
• Assess the patient's vital signs (for increased respiratory and heart rates and for narrowing pulse pressure) and mental status. Auscultate the heart for abnormal sounds and the lungs for crackles or rhonchi.
• Frequently monitor blood urea nitrogen and serum creatinine, potassium, sodium, chloride, and magnesium levels.
• Provide continuous cardiac monitoring during acute and advanced disease stages to identify and manage arrhythmias promptly.
• Watch for calf pain and tenderness.

Patient teaching
• Advise the patient to avoid foods high in sodium content, such as canned and commercially prepared foods and dairy products, to curb fluid overload.
• Teach the patient that he must replace the potassium lost through diuretic therapy by

DOSAGE FINDER

Identifying drug dosages in heart failure

The drugs listed below may be used to treat heart failure.

Amrinone
For short-term management of congestive heart failure (CHF) in patients unresponsive to digitalis glycosides, diuretics, and vasodilators, give an adult 0.75 mg/kg I.V. over 2 to 3 minutes. Follow this with a continuous infusion of 200 mg of amrinone in 250 ml of sodium chloride solution, delivered at an infusion rate of 5 to 10 mcg/kg/minute. Adjust the dosage according to the patient's clinical response. If necessary, give a bolus of 0.75 mg/kg 30 minutes after therapy starts.

The daily amrinone dosage shouldn't exceed 10 mg/kg, although some patients have received up to 18 mg/kg a day for short durations. The patient should maintain a steady state plasma level of 3 mcg/ml.

Digoxin
To treat CHF, atrial flutter and fibrillation, and atrial tachycardias, including paroxysmal atrial tachycardia, give an adult a loading dose of 0.5 to 1 mg I.V. or I.M. (or 0.008 to 0.012 mg/kg) and a maintenance dose of 0.125 to 0.5 mg daily. The usual maintenance dose is 0.25 mg.

Furosemide
To treat edema associated with CHF and pulmonary edema, give an adult initially 40 mg I.V. or I.M. After 1 hour, increase the dose to 80 mg, if needed.

taking a prescribed potassium supplement and eating potassium-rich foods, such as bananas, apricots, and oranges.
• Stress the need for regular medical checkups.
• Emphasize the importance of taking digitalis glycosides exactly as prescribed. Tell the patient to watch for and immediately report signs of toxicity, such as anorexia, vomiting, confusion, slow or irregular pulse rate and, in older patients, flulike symptoms.

• Tell the patient to notify the doctor if his pulse rate is unusually irregular or if it is less than 60 beats/minute; if he experiences dizziness, blurred vision, shortness of breath, persistent dry cough, palpitations, increased fatigue, paroxysmal nocturnal dyspnea, swollen ankles, or decreased urine output; or if he gains 3 to 5 lb (1.4 to 2.3 kg) in 1 week.

CARDIAC TAMPONADE

A rapid rise in intrapericardial pressure impairs diastolic filling of the heart in cardiac tamponade. The rise in pressure usually results from blood or fluid accumulation in the pericardial sac. If fluid accumulates rapidly, as little as 250 ml can create an emergency situation. Slow accumulation and rise in pressure, as in pericardial effusion associated with cancer, may not produce immediate signs and symptoms because the fibrous wall of the pericardial sac can gradually stretch to accommodate as much as 1 to 2 liters of fluid.

CAUSES

Cardiac tamponade may be idiopathic (Dressler's syndrome) or may result from:
• effusion (in cancer, bacterial infections, tuberculosis and, rarely, acute rheumatic fever)
• hemorrhage from trauma (such as gunshot or stab wounds of the chest, perforation by a catheter during cardiac or central venous catheterization, or cardiac surgery)
• hemorrhage from nontraumatic causes (such as rupture of the heart or great vessels or anticoagulant therapy in a patient with pericarditis)
• viral, postradiation, or idiopathic pericarditis
• acute myocardial infarction
• chronic renal failure during dialysis
• drug reaction (procainamide, hydralazine, minoxidil, isoniazid, penicillin, methysergide, and daunorubicin)
• connective tissue disorders (such as rheumatoid arthritis, systemic lupus erythematosus, rheumatic fever, vasculitis, and scleroderma).

COMPLICATIONS

Pressure resulting from fluid accumulation in the pericardium decreases ventricular filling and cardiac output, resulting in cardiogenic shock and death if untreated.

ASSESSMENT

The patient's history may show a disorder that can cause cardiac tamponade. He may report acute pain and dyspnea, which forces him to sit upright and lean forward to ease breathing and lessen the pain. He may be orthopneic, diaphoretic, anxious, restless, and pale or cyanotic. You may note neck vein distention produced by increased venous pressure, although this may not be present if the patient is hypovolemic.

Palpation of the peripheral pulses may disclose rapid, weak pulses. Palpation of the upper quadrant may reveal hepatomegaly.

Percussion may detect a widening area of flatness across the anterior chest wall, indicating a large effusion. Hepatomegaly may also be noted.

Auscultation of the blood pressure may demonstrate a decreased arterial blood pressure, pulsus paradoxus (an abnormal inspiratory drop in systemic blood pressure greater than 15 mm Hg), and narrow pulse pressure.

Heart sounds may be muffled. A quiet heart with faint sounds usually accompanies only severe tamponade and occurs within minutes of the tamponade, as happens with cardiac rupture or trauma. The lungs are clear.

DIAGNOSTIC TESTS

The following test results are characteristic:
• *Chest X-rays* show a slightly widened mediastinum and enlargement of the cardiac silhouette.
• *Electrocardiography (ECG)* is useful to rule out other cardiac disorders. The QRS amplitude may be reduced, and electrical alternans of the P wave, QRS complex, and T wave may be present. Generalized ST-segment elevation is noted in all leads.
• *Pulmonary artery pressure monitoring* detects increased right atrial pressure, right ventricular diastolic pressure, and central venous pressure (CVP).

• *Echocardiography* records pericardial effusion with signs of right ventricular and atrial compression.

TREATMENT

The goal of treatment is to relieve intrapericardial pressure and cardiac compression by removing accumulated blood or fluid. Pericardiocentesis (needle aspiration of the pericardial cavity) or surgical creation of an opening dramatically improves systemic arterial pressure and cardiac output with aspiration of as little as 25 ml of fluid. A drain may be inserted into the pericardial sac to drain the fluid. This may be left in until the effusion process stops or surgery (pericardial window) is performed. In the case of infection, antibiotics can be instilled through the drain, which is clamped and later opened to drain the antibiotic.

In the hypotensive patient, trial volume loading with I.V. 0.9% sodium chloride solution with albumin and perhaps an inotropic drug, such as dopamine, is necessary to maintain cardiac output.

Depending on the cause of tamponade, additional treatment may include:
• in traumatic injury, blood transfusion or a thoracotomy to drain reaccumulating fluid or to repair bleeding sites
• in heparin-induced tamponade, administering the heparin antagonist protamine
• in warfarin-induced tamponade, administering vitamin K.

KEY NURSING DIAGNOSES AND PATIENT OUTCOMES

Altered tissue perfusion (cerebral, renal, cardiopulmonary) related to decreased cardiac output caused by cardiac tamponade. Based on this nursing diagnosis, you'll establish these patient outcomes. The patient will:
• regain and maintain normal tissue perfusion
• remain alert and oriented to time, person, and place
• maintain normal renal function as exhibited by a urine output of at least 30 ml/hour
• not experience any cardiac arrhythmias.

*Decreased cardiac output related to im-*paired diastolic filling of the heart caused by increased intrapericardial pressure.* Based on this nursing diagnosis, you'll establish these patient outcomes. The patient will:
• exhibit a normal pulse and blood pressure
• maintain adequate cardiac output.

Ineffective breathing pattern related to chest pain caused by cardiac tamponade. Based on this nursing diagnosis, you'll establish these patient outcomes. The patient will:
• demonstrate a respiratory rate that fluctuates no more than 5 breaths/minute from the baseline
• maintain arterial blood gas values within the normal range
• be able to breathe easily.

NURSING INTERVENTIONS

• If the patient isn't in the intensive care unit already, transfer him there immediately.
• Infuse I.V. solutions and inotropic drugs such as dopamine, as ordered, to maintain the patient's blood pressure.
• Administer oxygen therapy as needed.
• Prepare the patient for pericardiocentesis, a thoracotomy, or CVP line insertion, as indicated.
• Provide supportive care as indicated by the patient's condition and the underlying cause of the tamponade.
• Reassure the patient to reduce anxiety.

Monitoring

• Check for signs of increasing tamponade, increasing dyspnea, and arrhythmias.
• After treatment, watch for a decrease in CVP and a concomitant rise in blood pressure, which indicate relief of cardiac compression.
• Monitor the patient's respiratory status for signs of respiratory distress, such as severe tachypnea or changes in level of consciousness.

Patient teaching

• If the patient is not acutely ill, briefly teach him about his condition and explain why it is occurring. Tell him how the condition will be treated, and explain each new procedure before beginning.

• Stress the importance of alerting the nurse if symptoms worsen.

MYOCARDIAL CONTUSION

Blunt chest trauma can result in a myocardial contusion when the force of the impact compresses the heart between the sternum and the spinal column, leading to bruising of the myocardium. This causes capillary hemorrhage, which varies in size from petechiae to hemorrhage of the full thickness of the myocardium. If myocardial function is seriously compromised, myocardial contusion can become life-threatening. It most often affects the right ventricle because of this chamber's location.

CAUSES
Commonly, the blunt chest trauma that causes myocardial contusion results from a motor vehicle accident that forces the chest wall against the steering wheel. It also can occur from a fall or any other direct blow that results in sternal or anterior thoracic compression.

COMPLICATIONS
A myocardial contusion can lead to several life-threatening complications, including cardiac arrhythmias and cardiac tamponade. Also, congestive heart failure (CHF) may result from disruption and separation of myocardial fibers associated with extravasation of blood and fluid.

ASSESSMENT
The patient's history typically reveals a recent accident or event involving blunt anterior chest trauma. The patient may report no history of cardiovascular disease or risk factors for myocardial infarction (MI). He may complain of palpitations, shortness of breath, and angina-like substernal chest pain not associated with movement or respirations.

Inspection of the patient may show ecchymoses over the sternum. Auscultation of the lungs may disclose crackles indicative of developing CHF. You may note a rapid heartbeat or an abnormal heart sound, such as an early pericardial friction rub. Heart auscultation also may reveal S_3 heart sounds. Blood pressure may be decreased. Be aware that myocardial contusion is sometimes overlooked in patients with multiple severe injuries who have no obvious thoracic trauma.

DIAGNOSTIC TESTS
The following findings support a diagnosis of myocardial contusion:
• With cardiac damage, *electrocardiography (ECG)* may show right bundle-branch block, arrhythmias, conduction abnormalities, a pattern of pericarditis, and ST-T wave changes.
• *Serum levels of aspartate aminotransferase (formerly SGOT), alanine aminotransferase (formerly SGPT), lactate dehydrogenase, creatine kinase (CK),* and the cardiac muscle *isoenzyme CK-MB* are elevated.
• *Echocardiography, computed tomography,* and *nuclear heart and lung scans* show the extent of injury.

TREATMENT
Overall, therapy for myocardial contusion is similar to that for MI. The treatment calls for intensive monitoring to detect arrhythmias and prevent cardiogenic shock. If an arrhythmia develops, antiarrhythmic agents may be necessary. A temporary pacemaker may be required for conduction defects. If the patient has severely decreased cardiac output, anticoagulant therapy may be prescribed to prevent embolus formation.

KEY NURSING DIAGNOSES AND PATIENT OUTCOMES
Decreased cardiac output related to ischemic areas of the myocardium. Based on this nursing diagnosis, you'll establish these patient outcomes. The patient will:
• maintain hemodynamic stability, as evidenced by normal pulse and blood pressure measurements
• remain alert and oriented to person, time, and place
• maintain normal renal function, as evidenced by a urine output of at least 30 ml/hour.

Altered cardiopulmonary tissue perfusion related to decreased cardiac output. Based on this nursing diagnosis, you'll establish these patient outcomes. The patient will:
• be free of cardiac arrhythmias and ischemic changes on his ECG
• regain and maintain normal cardiopulmonary tissue perfusion, as evidenced by the presence of palpable peripheral pulses and warm, dry skin.

Ineffective breathing pattern related to chest pain. Based on this nursing diagnosis, you'll establish these patient outcomes. The patient will:
• demonstrate a respiratory rate that fluctuates no more than 5 breaths/minute from the baseline
• maintain arterial blood gas values within the normal ranges
• report ease in breathing.

NURSING INTERVENTIONS

For suspected cardiac damage, care is essentially the same as for a patient with an MI.
• Expect the patient to be admitted to the intensive care unit for observation.
• Impose bed rest in semi-Fowler's position (unless the patient requires the Trendelenburg position).
• As needed, administer analgesics to control pain and supportive drugs, such as digitalis glycosides or other antiarrhythmic agents, as ordered, to control heart failure or arrhythmias. Administer medications P.O. or I.V., not I.M. as this will elevate CK levels.
• Administer supplemental oxygen, as ordered, to ensure adequate oxygenation of tissues.
• Administer I.V. fluids, as ordered, to maintain fluid balance.
• As ordered, assist with central venous line insertion to monitor central venous pressure, which reflects heart function and total circulating volume.
• Assist with insertion of a pulmonary artery catheter to measure pulmonary pressure, if cardiac output is severely reduced with inadequate peripheral perfusion.

Monitoring

• Continuously monitor the patient for changes in his condition, especially his cardiopulmonary function.
• Watch the cardiac monitor for any irregularities.
• Regularly reassess vital signs, mental status, and urine output.
• If hemodynamic monitoring is being performed, evaluate the results frequently to determine the status of cardiac output.
• Watch for complications, such as cardiac tamponade (muffled or distant heart sounds, jugular vein distention, orthopnea, dyspnea, tachypnea, restlessness or decreased mentation, pulsus paradoxus value above 12 mm Hg, hypotension, and lowered pulse pressure) and CHF (dyspnea, orthopnea, cough, cyanosis, restlessness, diaphoresis, pulsus alterans, S_3 or S_4 heart sounds, crackles, and edema).
• Frequently check arterial blood gas levels for hypoxemia. Also watch for signs and symptoms of hypoxemia, such as restlessness, anxiety, headache, confusion, hypotension, tachycardia, use of accessory muscles during respiration, dyspnea, and cyanosis.

Patient teaching

• Reinforce the doctor's explanation of the patient's condition and treatment plan. Make sure he and his family understand the care plan. Explain that treatment for myocardial contusion is similar to that required after an MI.
• Stress the importance of compliance with the prescribed treatment plan to prevent permanent heart damage.
• Advise the patient to alert the nurse or doctor if dyspnea, chest pain, or other symptoms develop or worsen.
• Tell the patient to avoid contact sports when discharged until the pain is resolved and the doctor permits him to resume such activities.

SYMPTOMATIC BRADYCARDIA

This disorder is characterized by a heart rate below 60 beats/minute and by signs and symptoms of decreased cardiac output. Symptomatic bradycardia can become fatal if the heart rate drops low enough to seriously compromise cardiac output or if the disorder induces an ectopic ventricular rhythm, such as ventricular fibrillation.

CAUSES

Symptomatic bradycardia results from increased vagal and decreased sympathetic stimulation that lowers the heart rate enough to cause symptoms of decreased cardiac output. This may occur in conditions such as acute myocardial infarction, sick sinus syndrome (Stokes-Adams syndrome), or hyperkalemia. Symptomatic bradycardia also may develop as an adverse reaction to certain drugs, such as calcium channel blockers, anticholinesterases, beta blockers, digitalis glycosides, and morphine. In susceptible patients, the disorder may be triggered by severe pain, vomiting, or straining during defecation.

COMPLICATIONS

Symptomatic bradycardia may allow an ectopic focus to take over as a pacemaker, leading to potentially serious ventricular arrhythmias, such as ventricular fibrillation. Because of reduced cardiac output, cerebral and coronary blood flow may become inadequate, causing syncope and angina.

ASSESSMENT

The patient's history may reveal a condition known to cause symptomatic bradycardia. The patient may report dizziness, light-headedness, blurred vision, and recent episodes of syncope.

On inspection, you may observe the patient to be pale and diaphoretic. Syncope may be evident. Palpation reveals a peripheral pulse rate lower than 60 beats/minute with a regular or irregular rhythm. Auscultation of the heartbeat also reveals a heart rate below 60 beats/minute and a regular or irregular rhythm. Auscultation of blood pressure may reveal hypotension.

DIAGNOSTIC TESTS

Symptomatic bradycardia is diagnosed by a heartbeat below 60 beats/minute coupled with signs and symptoms of decreased cardiac output. The electrocardiogram (ECG) supports a heart rate below 60 beats/minute. (See *ECG characteristics of symptomatic bradycardia.*)

TREATMENTS

For short-term management of symptomatic bradycardia, atropine is given rapidly by I.V. push. If atropine proves ineffective, isoproterenol may be given. (See *Identifying drug dosages in symptomatic bradycardia,* page 120.) If drug therapy fails, or if its effect is short-lived, temporary transvenous endocardial or transcutaneous pacing may be required to maintain a normal heart rate. For long-term management, permanent pacing is often indicated.

Drugs with known bradycardic effects, such as digitalis glycosides, reserpine, morphine, calcium channel blockers, or beta blockers, should be avoided or discontinued in the presence of symptomatic sinus bradycardia.

KEY NURSING DIAGNOSES AND PATIENT OUTCOMES

Anxiety related to the potential seriousness of symptomatic bradycardia. Based on this nursing diagnosis, you'll establish these patient outcomes. The patient will:
• express reasons for his anxiety
• express an understanding of symptomatic bradycardia and when to seek medical attention
• cope with having symptomatic bradycardia without demonstrating severe signs of anxiety.

Decreased cardiac output related to heart rate below 60 beats/minute. Based on this nursing diagnosis, you'll establish these patient outcomes. The patient will:
• regain and maintain hemodynamic stability, as evidenced by normal vital signs, urine output, and neurologic function

ECG characteristics of symptomatic bradycardia

In uncomplicated symptomatic bradycardia, the electrocardiogram (ECG) shows the distinguishing features given below.

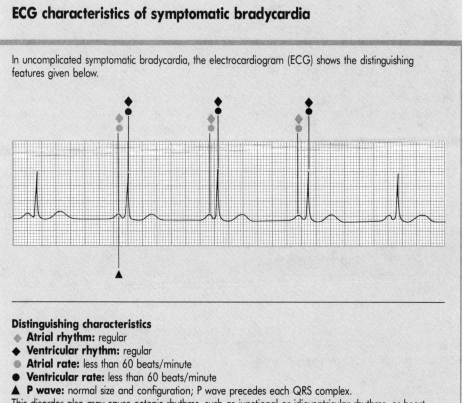

Distinguishing characteristics
- ◆ **Atrial rhythm:** regular
- ◆ **Ventricular rhythm:** regular
- ● **Atrial rate:** less than 60 beats/minute
- ● **Ventricular rate:** less than 60 beats/minute
- ▲ **P wave:** normal size and configuration; P wave precedes each QRS complex.

This disorder also may cause ectopic rhythms, such as junctional or idioventricular rhythms, or heart block.

- exhibit no other arrhythmias on his ECG or show ischemic changes
- report that symptoms of decreased cardiac output have disappeared.

NURSING INTERVENTIONS
- Notify the doctor immediately and obtain an ECG tracing to verify symptomatic bradycardia.
- Start an I.V. infusion for administration of emergency drug therapy.
- Have atropine available at the bedside and administer it as prescribed.
- Administer oxygen as needed, unless contraindicated.
- Prepare for temporary pacing or an isoproterenol infusion if atropine is not effective.

- When the patient's heart rate is stabilized, provide him with an opportunity to verbalize his feelings of anxiety and offer reassurance.

Monitoring
- Frequently check the patient's vital signs, mental status, and urine output for signs of improvement or deterioration.
- Monitor the patient's ECG for evidence of ectopic rhythms and rate.
- After atropine administration, observe the patient's condition for desired response and tachycardia.
- Check serum digoxin level and potassium concentration, as ordered.

Identifying drug dosages in symptomatic bradycardia

The drugs listed below may be used to treat symptomatic bradycardia.

Atropine
To treat symptomatic bradycardia during advanced cardiac life support, give an adult 0.5 mg I.V. or 1 to 2 mg endotracheally every 5 minutes until the heart rate increases to the desired rate (usually 80 beats/minute). Don't exceed a total dose of 2 mg.

Isoproterenol
For immediate temporary control of atropine-resistant, hemodynamically significant bradycardia, give an adult a continuous infusion of 2 to 10 mcg/minute titrated to patient response.

Patient teaching
• Teach the patient how to take his own pulse, what pulse rate needs to be reported to the doctor, and which symptoms to report, such as light-headedness and dizziness.
• Explain the need for temporary transvenous endocardial or transcutaneous pacing, if needed. Be sure to describe the procedure and aftercare.
• As needed, outline the need for permanent pacing. Teach the patient about the procedure, the need for bed rest for the first 24 hours following the procedure, precautions to follow after insertion, and the need for follow-up visits to the doctor.

SINOATRIAL ARREST

In sinoatrial arrest, the sinoatrial (SA) node fails to initiate an impulse at the expected time in the cardiac cycle. In the absence of an impulse, neither the atria nor the ventricles are stimulated and the entire PQRST complex drops for one or more beats on the electrocardiogram (ECG). In sinoatrial block (also called sinus exit block), the impulse is initiated nor-

mally but is blocked within the SA node and fails to reach the atria. Again, the entire PQRST complex is absent on the ECG. Because of its negative effect on cardiac output, sinoatrial arrest or block is potentially life threatening if it occurs frequently.

CAUSES
Sinoatrial arrest or block may result from any of the following: acute infection; coronary artery disease, degenerative heart disease, or acute inferior or posterior-lateral wall myocardial infarction; vagal stimulation, Valsalva's maneuver, or carotid sinus massage; digitalis, quinidine, or salicylate toxicity; pesticide poisoning; pharyngeal irritation caused by endotracheal intubation; sick sinus syndrome; or hypothermia.

COMPLICATIONS
If sinoatrial arrest occurs infrequently, it usually represents vagal overactivity. However, repeated episodes of SA arrest or very prolonged pauses can cause hypotension and syncope.

ASSESSMENT
The patient's history may reveal a disorder that can cause sinoatrial arrest. He may report feeling a prolonged pause in his heartbeat, which may be followed by a feeling of light-headedness, blurred vision, or syncope.

Palpation of the patient's pulse or auscultation of the heartbeat reveals an irregular rhythm. If the patient's heart rate becomes too slow, his blood pressure will fall.

DIAGNOSTIC TESTS
The diagnosis is based on typical ECG findings during episodes of sinoatrial arrest. (For more information, see *ECG characteristics of sinoatrial arrest.*)

TREATMENT
If sinoatrial arrest occurs infrequently, the condition is usually self-limiting and requires no treatment. For a symptomatic patient, treatment focuses on maintaining cardiac output and discovering the cause of the sinus arrest. Atropine (0.5 to 1 mg I.V.) is used to re-

ECG characteristics of sinoatrial arrest

In a patient with sinoatrial arrest, the electrocardiogram (ECG) characteristics shown below are typical.

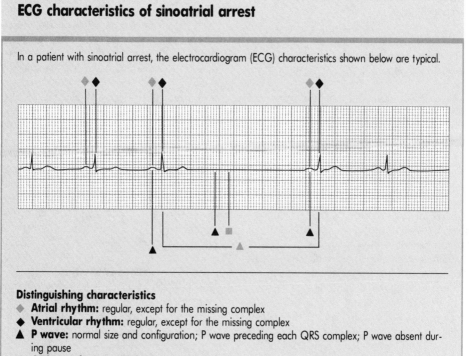

Distinguishing characteristics
♦ **Atrial rhythm:** regular, except for the missing complex
♦ **Ventricular rhythm:** regular, except for the missing complex
▲ **P wave:** normal size and configuration; P wave preceding each QRS complex; P wave absent during pause
■ **QRS complex:** normal duration and configuration; QRS complex missing during pause
▲ **Other:** pause doesn't equal a multiple of previous sinus rhythm.

store normal impulse formation or conduction at the SA node by inhibiting vagal effect on the SA node. Repeated episodes of sinus arrest may require a temporary or permanent pacemaker.

KEY NURSING DIAGNOSES AND PATIENT OUTCOMES

Anxiety related to potential seriousness of sinoatrial arrest. Based on this nursing diagnosis, you'll establish these patient outcomes. The patient will:
• express reasons for his anxiety
• express an understanding of sinoatrial arrest and when to seek medical attention
• cope with having sinoatrial arrest without demonstrating severe signs of anxiety.

Decreased cardiac output related to absence of myocardial contraction. Based on this

nursing diagnosis, you'll establish these patient outcomes. The patient will:
• maintain hemodynamic stability, as evidenced by normal vital signs, urine output, and neurologic function
• exhibit no other arrhythmias on his ECG and show no ischemic changes
• report no episodes of light-headedness, blurred vision, or syncope.

NURSING INTERVENTIONS

• Prepare to administer atropine I.V. as ordered if the patient experiences symptoms of decreased cardiac output (light-headedness, hypotension, syncope) during sinoatrial arrest.
• If the patient is receiving digitalis glycosides or quinidine, notify the doctor that the patient is experiencing episodes of sinoatrial arrest before administering these medications.

• Prepare for possible temporary transvenous endocardial or transcutaneous pacemaker insertion.

Monitoring

• Evaluate the patient's ECG and document sinoatrial arrest on an ECG strip when it occurs.
• Assess the frequency of sinoatrial arrest and evaluate the patient for potential causes.
• Monitor the patient for signs and symptoms of decreased cardiac output (light-headedness, hypotension, syncope) during each episode of sinoatrial arrest.

Patient teaching

• Show the patient how to take his own pulse rate, and advise him to notify his doctor if pauses are felt.
• Encourage the patient to remain on the medication dosage as prescribed and not to deviate from it without consulting the doctor.
• Review the signs and symptoms of decreased cardiac output and tell the patient what to do if any should occur.
• Explain the reason for a temporary transvenous endocardial or transcutaneous pacemaker, if needed. Describe the procedure and review any activity restrictions.
• Teach the patient about the reason for insertion of a permanent pacemaker, if needed. Describe the procedure, activity limitations (bed rest for the first 24 hours after insertion), precautions after insertion, and the need for follow-up doctor visits.

THIRD-DEGREE ATRIOVENTRICULAR BLOCK

In this potentially fatal arrhythmia, a total absence of atrioventricular (AV) conduction occurs. Also known as complete AV dissociation, this disorder is usually characterized by a slow, regular heartbeat (below 40 beats/minute) that shows no relationship between the atrial (P waves) and the ventricular (QRS complex) rhythms in the patient's electrocardiogram (ECG).

CAUSES

A temporary episode of third-degree AV block may result from severe digitalis toxicity or an inferior or anterior wall myocardial infarction. It may also occur transiently during cardiac catheterization, angioplasty, or atherectomy.

Chronic third-degree AV block most often results from widespread changes in the His-Purkinje system, leading to bilateral bundle-branch heart block. Other causes include a congenital abnormality, rheumatic fever, hypoxia, postsurgical complications of mitral valve replacement, Lev's disease (fibrosis and calcification that spreads from cardiac structures, such as the valves and septum, to the conductive tissue), and Lenegre's disease (conductive tissue fibrosis).

COMPLICATIONS

Third-degree AV block can lead to syncope, seizures, worsening angina pectoris, shock, left ventricular failure, and ventricular arrhythmias.

ASSESSMENT

The patient's history may disclose a disorder that may cause third-degree AV block. The patient may report a slow, regular pulse or a slow but irregular pulse if ventricular arrhythmias are occurring. He also may complain of generalized weakness, fatigue, chest pain, and dizziness. If the block is from a congenital abnormality or digitalis toxicity, he may be asymptomatic.

On inspection, you may note pale skin. If cerebral circulation is severely compromised, syncope may occur. Palpation of peripheral pulses may reveal a slow, regular pulse or a slow, irregular pulse. You also may detect cold, clammy extremities and reduced muscle strength. Auscultation of the heart may reveal a slow, regular heartbeat or an irregular heartbeat. Crackles and rhonchi may be present in the lung if heart failure is present. The patient's blood pressure may be low because of decreased cardiac output.

ECG characteristics of third-degree atrioventricular block

This arrhythmia, in which all atrioventricular impulses are prevented from reaching the ventricles, typically causes the electrocardiogram (ECG) changes shown below.

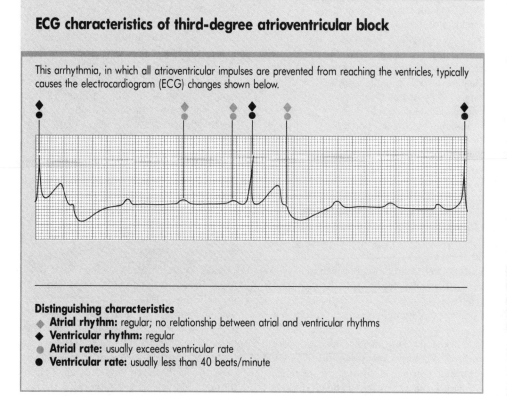

Distinguishing characteristics
- ◆ **Atrial rhythm:** regular; no relationship between atrial and ventricular rhythms
- ◆ **Ventricular rhythm:** regular
- ● **Atrial rate:** usually exceeds ventricular rate
- ● **Ventricular rate:** usually less than 40 beats/minute

DIAGNOSTIC TESTS

Third-degree AV block is diagnosed by ECG. (See *ECG characteristics of third-degree atrioventricular block.*)

TREATMENT

A patient who has third-degree AV block but adequate cardiac output may not require treatment. If, on the other hand, the patient has symptomatic bradycardia, the doctor will prescribe atropine or isoproterenol initially.

◆ NURSING ALERT. If the patient has suffered an acute MI, give isoproterenol cautiously and only as an emergency measure. That's because isoproterenol increases the heart rate and heightens myocardial oxygen demands, which could worsen myocardial ischemia. A temporary or permanent pacemaker may be required if decreased cardiac output continues.

KEY NURSING DIAGNOSES AND PATIENT OUTCOMES

Altered cerebral tissue perfusion related to decreased cardiac output. Based on this nursing diagnosis, you'll establish these patient outcomes. The patient will:
- maintain or exhibit improved mental function
- take appropriate action if dizziness or presyncope occurs
- remain safe and protected in his environment.

Decreased cardiac output related to bradycardia characteristic of third-degree AV block. Based on this nursing diagnosis, you'll establish these patient outcomes. The patient will:
- maintain hemodynamic stability, as evidenced by normal vital signs, urine output, and neurologic function

• exhibit no other arrhythmias on his ECG or show ischemic changes
• report no episodes of light-headedness, syncope, or chest pain.

Impaired gas exchange related to decreased cardiac output. Based on this nursing diagnosis, you'll establish these patient outcomes. The patient will:
• maintain adequate ventilation
• communicate an understanding to conserve energy and limit activities until cardiac output increases
• maintain normal arterial blood gas (ABG) values.

NURSING INTERVENTIONS

• Notify the doctor immediately when third-degree AV block occurs and place the patient on bed rest.
• Administer isoproterenol or atropine as ordered. Document the drug's effectiveness, if given.
• Prepare to administer transcutaneous pacing or assist the doctor with the insertion of a temporary transvenous endocardial pacemaker, if required.
• Document the patient's tolerance to the temporary pacemaker if inserted and its effectiveness on the heart block.
• Maintain the patient in a safe and protected environment if neurologic deficits occur.

Monitoring

• Continuously monitor the patient's clinical tolerance to third-degree AV block. (Remember that a ventricular response of more than 40 beats/minute may be adequate for systemic perfusion of the patient on bed rest.)
• Evaluate the patient for signs and symptoms associated with a slow heart rate and decreased cardiac output, including fatigue, light-headedness, mental confusion, Stokes-Adams attacks, or congestive heart failure.
• Frequently assess the patient's vital signs, neurologic status, and urine output for evidence of decreased cardiac output and shock.
• Observe the patient's ECG for ventricular arrhythmias or ischemic changes.
• Check the patient's ABG values for abnormalities.

• Assess patient discomfort during temporary pacing therapy.

Patient teaching

• If the patient is not acutely ill, teach him about third-degree AV block and how it is treated.
• If appropriate, explain to the patient why temporary pacing is being initiated. Review what happens during the procedure and the activity limitations while it's in place. Reinforce that it's a temporary measure.
• If a permanent pacemaker is required, teach the patient about the procedure, postoperative activity limitations, and the importance of follow-up doctor visits.

PREMATURE VENTRICULAR CONTRACTIONS

Also known as ventricular extrasystolic beats, premature ventricular contractions (PVCs) are among the most common arrhythmias. PVCs are ventricular contractions that occur earlier in the cardiac cycle than expected because an irritable focus within the ventricle fires before the arrival of the next anticipated impulse from the sinoatrial node. In many cases, a compensatory pause follows a PVC. On an electrocardiogram (ECG) strip, all PVCs may not look alike.

PVCs may potentially become life-threatening because they can alter cardiac output if frequent or induce more serious arrhythmias, such as ventricular tachycardia or fibrillation. Although PVCs can occur in both healthy and diseased hearts, they develop more frequently in patients with structural heart disease.

PVCs may occur singly, in pairs (couplets), or in threes (commonly referred to as a short run of ventricular tachycardia). They may also occur in various patterns, such as every other beat (bigeminal), every third beat (trigeminal), or every fourth beat (quadrigeminal).

CAUSES

PVCs may result from heart failure; old or acute myocardial ischemia, infarction, or contusion; myocardial irritation by a ventric-

ECG characteristics of PVCs

In a patient with premature ventricular contractions (PVCs), the electrocardiogram (ECG) typically exhibits the characteristics shown below.

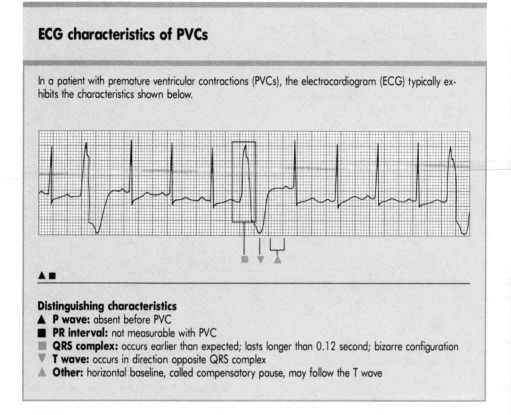

Distinguishing characteristics
▲ **P wave:** absent before PVC
■ **PR interval:** not measurable with PVC
▨ **QRS complex:** occurs earlier than expected; lasts longer than 0.12 second; bizarre configuration
▽ **T wave:** occurs in direction opposite QRS complex
△ **Other:** horizontal baseline, called compensatory pause, may follow the T wave

ular catheter, such as a pacemaker or pulmonary artery catheter; toxicity from drugs such as digitalis glycosides or theophylline; hypoxia; hypokalemia; or hypocalcemia. Other causes include mitral valve disease; caffeine, alcohol, or tobacco use; or sympathomimetic drugs that are given as sprays, inhalers, or nose drops. Because many antiarrhythmic drugs are proarrhythmic, they also can aggravate or increase the frequency of PVCs.

COMPLICATIONS
PVCs may lead to decreased cardiac output and the onset of potentially fatal arrhythmias, such as ventricular tachycardia or ventricular fibrillation. PVCs are more likely to cause these life-threatening arrhythmias if they occur in certain patterns. The patient is also at increased risk for sudden death when PVCs occur in conjunction with angina.

ASSESSMENT
The patient's history may disclose a disorder that can cause PVCs. He may report palpitations. If cardiac output decreases significantly, he also may complain of light-headedness, blurred vision, or episodes of syncope.

Palpation of peripheral pulses and cardiac auscultation reveals an irregular heartbeat. Blood pressure may be low because of decreased cardiac output.

DIAGNOSTIC TESTS
An ECG is the definitive test for PVCs. (See *ECG characteristics of PVCs.*)

TREATMENT
If the patient is asymptomatic, isn't known to have heart disease, and doesn't have frequent PVCs, treatment usually isn't required. If the patient is symptomatic, treatment typically

When PVCs signal danger

When you detect premature ventricular contractions (PVCs), you must determine whether they appear in a pattern that indicates danger. If they do, your patient will need immediate treatment. Here are some examples of dangerous PVC patterns.

Paired PVCs
Two PVCs in a row are called a pair or couplet (see highlighted area). A pair can produce ventricular tachycardia because the second PVC usually meets refractory tissue. Three or more PVCs in a row are considered a run of ventricular tachycardia.

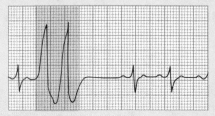

Bigeminy
PVCs that occur every other beat (bigeminy) or every third beat (trigeminy) can result in ventricular tachycardia or fibrillation (see highlighted areas).

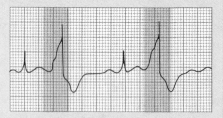

R-on-T phenomenon
In this phenomenon, the PVC occurs so early that it falls on the T wave of the preceding beat (see highlighted area). Because the cells haven't fully repolarized, ventricular tachycardia or fibrillation can result.

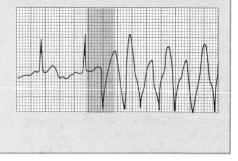

Multiform PVCs
PVCs that look different from one another arise from different ventricular sites or from the same site with abnormal conduction (see highlighted areas). They may indicate severe heart disease or digitalis toxicity.

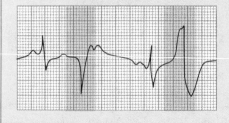

involves administration of antiarrhythmic drugs and appropriate treatment of the underlying cause.

PVCs may be frequent or dangerous. (See *When PVCs signal danger.*) For such PVCs, the most common drug therapy used to abolish them is a lidocaine bolus followed by a continuous lidocaine infusion. Other drugs, such as procainamide or bretylium, may be used if the PVCs don't respond to lidocaine. (See *Identi-*

fying drug dosages in PVCs.) After the patient's condition has stabilized or the danger has subsided, oral antiarrhythmic therapy is usually initiated.

When a patient's PVCs are thought to result from a noncardiac problem, treatment aims to correct the underlying cause. This could mean, for example, treating acid-base or electrolyte disturbances, discontinuing a particular drug, or performing surgery to repair an aneurysm or valvular defect. If the patient has a pacemaker, repositioning the electrode may correct the problem. If he has a displaced pulmonary artery catheter in the right ventricle, catheter repositioning may eliminate PVCs.

KEY NURSING DIAGNOSES AND PATIENT OUTCOMES

Anxiety related to potential seriousness of PVCs. Based on this nursing diagnosis, you'll establish these patient outcomes. The patient will:
• express reasons for his anxiety
• express an understanding of need to comply with antiarrhythmic drug therapy to prevent recurrence
• cope with having PVCs without demonstrating severe signs of anxiety.

Altered tissue perfusion (cardiopulmonary, cerebral, renal) related to decreased cardiac output. Based on this nursing diagnosis, you'll establish these patient outcomes. The patient will:
• maintain normal cardiopulmonary, cerebral, and renal function
• remain free of chest pain and other arrhythmias
• maintain a urine output of at least 30 ml/hour
• remain alert and oriented to time, person, and place.

Decreased cardiac output related to inadequate ventricular filling time during PVCs. Based on this nursing diagnosis, you'll establish these patient outcomes. The patient will:
• maintain or regain hemodynamic stability, as evidenced by normal vital signs, urine output, and neurologic function
• exhibit no signs and symptoms of decreased cardiac output.

NURSING INTERVENTIONS

• Notify the doctor if an irregular heartbeat is detected and the patient exhibits signs and symptoms of decreased cardiac output.
• Have an ECG done to confirm the diagnosis, and prepare the patient for transfer to the intensive care unit.

DOSAGE FINDER

Identifying drug dosages in PVCs

The drugs listed below may be used to treat premature ventricular contractions (PVCs).

Lidocaine
To treat acute ventricular arrhythmias associated with acute myocardial infarction, digitalis toxicity, cardioversion, cardiac manipulation from trauma or surgery, or adverse effects of drugs, give an adult 50 to 100 mg in an I.V. bolus or endotracheally. If the arrhythmias don't stop within 5 minutes, repeat the dose. Start a maintenance infusion of 20 to 50 mcg/kg/minute (1 to 4 mg/minute for a 155-lb [70-kg] adult). Don't administer more than 300 mg in 1 hour. In a patient with congestive heart failure or liver disease, don't exceed 30 mcg/kg/minute.

If you can't use the I.V. or endotracheal route, administer 300 mg (for a 155-lb adult) by I.M. injection initially. If necessary, repeat the dose in 60 to 90 minutes.

Procainamide
To treat arrhythmias, including paroxysmal atrial tachycardia, PVCs, ventricular tachycardia, and atrial fibrillation, give an adult an initial dose of 100 mg slowly by I.V. injection or infusion. (Don't exceed 50 mg/minute.) Repeat the dose as needed to control arrhythmias. The maximum dosage is 1 g by direct injection or 500 to 600 mg by infusion over 25 to 30 minutes at 2 to 6 mg/minute. To keep arrhythmias under control, administer a titrated maintenance dose of 1 to 6 mg/minute, or administer 500 mg to 1 g I.M. every 4 to 6 hours.

Bretylium
To treat ventricular tachycardia and other ventricular arrhythmias, give an adult an infusion of 5 to 10 mg/kg over 10 to 30 minutes. If needed, repeat the infusion after 1 or 2 hours. Give a maintenance dose of 5 to 10 mg/kg infused over 10 to 30 minutes every 6 hours or a continuous infusion of 1 to 2 mg/minute. As an alternative, give 5 to 10 mg/kg of undiluted drug I.M. Repeat the dose after 1 to 2 hours if necessary, and give the same dose every 6 to 8 hours.

• Start an I.V. infusion in anticipation of parenteral antiarrhythmic drug therapy, if indicated.
• Administer antiarrhythmic agents, as prescribed.
• Initiate oxygen therapy, as prescribed.
• Provide the patient with an opportunity to verbalize his anxieties and concerns about having PVCs and offer reassurance.

Monitoring

• Carefully assess the patient's cardiac, electrolyte, and overall clinical status to determine the PVCs' effect on cardiac output and whether they're life-threatening.
• Monitor the patient's ECG. Document the frequency of the PVCs, their number per minute, and their pattern of occurrence, such as multiform, bigeminy, or couplets.
• Assess the patient's emotional status for evidence of negative stress, such as anxiety and fear.
• Evaluate the patient's response to antiarrhythmic therapy.

Patient teaching

• Explain to the patient and his family what PVCs are and how they are treated.
• Teach the patient about the prescribed antiarrhythmics, such as their dosage and possible adverse effects and toxic reactions.
• Stress the importance of medication compliance.
• Advise the patient to stop smoking and to limit caffeine and alcohol intake.
• Explain the importance of follow-up care.

VENTRICULAR TACHYCARDIA

A serious arrhythmia that requires immediate treatment, ventricular tachycardia is a series of three or more consecutive premature ventricular contractions (PVCs) occurring at a rapid rate (more than 100 beats/minute). While it may be an isolated event, ventricular tachycardia is more likely to be a chronic problem.

CAUSES

Ventricular tachycardia usually results from electrical disturbances related to previous myocardial injury or disease. For most patients, ventricular tachycardia is a major complication of myocardial infarction and chronic ischemic heart disease. Other cardiovascular causes include ventricular aneurysm, coronary artery disease, rheumatic heart disease, mitral valve prolapse, heart failure, myocarditis, and cardiomyopathy. Additional causes are proarrhythmic effects of antiarrhythmic drugs; toxicity from certain drugs, such as digitalis glycosides, procainamide, quinidine, and epinephrine; metabolic disorders, such as hypokalemia and hypomagnesemia; anxiety; pulmonary embolism; and ventricular catheters.

In addition, ventricular tachycardia may result from a PVC occurring before the cells have fully repolarized – the R-on-T phenomenon. It is also associated with prolonged QT-interval syndrome caused by delayed ventricular repolarization.

Occasionally, ventricular tachycardia is found in normal hearts, extending over all age-groups – a condition that appears to be adrenergically facilitated. Ventricular tachycardia is rare in children unless they've had intracardiac surgery, a metabolic imbalance, drug toxicity, cardiomyopathy, or familial prolonged QT syndrome.

COMPLICATIONS

Ventricular tachycardia can lead to cardiovascular collapse, ventricular fibrillation, and sudden cardiac death.

ASSESSMENT

The patient's history may disclose a disorder that can cause ventricular tachycardia. If the patient can compensate for the decreased cardiac output stemming from ventricular tachycardia, he may have only mild signs and symptoms – or none at all.

Typically, however, inspection reveals that the patient with ventricular tachycardia becomes rapidly unresponsive. Palpation may reveal cold, clammy skin, and peripheral

ECG characteristics of ventricular tachycardia

In the patient with ventricular tachycardia, the electrocardiogram (ECG) typically exhibits the distinguishing features shown below.

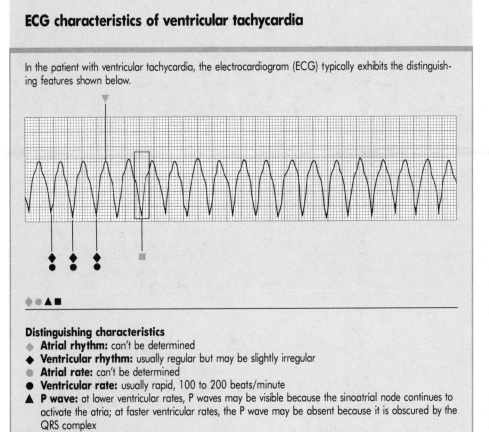

Distinguishing characteristics
- **Atrial rhythm:** can't be determined
- **Ventricular rhythm:** usually regular but may be slightly irregular
- **Atrial rate:** can't be determined
- **Ventricular rate:** usually rapid, 100 to 200 beats/minute
- **P wave:** at lower ventricular rates, P waves may be visible because the sinoatrial node continues to activate the atria; at faster ventricular rates, the P wave may be absent because it is obscured by the QRS complex
- **PR interval:** not measurable
- **QRS complex:** lasts longer than 0.12 second; bizarre appearance, usually with increased amplitude
- **T wave:** occurs in opposite direction of QRS complex

pulses may be absent because of a sudden decrease in peripheral perfusion. Auscultation of the heartbeat reveals the rate to be higher than 100 beats/minutes, if countable. Blood pressure drops as cardiac output decreases.

DIAGNOSTIC TESTS
Ventricular tachycardia is diagnosed by electrocardiography (ECG). (See *ECG characteristics of ventricular tachycardia*.) Two other forms of ventricular tachycardia, torsades de pointes and ventricular flutter, may also occur and are also diagnosed by ECG. (See *Recognizing other forms of ventricular tachycardia*, pages 130 and 131.)

Holter ECG monitoring, exercise stress testing, radionuclide ventriculography, and electrophysiologic testing may be used to assess the patient suspected of having ventricular tachycardia.

TREATMENT
Immediate treatment includes cardiopulmonary resuscitation (CPR) and other life-support measures. (See *Treating ventricular tachycardia: A step-by-step guide*, page 132.)

Recognizing other forms of ventricular tachycardia

Ventricular tachycardia can take two other forms — torsades de pointes and ventricular flutter.

Torsades de pointes
With this arrhythmia, the ventricular rate ranges from 150 to 250 beats/minute, and the QRS complexes are wide. Usually, they deflect downward for several beats and then upward for several beats. This arrhythmia may stop and start suddenly. Sometimes the sinus rhythm resumes spontaneously, but in other cases torsades de pointes degenerates into ventricular fibrillation.

Any condition that can cause a prolonged QT interval can cause torsades de pointes. These conditions include congenital prolonged QT syndrome (Romano-Ward syndrome), myocardial ischemia, sinoatrial disease that results in profound bradycardia, the vagal response, subarachnoid hemorrhage, atrioventricular block,

and Prinzmetal's angina. The arrhythmia may also result from electrolyte imbalance (hypokalemia, hypocalcemia, or hypomagnesemia), drug toxicity (particularly from quinidine, procainamide, disopyramide, or amiodarone), and an overdose of certain psychotropic drugs (such as phenothiazines and tricyclic antidepressants).

Although the patient with torsades de pointes will have signs and symptoms similar to those of ventricular tachycardia, the treatment is different. Quinidine, lidocaine, and tocainide aren't effective and may even worsen the arrhythmia. Isoproterenol is the drug of choice. Bretylium, propranolol, or phenytoin may also be used. Or the doctor may order mechanical overdrive pacing and treat the arrhythmia's cause.

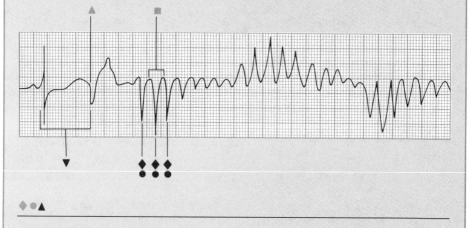

Distinguishing characteristics
- ♦ **Atrial rhythm:** can't be determined
- ♦ **Ventricular rhythm:** regular or irregular
- ● **Atrial rate:** can't be determined
- ● **Ventricular rate:** 150 to 250 beats/minute
- ▲ **P wave:** hidden in QRS complex; can't be identified
- ■ **QRS complex:** usually wide with phasic variation, complexes deflecting downward for several beats and then upward for several beats
- ■ **QT interval:** prolonged preceding arrhythmia
- ▲ **Other:** arrhythmia may start and stop suddenly

Recognizing other forms of ventricular tachycardia *(continued)*

Ventricular flutter

This arrhythmia is characterized by a ventricular rate that ranges between 150 and 300 beats/minute. Usually, the QRS complex is wide and continuous with a zigzag, helical pattern. The significance, signs and symptoms, and treatment for this arrhythmia are the same as for ventricular tachycardia. But ventricular flutter deteriorates quickly into ventricular fibrillation.

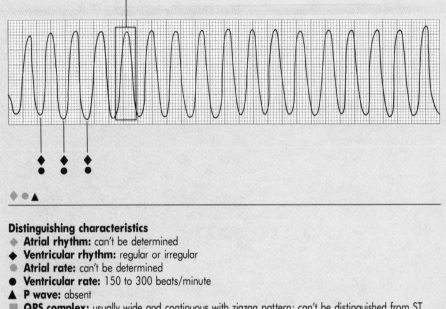

Distinguishing characteristics
- ♦ **Atrial rhythm:** can't be determined
- ◆ **Ventricular rhythm:** regular or irregular
- ● **Atrial rate:** can't be determined
- ● **Ventricular rate:** 150 to 300 beats/minute
- ▲ **P wave:** absent
- ■ **QRS complex:** usually wide and continuous with zigzag pattern; can't be distinguished from ST segment and T wave

KEY NURSING DIAGNOSES AND PATIENT OUTCOMES

Altered tissue perfusion (cardiopulmonary, cerebral, renal) related to decreased cardiac output. Based on this nursing diagnosis, you'll establish these patient outcomes. The patient will:
• maintain normal cardiopulmonary, cerebral, and renal function
• remain free of chest pain and other arrhythmias
• show no evidence of irreversible damage, such as altered mental status or renal failure.

Decreased cardiac output related to inadequate ventricular filling time caused by rapid ventricular rate. Based on this nursing diagnosis, you'll establish these patient outcomes. The patient will:
• maintain or regain hemodynamic stability, as evidenced by normal vital signs, urine output, and neurologic function
• attain normal cardiac output with cessation of ventricular tachycardia.

Impaired gas exchange related to decreased cardiac output caused by ventricular tachycardia. Based on this nursing diagnosis,

Treating ventricular tachycardia: A step-by-step guide

The advanced cardiac life support (ACLS) guidelines recommend a series of steps for treating sustained ventricular tachycardia (VT). They're not intended as a strict set of rules. Certain patients with sustained VT will require interventions not covered in these steps.

The flowchart below shows the steps recommended in the ACLS guidelines. Keep in mind that you'd continue following them only if VT persists.

You have two possible paths to follow if you detect a pulse: one for a stable patient, the other for an unstable one. Consider the patient unstable if he develops chest pain, dyspnea, hypotension, congestive heart failure, ischemia, or myocardial infarction. If he doesn't have hypotension or pulmonary edema and isn't unconscious, you can use a precordial thump before cardioversion.

If the patient is hypotensive or unconscious or has pulmonary edema, and cardioversion alone doesn't work, give lidocaine and then bretylium. For other patients, give lidocaine and then procainamide, followed by bretylium.

When VT resolves, infuse the antiarrhythmic drug that helped resolve the arrhythmia.

No pulse	**Pulse present**	
Treat as ventricular fibrillation.	**Stable patient**	**Unstable patient**
	Administer oxygen. Establish I.V. access.	Administer oxygen. Consider sedating patient. Establish I.V. access.
	Give lidocaine, 1 to 1.5 mg/kg.	Cardiovert with 100 joules.
	Give lidocaine 0.5 to 0.75 mg/kg every 5 to 10 minutes until VT resolves, or up to 3 mg/kg.	Cardiovert with 200 joules.
	Give procainamide 20 to 30 mg/ minute until VT resolves, or up to 17 mg/kg.	Cardiovert with 300 to 360 joules.
	Give bretylium 5 to 10 mg/kg over 8 to 10 minutes; maximum of 30 mg/kg over 24 hours.	If VT recurs, give lidocaine and cardiovert again starting at the energy level previously successful; then give procainamide or bretylium.
	Cardiovert if patient becomes unstable.	

you'll establish these patient outcomes. The patient will:
• regain and maintain adequate ventilation
• exhibit normal arterial blood gas values.

NURSING INTERVENTIONS
• Notify the doctor immediately.
• Initiate CPR.
• Expect to follow the advanced cardiac life

support guidelines for treating ventricular tachycardia.
• Prepare to assist the doctor with the insertion of a temporary transvenous endocardial pacemaker for overdrive pacing and suppression of tachycardia, if needed. Document the procedure, the patient's tolerance of the procedure, and the effect of the pacemaker on the arrhythmia.

Monitoring
• Continuously monitor the patient's ECG, noting the rate, duration, and morphology of the tachycardia as well as the beats that triggered it.
• Evaluate the patient's response to ventricular tachycardia and its treatment.
• Watch the patient for adverse treatment effects, such as drug reactions.

Patient teaching
• For the conscious patient, explain the arrhythmia and why intervention is necessary. Review the same information with the unconscious patient when he becomes alert.
• Teach the conscious patient the purpose and procedure of cardioversion, the need for sedation, and what he may feel.
• If a temporary pacemaker is needed, review the need for this procedure. Explain the procedure and activity limitations while the device is in place. Reinforce that this is a temporary measure.
• For a patient with chronic ventricular tachycardia, explain the prescribed antiarrhythmic drugs and stress the importance of compliance.
• Before discharge, review with the patient and family reportable symptoms, exercise restrictions, driving restrictions (if any), and follow-up clinic appointments. Also arrange for the family to learn CPR and the use of a defibrillator at home, if indicated.
• Advise the patient to obtain a medical identification bracelet if chronic ventricular tachycardia is present.

VENTRICULAR FIBRILLATION

Always an emergency, ventricular fibrillation is the most frequently recorded rhythm in survivors of sudden cardiac arrest. Most often, it begins as an episode of rapid, unrecorded ventricular tachycardia. Ventricular fibrillation occurs when individual muscle fibers depolarize rapidly in a disorganized fashion, resulting in multiple sites of reentrant activity. The result is inefficient and chaotic mechanical activity. Because the ventricle is unable to contract forcefully and synchronously, cardiac output falls to zero. (See *ECG characteristics of ventricular fibrillation*, page 134.)

Ventricular fibrillation is classified as primary or secondary. Primary ventricular fibrillation begins suddenly in patients without profound hypotension or cardiac failure. Secondary ventricular fibrillation occurs as a terminal rhythm in patients with circulatory failure. Primary ventricular fibrillation is much easier to correct with electrical intervention. (See *Treating ventricular fibrillation: A step-by-step guide*, page 135.)

CAUSES
Ventricular fibrillation usually results from myocardial ischemia or infarction. Other cardiac causes include untreated ventricular tachycardia, the R-on-T phenomenon, and a prolonged QT interval. Noncardiac causes of ventricular fibrillation include electrolyte imbalances (hypokalemia and hyperkalemia, hypocalcemia and hypercalcemia, hypomagnesemia), acid-base imbalances, hypothermia, electrocution, and anaphylaxis. Drugs that may cause the ventricle to fibrillate include cocaine, digitalis glycosides, antiarrhythmic drugs (typically class Ia medications, such as disopyramide, quinidine, or procainamide), phenothiazines, and tricyclic antidepressants.

Ventricular fibrillation can be initiated by reentry or rapid impulse formation. Fibrillation requires an initiating stimulus, myocardium involvement, and electrical instability. This electrical force arises within the ventri-

ECG characteristics of ventricular fibrillation

As shown in the electrocardiogram (ECG) strips below, ventricular fibrillation produces a waveform that is a wavy line. The characteristics shown below are typical.

Coarse

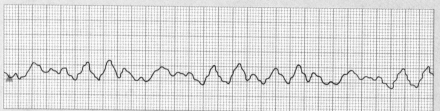

Fine

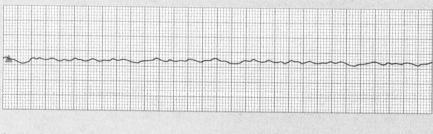

◆ ◆● ●▲■

Distinguishing characteristics
◆ **Atrial rhythm:** can't be determined
◆ **Ventricular rhythm:** no pattern or regularity
● **Atrial rate:** can't be determined
● **Ventricular rate:** can't be determined
▲ **P wave:** indiscernible
■ **QRS complex:** duration indiscernible
▲ **Other:** waveform is a wavy line; when the waves are large, the rhythm is coarse fibrillation; when the waves are small, the rhythm is fine fibrillation

cle and repeatedly stimulates the ventricular muscles at a rate so rapid that the recovery period disappears and the individual muscle fibers can only twitch continuously – unable to contract.

COMPLICATIONS

Because muscle twitching is completely ineffective in propelling blood from the ventricles, the circulation stops abruptly. Death ensues within minutes unless ventricular fibrillation is terminated and normal rhythm is restored.

ASSESSMENT

The patient's history may reveal a condition associated with the development of ventricular fibrillation. Inspection reveals the patient to be unresponsive and apneic or to have agonal respirations. Palpation discloses un-

Treating ventricular fibrillation: A step-by-step guide

The advanced cardiac life support guidelines recommend a series of steps for treating ventricular fibrillation (VF) or pulseless ventricular tachycardia (VT). The steps, shown in the flowchart, aren't intended as strict rules. Certain patients will require interventions not covered in the steps. Also, keep in mind that you'd continue following them only if VF or pulseless VT persists. Treat the two conditions the same way.

After each defibrillation attempt, assess the patient's pulse rate and rhythm. If the arrhythmia recurs after a transient conversion, apply the joule level that produced the conversion.

If possible, intubate the patient earlier than shown on the flowchart, but only if it can be done during the other interventions. If he can be ventilated without being intubated, however, defibrillate and give epinephrine first.

Keep in mind that some doctors prefer administering lidocaine in 0.5 mg/kg boluses every 5 to 10 minutes to a total dose of 3 mg/kg. Also keep in mind that sodium bicarbonate isn't recommended for a routine cardiac arrest.

Witnessed cardiac arrest

Check pulse. If absent, administer precordial thump and check pulse again.

Unwitnessed cardiac arrest

Check pulse.

If absent, perform cardiopulmonary resuscitation (CPR) until a defibrillator is available.
Check cardiac monitor to detect VF or VT.

Defibrillate with 200 joules.
If unsuccessful, defibrillate with 200 to 300 joules.
If unsuccessful, defibrillate with up to 360 joules.

Check pulse; if absent, perform CPR.
Establish I.V. access.
Intubate when possible.

Give epinephrine 1:10,000, 1.0 mg I.V. push, every 3 to 5 minutes.

Defibrillate with up to 360 joules.

Give lidocaine, 1 to 1.5 mg/kg I.V. push.

Defibrillate with up to 360 joules.

Give bretylium, 5 mg/kg I.V. push.
(Consider giving sodium bicarbonate.)

Defibrillate with up to 360 joules.

Give bretylium, 10 mg/kg I.V. push.

Defibrillate with up to 360 joules.

Repeat lidocaine or bretylium.

Defibrillate with up to 360 joules.

detectable peripheral pulses, and auscultation confirms the absence of a heartbeat.

DIAGNOSTIC TESTS

Electrocardiography (ECG), which reveals a wavy line with no recognizable pattern, confirms the diagnosis.

TREATMENT

Immediate treatment includes defibrillation, cardiopulmonary resuscitation (CPR), and other life-support measures.

KEY NURSING DIAGNOSES AND PATIENT OUTCOMES

Altered tissue perfusion (cardiopulmonary, cerebral, renal) related to decreased cardiac output. Based on this nursing diagnosis, you'll establish these patient outcomes. The patient will:
• maintain normal cardiopulmonary, cerebral, and renal function
• remain free of chest pain and other arrhythmias
• show no evidence of irreversible damage, such as altered mental status or renal failure.

Decreased cardiac output related to cessation of ventricular contraction. Based on this nursing diagnosis, you'll establish these patient outcomes. The patient will:
• maintain or regain hemodynamic stability exhibited by normal vital signs, urine output, and neurologic function
• attain normal cardiac output with cessation of ventricular fibrillation.

Impaired gas exchange related to decreased cardiac output. Based on this nursing diagnosis, you'll establish these patient outcomes. The patient will:
• regain and maintain adequate ventilation
• exhibit normal arterial blood gas values.

NURSING INTERVENTIONS

• Notify the doctor immediately and begin CPR if the patient's pulse is absent.
• Perform direct current countershock (defibrillation) as soon as possible. (Remember that the longer ventricular fibrillation persists, the more resistant it is to electric shock.)

• Continue CPR if defibrillation is unsuccessful.
• Expect to follow advanced cardiac life support guidelines for treating ventricular fibrillation.
• Establish or maintain I.V. access.
• Administer medications as ordered.
• Assist with intubation, if indicated.

Monitoring

• Continuously monitor the patient's ECG pattern for evidence of resolution of ventricular fibrillation.
• Assess the patient's response to treatment measures.
• Evaluate the patient for neurologic deficits following successful resolution of ventricular fibrillation.
• Check urine output and blood urea nitrogen and creatinine levels for evidence of renal dysfunction.

Patient teaching

• Once the patient is stable and able to comprehend teaching, explain what happened and offer reassurance to the patient and family.
• Teach the patient about prescribed antiarrhythmic medications, and stress the importance of compliance.

ASYSTOLE

Also known as ventricular standstill, asystole occurs when electrical activity in the ventricles stops. Asystole can be transient, causing syncope or near syncope, or it can be a terminal cardiac event unless immediate emergency treatment is given.

CAUSES

Asystole can stem from cardiac or noncardiac causes. Cardiac causes include myocardial ischemia or infarction, aortic valve disease, heart failure, ventricular arrhythmias, atrioventricular block, heart rupture, cardiac tamponade, pacemaker failure, or electromechanical dissociation. Noncardiac causes include hypoxemia, hypokalemia or hyperkale-

ECG characteristics of asystole

In the patient with asystole, the electrocardiogram (ECG) exhibits the distinguishing features shown below.

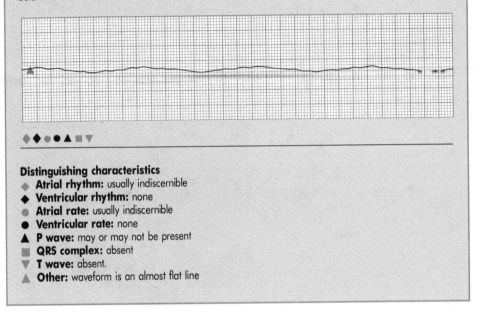

◆◆●●▲■▼

Distinguishing characteristics
◆ **Atrial rhythm:** usually indiscernible
◆ **Ventricular rhythm:** none
● **Atrial rate:** usually indiscernible
● **Ventricular rate:** none
▲ **P wave:** may or may not be present
■ **QRS complex:** absent
▼ **T wave:** absent.
▲ **Other:** waveform is an almost flat line

mia, severe acidosis, electric shock, pulmonary embolism, or cocaine overdose.

COMPLICATIONS
Asystole rapidly results in death if the arrhythmia is not terminated.

ASSESSMENT
The patient's history may reveal a condition associated with the development of asystole. Inspection reveals the patient quickly becoming unresponsive and apneic. Peripheral pulses are undetectable on palpation, and auscultation confirms the absence of a heartbeat.

DIAGNOSTIC TESTS
Asystole is diagnosed by the absence of a heartbeat and the absence of electrical activity on the electrocardiogram (ECG). (See *ECG characteristics of asystole*.)

TREATMENT
A patient with asystole requires immediate treatment including cardiopulmonary resuscitation (CPR) and other life-support measures. (See *Treating asystole: A step-by-step guide*, page 138.)

KEY NURSING DIAGNOSES AND PATIENT OUTCOMES
Altered tissue perfusion (cardiopulmonary, cerebral, renal) related to decreased cardiac output. Based on this nursing diagnosis, you'll establish these patient outcomes. The patient will:
• maintain normal cardiopulmonary, cerebral, and renal function
• remain free of chest pain and other arrhythmias
• show no evidence of irreversible damage, such as altered mental status or renal failure.

Treating asystole: A step-by-step guide

The advanced cardiac life support (ACLS) guidelines recommend a series of steps for treating asystole. These steps aren't intended as a strict set of rules. Certain patients with asystole will require interventions not covered in these steps.

This flowchart shows the steps recommended in the ACLS guidelines. Keep in mind that you'd continue following them only if asystole persists. On the flowchart, VF indicates ventricular fibrillation.

If possible, intubate the patient earlier than shown on the flowchart, but only if it can be done during the other interventions. If he can be ventilated without being intubated, however, cardiopulmonary resuscitation (CPR) and epinephrine administration assume higher initial priorities. The doctor may order epinephrine endotracheally.

Keep in mind that sodium bicarbonate isn't recommended for a routine cardiac arrest.

If rhythm is unclear but VF may be present, defibrillate the patient. If asystole appears, confirm its presence in two leads.

▼

Continue CPR.

▼

Establish I.V. access.

▼

Intubate when possible.

▼

Consider immediate transcutaneous pacing.

▼

Give epinephrine 1:10,000, 1 mg I.V. push, every 3 to 5 minutes.

▼

Give atropine 1 mg I.V. push (repeat in 3 to 5 minutes) up to 0.04 mg/kg

▼

Consider terminating efforts.

Decreased cardiac output related to cessation of ventricular contraction caused by asystole. Based on this nursing diagnosis, you'll establish these patient outcomes. The patient will:
• maintain or regain hemodynamic stability, as evidenced by normal vital signs, urine output, and neurologic function
• attain normal cardiac output with resolution of asystole.

Impaired gas exchange related to decreased cardiac output. Based on this nursing diagnosis, you'll establish these patient outcomes. The patient will:
• regain and maintain adequate ventilation
• exhibit normal arterial blood gas values with adequate spontaneous or mechanical ventilation.

NURSING INTERVENTIONS
• Notify the doctor immediately.
• Initiate CPR.
• Expect to follow advanced cardiac life support guidelines for treating asystole. Check two ECG leads to rule out fine ventricular fibrillation. If determining the type of arrhythmia—asystole or fine ventricular fibrillation—is still difficult, treat as ventricular fibrillation.
• Prepare to administer transcutaneous pacing or assist the doctor to insert a temporary transvenous endocardial pacemaker. Document the procedure, how the patient tolerated it, and how the pacemaker affects the arrhythmia.

Monitoring
• Continuously monitor the patient's ECG pattern for evidence of electrical activity.
• Assess the patient's response to treatment.

• Evaluate the patient for neurologic deficits following successful resolution of asystole.

• Check renal function by measuring urine output and serum blood urea nitrogen and creatinine levels.

Patient teaching

• Once the patient is stable and able to comprehend teaching, explain to him and his family what happened and offer reassurance.

• Explain the treatments and how they will affect the patient's recovery.

• If applicable, begin discharge teaching to the patient and his family, including any medications and the possible need for a permanent pacemaker.

ELECTROMECHANICAL DISSOCIATION

Always a medical emergency, electromechanical dissociation occurs when the electrical activity of the heart has no association with evidence of effective myocardial contraction. In other words, the heart stops contracting effectively despite the presence of a normal electrocardiogram (ECG) rhythm or a rhythm expected to produce a heartbeat.

Electromechanical dissociation is sometimes classified as primary or secondary. The primary form, which is more common, may occur when the heart's ability to contract is seriously impaired (for example, with acute ischemic heart disease or with prolonged resuscitation during cardiac arrest). The secondary form may result from another life-threatening disorder, such as massive pulmonary embolus, cardiac tamponade, severely defective prosthetic heart valve, massive hemorrhage, or tension pneumothorax.

A rare, transient form of electromechanical dissociation may develop during an invasive cardiac procedure, such as angioplasty or atherectomy.

Although sometimes incorrectly referred to as an arrhythmia, electromechanical dissociation is actually a state of cardiovascular collapse that requires immediate attention.

Unfortunately, even with prompt treatment, the disorder is frequently fatal.

CAUSES

Electromechanical dissociation results from mechanical failure or diminished venous return to the right atrium. It is not caused by electrical failure, as seen in ventricular fibrillation or asystole. Although not completely understood, abnormal intracellular calcium, acidosis, or depletion of adenosine triphosphate (the intracellular energy source) is believed to contribute to the primary form. In the secondary form, the rapid cessation of venous blood return to the heart is thought to precipitate mechanical failure. The rare transient form of this disorder may result from temporary restriction of blood flow, related to placement of intracoronary devices.

COMPLICATIONS

Except for the rare transient form, electromechanical dissociation is usually fatal.

ASSESSMENT

The patient's history may reveal conditions that may lead to secondary electromechanical dissociation, such as the presence of a prosthetic heart valve or tension pneumothorax. The patient may complain of shortness of breath, chest pain, and numbness just before unresponsiveness and apnea occur.

Because little or no warning precedes electromechanical dissociation, inspection usually reveals the patient to be unresponsive with no visible respiratory effort. Inspection of the cardiac rhythm shows sinus rhythm at a normal rate or at least a rhythm normally associated with a heartbeat. However, peripheral pulses cannot be palpated nor heart sounds auscultated. Blood pressure and respiratory rate are unobtainable.

DIAGNOSTIC TESTS

The diagnosis of electromechanical dissociation is based on the absence of a heartbeat despite an ECG showing a viable rhythm. (See *ECG characteristics of electromechanical dissociation,* page 140.)

ECG characteristics of electromechanical dissociation

In electromechanical dissociation, isolated electrical activity occurs sporadically without evidence of effective myocardial contraction. The electrocardiogram (ECG) strip may show sinus tachycardia or a variety of other arrhythmias, such as sinus node arrhythmias, atrial arrhythmias, or atrioventricular-conduction disturbances.

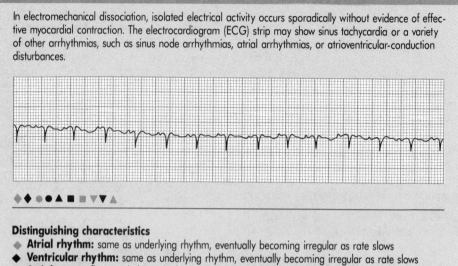

♦♦ ⦁●▲■▨▽▼▲

Distinguishing characteristics
- ♦ **Atrial rhythm:** same as underlying rhythm, eventually becoming irregular as rate slows
- ♦ **Ventricular rhythm:** same as underlying rhythm, eventually becoming irregular as rate slows
- ● **Atrial rate:** reflects underlying rhythm
- ● **Ventricular rate:** reflects underlying rhythm but gradually decreasing
- ▲ **P wave:** same as underlying rhythm, but gradually flattens and disappears
- ■ **PR interval:** same as underlying rhythm, but eventually disappears as P wave disappears
- ▨ **QRS complex:** same as underlying rhythm, but eventually becomes progressively wider
- ▽ **T wave:** same as underlying rhythm, but eventually becomes indiscernible
- ▼ **QT interval:** same as underlying rhythm, but eventually becomes indiscernible
- ▲ **Other:** usually within several minutes, a flat line tracing indicating asystole

TREATMENT

Emergency measures aim to restore myocardial contractility through cardiopulmonary resuscitation (CPR) measures.

KEY NURSING DIAGNOSES AND PATIENT OUTCOMES

Altered tissue perfusion (cerebral, cardiopulmonary, renal, gastrointestinal, peripheral) related to cardiovascular collapse. Based on this nursing diagnosis, you'll establish these patient outcomes. The patient will:
- regain and maintain normal tissue perfusion
- exhibit no evidence of residual damage.

Decreased cardiac output related to cardiovascular collapse. Based on this nursing diagnosis, you'll establish these patient outcomes. The patient will:
- develop and sustain a heartbeat with effective CPR
- regain and maintain adequate cardiac output, as evidenced by normal vital signs, mental status, and adequate urine output.

Fear related to threat of death from possible recurrence of electromechanical dissociation. Based on this nursing diagnosis, you'll establish these patient outcomes. The patient will:
- identify and verbalize his fears
- use support systems to diminish his fears
- exhibit fewer physical signs of fear.

NURSING INTERVENTIONS

• Initiate CPR while second staff member notifies the doctor. Continue CPR if the patient has no palpable pulses despite the presence of cardiac rhythm on an ECG.
• Insert a peripheral I.V. line, if not already present.
• Be prepared to administer epinephrine, isoproterenol, sodium bicarbonate and, possibly, calcium chloride, as ordered.
• Administer oxygen to ensure adequate oxygenation of tissues.
• Transfer the patient to the intensive care unit (ICU) if he survives.
• Provide the patient with an opportunity to verbalize his fears about recurrence and offer support after electromechanical dissociation has been resolved.

Monitoring

• Continuously monitor the patient's cardiopulmonary status (ECG, pulse and heart rate, and blood pressure). Watch for and note the presence of an actual heartbeat.
• Evaluate arterial blood gas values for acid-base balance if heartbeat is established.
• Assess the patient's emotional response to electromechanical dissociation if he survives.

Patient teaching

• If the patient survives, explain electromechanical dissociation to him and his family.
• Because the patient and family may be anxious about the ICU and emergency treatment measures, offer explanations and reassurance.
• Prepare the family for a probable fatal outcome and help them find effective coping strategies.

HYPERTENSIVE CRISIS

Characterized by a rapid, sharp rise in blood pressure, hypertensive crisis can be fatal unless treated promptly. In most patients, blood pressure is considered excessively elevated when mean systolic pressure exceeds 180 mm Hg and mean diastolic pressure ex-

Classifying blood pressure

The Joint National Committee on the Detection, Evaluation, and Treatment of High Blood Pressure recently revised its guidelines for classifying hypertension. The terms *mild, moderate,* and *severe* have been replaced with *normal* (systolic pressure below 130 mm Hg and diastolic pressure below 85 mm Hg), *high normal* (130 to 139 mm Hg systolic and 85 to 89 mm Hg diastolic), and *four stages* of hypertension, in order of increasing severity. They are:
• *Stage 1:* 140 to 159 mm Hg systolic and 90 to 99 mm Hg diastolic
• *Stage 2:* 160 to 179 mm Hg systolic and 100 to 109 mm Hg diastolic
• *Stage 3:* 180 to 209 mm Hg systolic and 110 to 119 mm Hg diastolic
• *Stage 4:* more than 210 mm Hg systolic and more than 120 mm Hg diastolic.

Diuretics and beta blockers represent the drugs of choice for initial therapy. Alternative drugs, reserved for patients for whom diuretics and beta blockers are contraindicated, include angiotensin-converting enzyme inhibitors, alpha blockers, alpha-beta blockers, and calcium channel blockers.

ceeds 120 mm Hg. However, keep in mind that hypertensive crisis isn't a particular blood pressure reading but a clinical state. (See *Classifying blood pressure.*)

In hypertensive crisis, the speed and severity of the increase in blood pressure can compromise the patient's cerebral, renal, and cardiovascular functions. Unless treated promptly, hypertensive crisis can lead to death.

CAUSES

Hypertensive crisis can result from:
• untreated or inadequately treated essential hypertension
• renal disease, such as acute or chronic glomerulonephritis, pyelonephritis, and renal vascular disease
• eclampsia
• intracerebral hemorrhage
• acute left ventricular failure

Recognizing and treating malignant hypertension

Another medical emergency, malignant hypertension is characterized by the following signs and symptoms:
• marked blood pressure elevation
• papilledema
• retinal hemorrhages and exudates
• manifestations of hypertensive encephalopathy, such as severe headache, vomiting, visual disturbances, transient paralysis, seizures, stupor, and coma.

In addition, cardiac decompensation and acute renal failure may develop in this disorder.

The average age at diagnosis is 40, and the disorder affects more men than women. Before the availability of effective antihypertensives, most patients died within 2 years. Even with effective treatment, however, at least half the patients die within 5 years.

Causes
The cause of malignant hypertension isn't known. However, studies do show that dilation

of cerebral arteries and generalized arteriolar fibrinoid necrosis contribute to the disorder. The cerebral arteries dilate because markedly high arterial pressure prevents normal regulation of cerebral blood flow. The resulting excess in cerebral blood flow produces encephalopathy.

Treatment
Emergency treatment aims to quickly reduce blood pressure and identify the underlying cause.
• Diazoxide given rapidly I.V. can begin to reduce blood pressure in 1 to 3 minutes. Nitroprusside and trimethaphan, given by continuous infusion, may be tried. Other drugs for maintaining long-term control of blood pressure include hydralazine and methyldopa.
• With suspected pheochromocytoma, drugs that release additional catecholamines — such as methyldopa, reserpine, and guanethidine — are contraindicated.
• Furosemide and digitalis glycosides may be used to treat associated heart failure.

• polycythemia
• pituitary tumors
• coarctation of the aorta
• adrenocortical hyperfunction
• monoamine oxidase inhibitor interactions.

Two distinct but usually concurrent mechanisms occur in hypertensive crisis: dilation of cerebral arterioles and damage to the arteriolar wall. With normal fluctuations in blood pressure, the brain maintains adequate perfusion through autoregulation. When blood pressure drops, the cerebral arterioles dilate; when it rises, these arterioles constrict to maintain constant cerebral blood flow.

However, in hypertensive crisis, blood pressure climbs so high that the arterioles, already constricted, can no longer withstand the pressure and dilate suddenly. With the brain hyperperfused under such high pressure, fluid moves into the interstitial spaces, causing cerebral edema, hemorrhage, or both.

COMPLICATIONS
Without prompt treatment, hypertensive crisis can lead to rapid death from brain damage or cerebrovascular accident (CVA) or to a more gradual death from renal impairment.

Hypertensive encephalopathy may also occur as a result of cerebral edema or hemorrhage or both caused by an excessive mean arterial pressure. In addition, necrotizing arteriolitis (arteriolar inflammation) can occur within hours. The inflamed, damaged vessels affect target organs in the following pattern:
• In the eyes, the retinal arteries become severely constricted, leading to retinopathy.
• In the kidneys, severe arteriolar constriction impairs circulation and may cause renal failure. During hypertensive crisis, arteriolar changes are accelerated and malignant hypertension ensues. (See *Recognizing and treating malignant hypertension.*)

• In the heart, excessively high pressure in the aorta at the end of diastole impedes systolic ejection. With intra-aortic pressure so high, the left ventricle must generate more wall tension or work harder to open the aortic valve when systole begins. This high afterload increases oxygen demand and the heart's workload. And the imbalance between oxygen demand and supply may cause myocardial ischemia, leading to myocardial infarction (MI), pulmonary edema, or both.

ASSESSMENT

The patient's history usually reveals hypertension treated inadequately or managed poorly because of noncompliance with the prescribed hypertension regimen. The history may also reveal a concurrent condition known to cause hypertensive crisis. In addition, the medication history may reveal the patient has been recently taking certain drugs, such as cough medicines and analgesics, that may raise blood pressure.

The patient usually reports obvious symptoms, such as severe headache, nausea, dizziness, shortness of breath, anginal pain, and visual disturbances. However, some patients may be asymptomatic and unaware of a blood pressure problem until they are diagnosed with hypertensive crisis during a routine examination.

Routine inspection of the chest may exhibit a precordial heave and a lateral displacement of the point of maximal impulse (indicating cardiomegaly, which can trigger or result from hypertensive crisis). Dependent edema may be visible. The patient may demonstrate an altered level of consciousness (LOC), as indicated by confusion, somnolence, or stupor. Oliguria and azotemia may be present. Inspection of the eye during the funduscopic examination may show arteriolar narrowing, arteriovenous compression, hemorrhaging, exudates, and papilledema—possible signs of hypertensive crisis.

Weak peripheral pulses may be palpated. Auscultation of the heart may reveal tachycardia, murmur of aortic insufficiency, a third heart sound (S_3, usually accompanying congestive heart failure), a fourth heart sound (S_4,

signifying a rigid left ventricle), and arrhythmias. A bruit may be auscultated over the flanks or anteriorly over the renal vasculature. The blood pressure is excessively elevated, especially the diastolic, which is 120 mm Hg or greater.

DIAGNOSTIC TESTS

Although blood pressure measurement is the critical diagnostic parameter in the diagnosis of hypertensive crisis, the doctor will order the following tests to identify the cause of hypertension and evaluate the effects of hypertensive crisis on target organs:

• *Complete blood count* typically shows polycythemia.
• *Hematocrit* is decreased and may signal renal failure.
• *Serum potassium level* will decrease if primary aldosteronism causes the hypertension.
• *Blood urea nitrogen and creatinine clearance tests* help detect renal causes of hypertension.
• *Serum glucose level* will be elevated if hypertension results from diabetes mellitus, Cushing's syndrome, or pheochromocytoma.
• *Serum uric acid test* may reveal hyperuricemia associated with hypertension.
• *Urinary vanillylmandelic acid level* may be elevated in pheochromocytoma.
• *Urinalysis* may reveal proteinuria and hematuria if renal dysfunction causes the hypertension.
• *Renal arteriography* may identify renal artery stenosis as the cause of hypertension.
• *Excretory urography* may indicate renal disease (although it can't pinpoint the underlying cause).
• *Chest X-ray* identifies cardiomegaly.
• *Electrocardiography (ECG)* may indicate left ventricular hypertrophy or ischemia from hypertension.

TREATMENT

Emergency treatment of hypertensive crisis centers on I.V. drug therapy to reduce blood pressure quickly but cautiously. Drugs may include diazoxide, hydralazine, or nitroprusside (vasodilators); trimethaphan (a ganglionic blocking agent), or phentolamine (an al-

DOSAGE FINDER

Identifying drug dosages in hypertensive crisis

The drugs listed below may be used to treat hypertensive crisis.

Diazoxide
To treat malignant hypertension or hypertensive crisis, give an adult 1 to 3 mg/kg I.V. up to a total of 150 mg. Repeat every 5 to 15 minutes as needed. Administer maintenance doses every 4 to 24 hours as needed up to 1.2 g/day.

Hydralazine
To treat hypertension, give an adult 10 to 20 mg I.V. or 20 to 40 mg I.M., as needed, usually every 4 to 6 hours.

Nitroprusside
To rapidly reduce blood pressure in hypertensive emergencies, give an adult not receiving other hypotensive drugs 0.5 to 10 mcg/kg/minute by continuous infusion. The average dose is 3 mcg/kg/minute. Discontinue the drug if 10 mcg/kg/minute for 10 minutes doesn't produce an adequate blood pressure reduction.

Trimethaphan
To treat hypertensive crisis and control hypotension during surgery, give an adult 500 mg (10 ml) in 500 ml of dextrose 5% in water to yield concentration of 1 mg/ml I.V. Start I.V. drip at 1 to 2 mg/minute and titrate to achieve desired hypotensive response. Range is 0.3 to 6 mg/minute.

Phentolamine
To treat hypertensive crisis resulting from an interaction between a monoamine oxidase inhibitor and sympathomimetic amines, give an adult 5 to 10 mg I.V. or I.M.

pha-adrenergic blocking agent). The dosage is titrated to the patient's response. (See *Identifying drug dosages in hypertensive crisis.*)

Other drugs, such as I.V. nitroglycerin, I.M. reserpine, I.V. methyldopa, or I.V. labetalol (first by bolus, then by continuous infusion), may also be administered to reduce preload

and afterload as well as blood pressure. When the patient's blood pressure stabilizes at the desired level, the doctor will start the transition from I.V. to oral drug administration.

KEY NURSING DIAGNOSES AND PATIENT OUTCOMES
Altered cerebral tissue perfusion related to dilation of cerebral arterioles. Based on this nursing diagnosis, you'll establish these patient outcomes. The patient will:
• regain and maintain normal LOC as blood pressure is reduced
• show no signs and symptoms of cerebral deficits
• report headache is alleviated.

Anxiety related to threat of death caused by situational crisis. Based on this nursing diagnosis, you'll establish these patient outcomes. The patient will:
• state feelings of anxiety
• use available support systems to assist with coping
• demonstrate abated physical symptoms of anxiety.

High risk for injury related to adverse effects of hypertensive crisis on target organs. Based on this nursing diagnosis, you'll establish these patient outcomes. The patient will:
• maintain normal organ function
• regain and maintain stable blood pressure at desired level.

NURSING INTERVENTIONS
• Prepare and administer emergency antihypertensive drugs I.V. as prescribed. Titrate the dosage according to the patient's response.
• Assist with insertion of an arterial line for monitoring blood pressure.
• Keep the patient on bed rest until blood pressure has stabilized. Also keep his environment quiet and as stress-free as possible.
• Answer all questions and address all concerns the patient and family may have to allay anxiety that may be a factor in keeping the patient's blood pressure elevated.
• Be prepared to administer supportive care if target organ dysfunction occurs.

Monitoring

• Measure the patient's blood pressure every 5 minutes or as often as ordered. When his blood pressure is stable, monitor it every 15 minutes for 1 hour, then hourly thereafter as ordered. When I.V. antihypertensive drug therapy has been converted to oral therapy, take vital signs every 2 to 4 hours and then every 8 hours if no significant change is noted.
• Monitor the rate of drug infusions closely using an infusion pump to prevent hypotension.
• Observe the patient for adverse drug reactions.
• Assess the patient for adverse effects of hypertensive crisis on target organs as well as for complications. Be especially alert for signs and symptoms of heart failure, MI, and CVA.

Patient teaching

• Tell the patient and his family what hypertensive crisis is and how it happens. Explain the need for emergency drug therapy and the need to monitor him and his blood pressure closely to gauge drug effectiveness and detect adverse drug reactions.
• After the immediate crisis, focus on ensuring compliance with therapy – a challenge for many hypertensive patients.
• Teach the patient about hypertension. Emphasize that he needs long-term treatment and follow-up care, even if his symptoms disappear. Warn him that although treatment can control hypertension, it won't cure it. Stress that he can help ensure an excellent prognosis by following the prescribed treatment regimen.
• Encourage the patient to participate in follow-up care. Urge him to obtain a blood pressure kit, and teach him how to use it to check his blood pressure periodically.
• Encourage the patient to keep a record of his home blood pressure readings and to bring the records to all doctor appointments.
• If necessary and appropriate, arrange for a home health nurse to make periodic follow-up visits to monitor the patient's blood pressure and evaluate his blood pressure measurement technique.

DISSECTING AORTIC ANEURYSM

Also called aortic dissection, dissecting aortic aneurysm is a localized dilation of the aorta characterized by a separation between the layers of the vascular wall. This separation allows blood to accumulate between the layers, forming an aneurysm. Dissection is most common in the ascending aorta but also occurs in the transverse and descending aorta. (See *Classifying dissecting aortic aneurysm*, page 146.) A surgical emergency, it causes death if the aneurysm ruptures.

Dissecting aortic aneurysm most commonly affects men between ages 45 and 70 – especially those with Marfan's syndrome or congenital heart disease.

CAUSES

Although trauma may cause a dissecting aortic aneurysm, it more commonly occurs with disorders that increase hemodynamic stress on the aorta, such as hypertension, arteriosclerosis, infection, coarctation, or Marfan's syndrome. The disorder also may result from damage to the aorta's middle layer (media), causing separation of the intima from the media.

As the aorta weakens and becomes less elastic, the media and adventitia (outermost layer) stretch outward. Blood flow pressure on the weakened wall ultimately leads to an intimal tear, with hemorrhagic separation of the aortic wall. Blood enters the media, forming an outpouching, or dilation. Stress from the resulting turbulent blood flow then dissects the layers of the media, forming a false channel between it and the intima. The heart's contractile force extends the dissection distally and proximally. The column of blood may extend varying distances along the length of the aorta.

COMPLICATIONS

Rupture of an aortic aneurysm into the pericardium leads to acute cardiac tamponade. Even with prompt surgical intervention, this crisis proves fatal in more than 50% of patients.

Classifying dissecting aortic aneurysm

These drawings illustrate the DeBakey system of classifying dissecting aortic aneurysm (shaded areas) according to location. Dissections can also be classified by their location relative to the aortic valve. Thus, types I and II are proximal; type III is distal.

Type I
In this type of dissection, the most common and lethal, intimal tearing occurs in the ascending aorta, and the dissection extends into the descending aorta.

Type II
In this type of dissection, which occurs most commonly with Marfan's syndrome, dissection is limited to the ascending or transverse aorta.

Type III
In this form of dissection, the intimal tear is located in the descending aorta and expands distally.

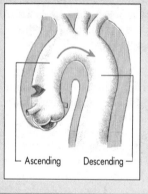

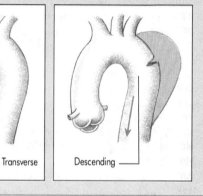

ASSESSMENT

The patient's history may reveal the cause of a dissecting aortic aneurysm. The patient reports a sudden onset of intense pain (from compression of surrounding structures, from the dissection itself, or both). He may describe the pain as a severe tearing or stabbing pain that may radiate from its point of origin in the direction of the dissection. He may indicate the location of the pain as being in the scapular area (suggesting dissection in the descending aorta), in the anterior chest area (suggesting dissection in the ascending aorta), or in the neck, throat, jaw, or teeth (suggesting an ascending or transverse dissection).

On inspection, the patient with an aortic dissection appears pale or cyanotic, diaphoretic, and acutely dyspneic. In addition, he may exhibit syncope, transient paralysis, weakness, or even an altered level of consciousness.

Palpation of peripheral pulses may reveal an absence of carotid, radial, and femoral pulses in an ascending dissection. In a descending dissection, peripheral pulse deficits are less likely detected. When they occur, they usually involve the left subclavian and femoral pulses with the carotid and radial pulses being present and equal bilaterally.

Auscultation of the heart may reveal a diastolic murmur, reflecting aortic insufficiency in ascending dissection. The murmur, which may have a musical quality, may be more audible in the right sternal border at the second intercostal space.

Elevated blood pressure is usually detected in a descending dissection with a significant differential in systolic pressure between the right and left arms (from occlusion of the brachial arteries). In an ascending dissection, systolic blood pressure is equal bilaterally. The patient may be hypotensive if cardiac tamponade, aneurysm rupture, or dissection of the brachiocephalic vessels occurs.

DIAGNOSTIC TESTS

In an asymptomatic patient, aortic dissection is usually diagnosed incidentally, through posteroanterior and oblique chest X-rays that show widening of the aorta and mediastinum.

Aortography (aortic angiography) is the most important diagnostic tool in confirming dissection because it identifies the tear site and determines the extent of the dissection.

Other tests may include magnetic resonance imaging and computed tomography scans to help confirm and locate the dissection.

TREATMENT

A dissecting aortic aneurysm requires emergency surgery to repair the aorta. The surgical procedure usually involves excision of the aneurysm followed by vascular repair with a preclotted Dacron or Teflon graft sutured in end-to-end fashion.

Antihypertensive drugs, such as nitroprusside, may be given to reduce and maintain the systolic pressure below 120 mm Hg. Isotonic fluids or colloids may be used to maintain pulmonary artery wedge pressure between 12 and 15 mm Hg.

KEY NURSING DIAGNOSES AND PATIENT OUTCOMES

Anxiety related to threat of death caused by a dissecting aortic aneurysm. Based on this nursing diagnosis, you'll establish these patient outcomes. The patient will:
• state feelings of anxiety
• use available support systems to cope with situational crisis
• demonstrate abated physical signs of anxiety.

High risk for injury related to possible aneurysm rupture. Based on this nursing diagnosis, you'll establish these patient outcomes. The patient will:
• have a dissecting aortic aneurysm identified immediately and treated promptly

• maintain normal body function
• experience no lasting deficits as a result of the dissecting aneurysm.

Fluid volume deficit related to hemorrhage caused by aneurysm rupture. Based on this nursing diagnosis, you'll establish these patient outcomes. The patient will:
• recover and maintain a normal fluid and blood volume
• maintain hemodynamic stability, as evidenced by stable vital signs, urine output of at least 30 ml/hour, and an alert and oriented mental presentation.

NURSING INTERVENTIONS

• Notify the doctor immediately and place the patient on strict bed rest.
• Administer oxygen therapy as prescribed.
• Insert an I.V. line peripherally, if not already in place. Assist with placement of a pulmonary artery catheter or central venous catheter, if time permits.
• Be prepared to administer nitroprusside or other antihypertensive agents to reduce blood pressure.
• Administer isotonic fluids or colloids, as ordered, to maintain pulmonary artery wedge pressure between 12 and 15 mm Hg. This pressure, slightly higher than normal, maximizes cardiac output.
• Prepare the patient for emergency surgery. Answer his questions and address his and his family's concerns to help alleviate anxiety.
• Care for the patient following surgery as for any patient undergoing a thoracotomy or abdominal surgery. Administer pain medications and care for incision and drainage tubes as needed.

Monitoring

• Assess and record the patient's blood pressure, pulse rate, and respiratory rate every 5 minutes or as often as ordered. Palpate all peripheral pulses frequently for quality and amplitude.
• Assess skin color and capillary refill.
• Evaluate the patient for signs of hemorrhage, such as hypotension, tachycardia, and tachypnea. Check urine output hourly.

• Measure pulmonary artery pressure and central venous pressure, if possible.
• Monitor drug infusions carefully. Use a pump to ensure accurate dosage.
• Evaluate the patient's emotional response to this situational crisis.
• Postoperatively, watch the patient closely for complications, such as shock, excessive bleeding, renal dysfunction, or infection.

Patient teaching

• Before discharge, teach the patient why he must comply with antihypertensive therapy. Describe posssible effects of antihypertensive medication.
• Teach the patient how to monitor his blood pressure.
• Instruct the patient to call the doctor immediately if he has a sharp pain in his chest or the back of his neck, which may indicate a recurrence of aortic dissection.

ACUTE ARTERIAL OCCLUSION

Potentially life-threatening, an acute arterial occlusion occurs when an obstruction in an artery interrupts vital blood flow. Major arteries that may be affected include the carotid, vertebral, innominate, subclavian, mesenteric, and celiac arteries.

The prognosis depends on the location of the occlusion, the development of collateral circulation to counteract reduced blood flow, and the time elapsed between the development of the occlusion and its removal.

CAUSES

The most common cause of acute arterial occlusion is obstruction of a major artery by a clot. The occlusive mechanism may be endogenous, resulting from emboli formation, thrombosis, or plaques, or exogenous, resulting from trauma or fracture.

Predisposing factors include smoking; aging; conditions such as hypertension, hyperlipidemia, and diabetes mellitus; and family history of vascular disorders, myocardial infarction, or cerebrovascular accident.

COMPLICATIONS

An acute arterial occlusion often causes severe ischemia, skin ulceration, and gangrene.

ASSESSMENT

The patient's history may reveal the presence of arterial occlusive disease. Varied assessment findings can be present depending on the vessel involved. (See *Signs and symptoms of arterial occlusive disease.*)

Acute arterial occlusion occurs suddenly, often without warning. However, peripheral occlusion can often be recognized by the five Ps:
• Pain, the most common symptom, occurs suddenly and is localized to the affected arm or leg.
• Pallor results from vasoconstriction distal to the occlusion.
• Pulselessness occurs distal to the occlusion.
• Paralysis and paresthesia occur in the affected arm or leg from disturbed nerve endings or skeletal muscles.

A sixth P, known as poikilothermy, refers to temperature changes that occur distal to the occlusion, making the skin feel cool.

DIAGNOSTIC TESTS

• *Arteriography* demonstrates the type, location, and degree of obstruction and the establishment of collateral circulation. It is particularly useful in evaluating candidates for reconstructive surgery.
• *Ultrasonography* and *plethysmography* show decreased blood flow distal to the occlusion.
• *Doppler ultrasonography* typically reveals a relatively low-pitched sound and a monophasic waveform.
• *Segmental limb pressures* and *pulse volume measurements* help evaluate the location and extent of the occlusion.
• *Ophthalmodynamometry* helps determine the degree of obstruction in the internal carotid artery by comparing ophthalmic artery pressure with brachial artery pressure on the affected side. More than a 20% difference between pressures suggests arterial insufficiency.

Signs and symptoms of arterial occlusive disease

A patient with arterial occlusive disease may have a wide variety of signs and symptoms, depending on which portion of the vasculature is affected by the disorder.

SITE OF OCCLUSION	SIGNS AND SYMPTOMS
Internal and external carotid arteries	Transient ischemic attacks (TIAs) due to reduced cerebral circulation produce unilateral sensory or motor dysfunction (transient monocular blindness, hemiparesis), possible aphasia or dysarthria, confusion, decreased mentation, and headache. These recurrent clinical features usually last for 5 to 10 minutes but may persist for up to 24 hours and may herald a cerebrovascular accident. Absent or decreased pulsation with a bruit that can be auscultated over the affected vessels.
Vertebral and basilar arteries	TIAs of brain stem and cerebellum produce binocular visual disturbances, vertigo, dysarthria, and "drop attacks" (falling down without loss of consciousness). Less common than carotid TIA.
Innominate (brachiocephalic) artery	Signs and symptoms of vertebrobasilar occlusion. Indications of ischemia (claudication) of right arm; possible bruit over right side of neck.
Subclavian artery	Subclavian steal syndrome characterized by the backflow of blood from the brain through the vertebral artery on the same side as the occlusion, into the subclavian artery distal to the occlusion; clinical effects of vertebrobasilar occlusion and exercise-induced arm claudication. Possible gangrene, usually limited to the digits.
Mesenteric artery	Bowel ischemia, infarct necrosis, and gangrene; sudden, acute abdominal pain; nausea and vomiting; diarrhea; leukocytosis; and shock due to massive intraluminal fluid and plasma loss.
Aortic bifurcation (saddle-block occlusion, a medical emergency associated with cardiac embolization)	Sensory and motor deficits (muscle weakness, numbness, paresthesia, paralysis) and signs of ischemia (sudden pain; cold, pale legs with decreased or absent peripheral pulses) in both legs.
Iliac artery (Leriche's syndrome)	Intermittent claudication of lower back, buttocks, and thighs, relieved by rest; absent or reduced femoral or distal pulses; shiny, scaly skin, subcutaneous tissue loss, and no body hair on affected limb; nail deformities; increased capillary refill time; blanching of feet on elevation; possible bruit over femoral arteries; impotence in males.
Femoral and popliteal arteries (associated with aneurysm formation)	Intermittent claudication of the calves on exertion; ischemic pain in feet; pretrophic pain (heralds necrosis and ulceration); leg pallor and coolness; shiny, scaly skin, subcutaneous tissue loss, and no body hair on affected limb; nail deformities; increased capillary refill time; blanching of feet on elevation; gangrene; no palpable pulses distal to occlusion. Auscultation over affected area may reveal a bruit.

• *Electroencephalography* and a *computed tomography scan* may be necessary to rule out brain lesions.

TREATMENT

Acute arterial occlusive disease usually requires surgery, such as the following:

Identifying drug dosages in acute arterial occlusion

The drugs listed below may be used to treat acute arterial occlusion.

Alteplase

For lysis of thrombi obstructing coronary arteries in acute myocardial infarction, give an adult weighing 143 lb (65 kg) or more 100 mg over 3 hours.

In the first hour, give 60 mg — 6 to 10 mg as a bolus in the first 1 to 2 minutes, and the rest as a diluted continuous infusion over the rest of the hour. Then administer 20 mg/hour as a continuous infusion for the next 2 hours. Don't exceed the recommended dosage of 100 mg over 3 hours; higher dosages may lead to intracranial bleeding.

Give an adult weighing under 143 lb 1.25 mg/kg over 3 hours.

In the first hour, give 60% of the total dose — 10% as a bolus in the first 1 to 2 minutes and the rest as a diluted continuous infusion. Then give the remaining 40% of the total dose over the next 2 hours, 20% each hour.

Streptokinase

To treat arterial embolism or thrombosis, give an adult a loading dose of 250,000 IU infused over 30 minutes. Set the rate at 30 ml/hour (for a 750,000 IU vial) or 90 ml/hour (for a 250,000 IU vial). Follow this with a maintenance dose of 100,000 IU/hour, administered by continuous infusion. Continue the infusion for 24 to 72 hours.

Urokinase

For lysis of coronary artery thrombosis, give an adult 6,000 IU/minute of urokinase intra-arterially via coronary artery catheter until artery opens maximally, usually within 15 to 30 minutes. Drug administration may prove necessary for up to 2 hours. Average total dose amounts to 500,000 IU.

• *Embolectomy.* A balloon-tipped Fogarty catheter is used to remove thrombotic material from the artery. Embolectomy is used mainly for mesenteric, femoral, or popliteal artery occlusion.

• *Thromboendarterectomy.* This involves the opening of the artery and removal of the obstructing thrombus and the medial layer of the arterial wall. Plaque deposits will remain intact. Thromboendarterectomy is usually performed after angiography and is often used in conjunction with autogenous vein or Dacron bypass surgery (femoropopliteal or aortofemoral).

• *Percutaneous transluminal coronary angioplasty (PTCA).* Using fluoroscopy and a special balloon catheter, PTCA dilates the stenosis or occluded artery to a predetermined diameter without overdistending it.

• *Laser surgery.* An excimer or a hot-tip laser obliterates the clot and plaque by vaporizing it.

• *Patch grafting.* This involves removal of the thrombosed arterial segment and replacement with an autogenous vein or Dacron graft.

• *Bypass graft.* Blood flow is diverted through an anastomosed autogenous or woven Dacron graft to bypass the thrombosed arterial segment.

• *Lumbar sympathectomy.* Depending on the condition of the sympathetic nervous system, this procedure may be an adjunct to reconstructive surgery.

• *Amputation.* This may be necessary if arterial reconstructive surgery fails or if gangrene, uncontrollable infection, or intractable pain develops.

Thrombolytics, such as alteplase, streptokinase, urokinase, and activase, may be used to dissolve clots and relieve an obstruction caused by a thrombus. (See *Identifying drug dosages in acute arterial occlusion.*)

Other therapy includes heparin to prevent emboli (for embolic occlusion) and bowel resection after restoration of blood flow (for mesenteric artery occlusion). Supportive treatment may include elimination of smoking, hypertension control, walking exercise, and foot and leg care. In carotid artery occlusion, antiplatelet therapy may begin with dipyridamole and aspirin.

KEY NURSING DIAGNOSES
AND PATIENT OUTCOMES

Altered peripheral or cerebral tissue perfusion related to cessation of blood flow caused by an acute arterial occlusion. Based on this nursing diagnosis, you'll establish these patient outcomes. The patient will:
• have his changed condition identified quickly and treated promptly
• regain adequate tissue perfusion, as evidenced by the presence of peripheral pulses, normal skin temperature and color in extremities, absence of pain, and orientation to time, person, and place.

High risk for injury related to loss of blood flow distal to site of arterial occlusion. Based on this nursing diagnosis, you'll establish these patient outcomes. The patient will:
• recognize seriousness of his condition and seek emergency care immediately at the onset of the occlusion
• demonstrate no residual deficits following alleviation of the occlusion.

Pain related to ischemia caused by the acute arterial occlusion. Based on this nursing diagnosis, you'll establish these patient outcomes. The patient will:
• attain temporary pain relief with analgesics
• become pain-free with surgical or drug therapy.

NURSING INTERVENTIONS

• Notify the doctor immediately if an acute arterial occlusion is suspected.
• Establish a peripheral I.V. line.
• If the patient has experienced an emboli occlusion, expect to administer heparin or thrombolytics by continuous I.V. drip, as ordered. Use an infusion monitor or pump to ensure the proper flow rate.
• If the occlusion has occurred in a lower extremity, wrap the patient's affected foot in soft cotton batting, and reposition it frequently to prevent pressure on any one area until surgery is performed.

◆ NURSING ALERT. Strictly avoid elevating or applying heat to the affected leg.
• Prevent trauma to the affected extremity. Use minimal-pressure mattresses, heel protec-

tors, a foot cradle, or a footboard to reduce pressure that could lead to skin breakdown. Keep the arm or leg warm but never use heating pads. If the patient is wearing socks, remove them frequently to check the skin.
• Avoid using restrictive clothing, such as antiembolism stockings.
• Administer analgesics to relieve pain.
• Prepare the patient for surgery. Explain the surgical procedure to the patient and family.

Monitoring

• Frequently assess the patient's circulatory status by checking for the most distal pulses and inspecting his skin color and temperature for evidence of aortic, iliac, femoral, or popliteal artery involvement. Compare findings to earlier assessments and observations.
• Evaluate the patient's neurologic status frequently for evidence of carotid, innominate, vertebral, or subclavian artery involvement. Watch for changes in level of consciousness, pupil size, and muscle strength.
• Monitor the patient for severe abdominal pain and change in bowel function by regularly performing an abdominal assessment for evidence of mesenteric artery involvement. Increasing abdominal distention and tenderness may indicate extension of bowel ischemia with resulting gangrene, or it may indicate peritonitis.
• Check the patient for signs of fluid and electrolyte imbalance. Monitor his intake and output for signs of renal failure (urine output of less than 30 ml/hour) in an acute arterial occlusive episode involving the mesenteric artery or aorta.
• Monitor any prescribed thrombolytic therapy closely. Maintain continuous infusions on a pump for accurate and safe delivery of the drug.
• Observe the patient receiving thrombolytic or anticoagulant therapy for signs of bleeding (I.V. site oozing, nosebleed, hematuria, bruising, and gum bleeding).

Patient teaching

• When preparing the patient for discharge, instruct him to watch for signs of recurrence (pain, pallor, numbness, paralysis, absence of

pulse) that can result from graft occlusion or occlusion at another site. Caution against wearing constrictive clothing, crossing his legs, or wearing garters. Tell him to avoid "bumping" injuries to affected limbs.
• Warn the patient to avoid all tobacco products.
• Tell the patient to avoid temperature extremes. If he must go outside in the cold, remind him to dress warmly and take special care to keep his feet warm.

CARDIOGENIC SHOCK

Sometimes called pump failure, cardiogenic shock is a condition of diminished cardiac output that severely impairs tissue perfusion. Cardiogenic shock occurs as a serious complication in nearly 15% of all patients who are hospitalized with acute myocardial infarction (MI). It typically affects patients whose area of infarction involves 40% or more of left ventricular muscle mass; in such patients, mortality may exceed 85%. Most patients with cardiogenic shock die within 24 hours of onset. The prognosis for those who survive is poor.

CAUSES
Cardiogenic shock can result from any condition that causes significant left ventricular dysfunction with reduced cardiac output, such as MI (most common), myocardial ischemia, papillary muscle dysfunction, and end-stage cardiomyopathy.

Other causes include myocarditis and depression of myocardial contractility after cardiac arrest and prolonged cardiac surgery. Mechanical abnormalities of the ventricle, such as acute mitral or aortic insufficiency or an acutely acquired ventricular septal defect or ventricular aneurysm, may also result in cardiogenic shock.

Regardless of the cause, left ventricular dysfunction initiates a series of compensatory mechanisms that attempt to increase cardiac output and, in turn, maintain vital organ function. As cardiac output falls, aortic and carotid baroreceptors activate sympathetic nervous responses. These compensatory responses increase heart rate, left ventricular filling pressure, and peripheral resistance to flow to enhance venous return to the heart. The action initially stabilizes the patient but later causes deterioration with rising oxygen demands on the already compromised myocardium. These events constitute a vicious circle of low cardiac output, sympathetic compensation, myocardial ischemia, and even lower cardiac output.

COMPLICATIONS
Death usually ensues because the vital organs can't overcome the deleterious effects of extended hypoperfusion.

ASSESSMENT
Typically, the patient's history includes a disorder (such as MI or cardiomyopathy) that severely decreases left ventricular function. Patients with underlying cardiac disease may complain of anginal pain because of decreased myocardial perfusion and oxygenation. Urine output is usually less than 20 ml/hour.

Inspection usually reveals pale skin, decreased sensorium, and rapid, shallow respirations. Palpation of peripheral pulses may detect a rapid, thready pulse. The skin feels cold and clammy.

Auscultation of blood pressure usually discloses a mean arterial pressure of less than 60 mm Hg and a narrowing pulse pressure. In a patient with chronic hypotension, the mean pressure may fall below 50 mm Hg before he exhibits any signs of shock. Auscultation of the heart detects gallop rhythm, faint heart sounds and, possibly (if shock results from rupture of the ventricular septum or papillary muscles), a holosystolic murmur.

Although many of these clinical features also occur in heart failure and other shock syndromes, they are usually more profound in cardiogenic shock. Patients with pericardial tamponade may have distant heart sounds.

DIAGNOSTIC TESTS

• *Hemodynamic monitoring* helps determine the severity of cardiogenic shock. (See *Understanding hemodynamic terms*, page 154, and *Hemodynamic values in cardiogenic shock*, page 155.)

• *Invasive arterial pressure monitoring* shows systolic arterial pressure less than 80 mm Hg caused by impaired ventricular ejection.

• *Arterial blood gas analysis* may show metabolic and respiratory acidosis and hypoxia.

• *Electrocardiography (ECG)* demonstrates possible evidence of acute MI, ischemia, or ventricular aneurysm.

• *Serum enzyme measurements* display elevated levels of creatine kinase (CK), lactate dehydrogenase (LD), aspartate aminotransferase (formerly SGOT), and alanine aminotransferase (formerly SGPT), which point to MI or ischemia and suggest heart failure or shock. CK and LD isoenzyme levels may confirm acute MI.

• *Cardiac catheterization* and *echocardiography* reveal other conditions that can lead to pump dysfunction and failure, such as cardiac tamponade, papillary muscle infarct or rupture, ventricular septal rupture, pulmonary emboli, venous pooling (associated with venodilators and continuous or intermittent positive-pressure breathing), and hypovolemia.

TREATMENT

The goal of therapy is to enhance cardiovascular status by increasing cardiac output, improving myocardial perfusion, and decreasing cardiac workload with combinations of cardiovascular drugs and mechanical assist techniques.(See *Devices used to treat cardiogenic shock*, page 156.)

I.V. drugs may include dopamine, a vasopressor that increases cardiac output, blood pressure, and renal blood flow; amrinone or dobutamine, inotropic agents that increase myocardial contractility; and norepinephrine, when a more potent vasoconstrictor is necessary. (See *Identifying dopamine dosage in cardiogenic shock*, page 157.) Nitroprusside, a vasodilator, may be used with a vasopressor to further improve cardiac output by decreasing peripheral vascular resistance (afterload) and reducing left ventricular end-diastolic pressure (preload). However, the patient's blood pressure must be adequate to support nitroprusside therapy and must be monitored closely.

Treatment may also include the intra-aortic balloon pump (IABP), a mechanical assist device that attempts to improve coronary artery perfusion and decrease cardiac workload. When drug therapy and IABP insertion fail, a ventricular assist pump (an experimental device) may be used.

KEY NURSING DIAGNOSES AND PATIENT OUTCOMES

Altered cardiopulmonary tissue perfusion related to decreased cardiac output caused by left ventricular dysfunction. Based on this nursing diagnosis, you'll establish these patient outcomes. The patient will:
• not exhibit cardiac arrhythmias
• remain free of chest pain
• exhibit arterial blood gas values within the normal range.

Decreased cardiac output related to left ventricular dysfunction caused by myocardial injury. Based on this nursing diagnosis, you'll establish these patient outcomes. The patient will:
• have a heart rate and blood pressure within the normal range
• regain and maintain a normal cardiac output.

Fear related to threat of death caused by cardiogenic shock. Based on this nursing diagnosis, you'll establish these patient outcomes. The patient will:
• identify and verbalize his fears
• use support systems to diminish his fears
• exhibit fewer physical symptoms of fear.

NURSING INTERVENTIONS

• In the intensive care unit (ICU), start I.V. infusions of 0.9% sodium chloride or lactated Ringer's solution using a large-bore (14G to 18G) catheter, which allows easier administration later of blood transfusions.

♦ NURSING ALERT. Don't start an I.V. infusion in the leg of a patient who is in shock and

Understanding hemodynamic terms

Become familiar with hemodynamic evaluation terms by reviewing the following descriptions.

Cardiac output refers to the volume of blood ejected by the heart each minute. Normally, it measures 4 to 6 liters/minute. If your patient has a pulmonary artery catheter equipped with a thermistor, you can use the thermodilution technique to determine cardiac output. You can also determine cardiac output indirectly from your patient's mixed venous oxygen saturation. Otherwise, calculate cardiac output using mean arterial pressure (MAP), central venous pressure (CVP), and systemic vascular resistance (SVR). Follow this formula:

$$\text{Cardiac output} = \frac{\text{MAP} - \text{CVP}}{\text{SVR}}$$

Cardiac index takes body size into account. By calculating this parameter, you can determine if your patient's cardiac output meets his needs. Cardiac index normally ranges from 2.5 to 4.2 liters/minute/m². Use this formula to calculate cardiac index:

$$\text{Cardiac index} = \frac{\text{cardiac output}}{\text{body surface area (m}^2)}$$

Preload indicators

Preload, which refers to ventricular volume plus pressure at the end of diastole, determines the length of muscle fibers when contraction begins. This length, in turn, determines contractile force and the velocity of muscle fiber shortening.

CVP reflects right atrial pressure and thus helps gauge right ventricular preload. Normal CVP measures 4 to 12 cm H_2O, or 1 to 6 mm Hg.

Pulmonary artery diastolic pressure (PADP) reflects left ventricular preload. PADP approximates left ventricular pressures in a patient who doesn't have pulmonic or mitral valve disease. Normal PADP measures 8 to 15 mm Hg.

Pulmonary artery wedge pressure (PAWP) also reflects left ventricular preload. PAWP is more accurate than PADP if the patient has pulmonic or mitral valve disease. Normal PAWP is 4 to 12 mm Hg; a value above 28 mm Hg usually constitutes pulmonary edema.

Afterload indicators

Afterload is the resistance the ventricle works against to eject blood during systole. Resistance depends on arterial blood pressure, valve characteristics, ventricular radius, and wall thickness.

SVR helps gauge left ventricular afterload. Normal SVR is 900 to 1,200 dynes/second/cm^{-5} or absolute units. An indirect measurement, it's commonly calculated by the hemodynamic monitoring system. Or you may calculate it using this formula:

$$\text{SVR} = \frac{\text{MAP} - \text{CVP}}{\text{cardiac output}} \times \text{a constant of 80}$$

Pulmonary vascular resistance (PVR), which reflects right ventricular afterload, is the total resistance to blood flow in the pulmonary circulation. Normal PVR is 20 to 120 dynes/second/cm^{-5} or absolute units. PVR is derived from other hemodynamic measurements, including pulmonary artery pressure (PAP). To calculate PVR, use this formula:

$$\text{PVR} = \frac{\text{mean PAP} - \text{PAWP}}{\text{cardiac output}} \times \text{a constant of 80}$$

Contractility indicators

Contractility refers to ventricular contractility. *Stroke volume* is the difference between volume at the end of diastole and left ventricular volume at the end of systole, which is the volume ejected with each heartbeat. Normal stroke volume is approximately 70 ml. You can calculate it using this formula:

$$\text{Stroke volume} = \frac{\text{cardiac output}}{\text{heart rate}}$$

Stroke volume index, which relates stroke volume to body size, produces a more accurate measurement than stroke volume. Normal stroke volume index is 40 ml/beat/m². To calculate it, divide the cardiac index by the heart rate.

Left ventricular stroke work (LVSW) reflects myocardial contractility. The normal range is 35 to 85 g/m²/beat. To calculate LVSW, use this formula:

$$\text{LVSW} = \frac{\text{cardiac output} \times \text{MAP}}{\text{heart rate}} \times \frac{\text{a constant}}{\text{of 13.6}}$$

Hemodynamic values in cardiogenic shock

This chart compares normal hemodynamic values to the hemodynamic values seen in patients with cardiogenic shock. Note that these values should be interpreted as general guidelines; each patient's trends will be distinct.

MEASUREMENT	NORMAL VALUE	VALUE IN CARDIOGENIC SHOCK
Systolic blood pressure	120 mm Hg	Low
Pulse pressure	40 mm Hg	Narrow
Cardiac output	4 to 6 liters/minute	Less than 2.5 liters/minute
Cardiac index	2.5 to 4.2 liters/minute/m²	Less than 2.0 liters/minute/m²
Stroke volume	70 ml	Low
Heart rate	60 to 100 beats/minute	More than 100 beats/minute
Pulmonary artery diastolic pressure	8 to 15 mm Hg	High
Pulmonary artery wedge pressure	4 to 12 mm Hg	More than 30 mm Hg
Central venous pressure	4 to 12 cm H_2O or 1 to 6 mm Hg (depending on device)	High
Systemic vascular resistance	900 to 1,200 absolute units	More than 1,400 absolute units
Pulmonary vascular resistance	20 to 120 absolute units	More than 120 absolute units
Left ventricular stroke work index	35 to 85 g/m²/beat	High

who has sustained abdominal trauma. The infused fluid may escape into the abdomen through a ruptured blood vessel.

• Administer oxygen by face mask or artificial airway to ensure adequate oxygenation of tissues. Adjust the oxygen flow rate to a higher or lower level, as arterial blood gas (ABG) measurements indicate. Many patients will need 100% oxygen, and some will require 5 to 15 cm H_2O of positive end-expiratory or continuous positive airway pressure ventilation.

• Administer an osmotic diuretic, such as mannitol, if ordered, to increase renal blood flow and urine output.

• When a patient is on the IABP, move him as little as possible.

◆ NURSING ALERT. Never flex the patient's "ballooned" leg at the hip because this may displace or fracture the catheter. Also never place the patient in a sitting position for any reason (including chest X-rays) while the balloon is inflated; the balloon will tear through the aorta and result in immediate death.

• If the patient becomes hemodynamically stable, gradually reduce the frequency of balloon inflation to wean him from the IABP.

• To ease emotional stress, plan your care to allow frequent rest periods and provide as much privacy as possible. Allow family members to visit and comfort the patient as much as possible.

• Allow the family members to express their anger, anxiety, and fear.

Devices used to treat cardiogenic shock

To improve the recovery chances of a patient with cardiogenic shock, the doctor may use an intra-aortic balloon pump (IABP) or a ventricular assist device (VAD).

Intra-aortic balloon pump

Placed in the descending thoracic aorta, the IABP pumps or propels blood in counterpoint to the heart's cycle of systole and diastole. After the balloon's catheter is connected to a pump console, the balloon is inflated and deflated automatically according to the patient's electrocardiogram or arterial waveform. Inflated during diastole, the balloon increases aortic diastolic pressure, which enhances coronary artery and peripheral perfusion.

The balloon is deflated immediately before systole, allowing the aortic valve to open under less pressure. This results in less work, less afterload, and less oxygen consumption.

Descending
thoracic
aorta

Ventricular assist device

A VAD may be used temporarily to pump the heart's blood. Types of VADs include the left ventricular assist device, right ventricular assist device, and biventricular assist device. Battery operated, the VAD diverts blood from the ventricular apex to the ascending aorta via surgically implanted outflow and inflow lines. VADs allow the failing heart to rest while recovering. They almost completely control stroke volume, reducing left ventricular workload while maintaining adequate perfusion.

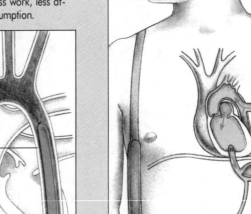

Monitoring

• Assess and record blood pressure, pulse, respiratory rate, and peripheral pulses every 1 to 5 minutes until the patient stabilizes. Record hemodynamic pressure readings every 15 minutes. Monitor cardiac rhythm continuously. Systolic blood pressure less than 80 mm Hg usually results in inadequate coronary artery blood flow, cardiac ischemia, arrhythmias, and further complications of low cardiac output. When blood pressure drops below 80 mm Hg, increase the oxygen flow rate and notify the doctor immediately.

♦ NURSING ALERT. A progressive drop in blood pressure accompanied by a thready pulse generally signals inadequate cardiac output from reduced intravascular volume. Notify the doctor, and increase the I.V. infusion rate.

• Using a pulmonary artery catheter, closely monitor pulmonary artery pressure, pulmonary artery wedge pressure (PAWP) and, if equipment is available, cardiac output A high PAWP indicates heart failure, increased systemic vascular resistance, decreased cardiac output, and decreased cardiac index and should be reported immediately.

• Insert an indwelling urinary catheter if necessary to measure hourly urine output. If output is less than 30 ml/hour (in adults), increase the fluid infusion rate but watch for signs of fluid overload, such as an increase in PAWP. Notify the doctor if urine output doesn't improve.

• Determine how much fluid to give by checking blood pressure, urine output, central venous pressure (CVP), or PAWP. (To increase accuracy, measure CVP at the level of the right atrium, using the same reference point on the chest each time.) Whenever the fluid infusion rate is increased, watch for signs of fluid overload, such as an increase in PAWP.

• Monitor ABG values, complete blood count, and electrolyte levels.

• During therapy, assess skin color and temperature and note any changes. Cold, clammy skin may be a sign of continuing peripheral vascular constriction, indicating progressive shock.

• During use of the IABP, assess pedal pulses and skin temperature and color to ensure adequate peripheral circulation. Check the dressing over the insertion site frequently for bleeding, and change it according to hospital policy. Also check the site for hematoma or signs of infection, and culture any drainage.

• When weaning the patient from the IABP, watch for ECG changes, chest pain, and other signs of recurring cardiac ischemia as well as for shock.

Patient teaching

• Because the patient and his family may be anxious about the ICU and about the IABP and other devices, offer explanations and reassurance.

DOSAGE FINDER

Identifying dopamine dosage in cardiogenic shock

For adjunctive treatment in cardiogenic shock, give an adult an infusion of 1 to 5 mcg/kg/minute initially. Increase the dosage by 1 to 4 mcg/kg/minute at 10- to 30-minute intervals until the desired response is achieved. The maintenance dosage is usually less than 20 mcg/kg/minute.

• Prepare the patient and his family for a probable fatal outcome, and help them find effective coping strategies.

HYPOVOLEMIC SHOCK

When intravascular blood volume drops dangerously low, hypovolemic shock ensues, leading to decreased cardiac output and inadequate tissue perfusion. The subsequent tissue anoxia prompts a shift in cellular metabolism from aerobic to anaerobic pathways. This results in an accumulation of lactic acid, which produces metabolic acidosis.

Without sufficient blood or fluid replacement, hypovolemic shock may lead to irreversible cerebral and renal damage, cardiac arrest and, ultimately, death. (See *How hypovolemic shock progresses,* page 158.)

CAUSES

Hypovolemic shock most commonly results from acute blood loss – about 20% of total volume. Massive blood loss may result from GI bleeding, internal or external hemorrhage, or any condition that reduces circulating intravascular volume or other body fluids.

Other causes include intestinal obstruction, peritonitis, acute pancreatitis, ascites, and dehydration from excessive perspiration, severe diarrhea or protracted vomiting, diabetes insipidus, diuresis, and inadequate fluid intake.

How hypovolemic shock progresses

Vascular fluid volume loss causes the extreme tissue hypoperfusion that characterizes hypovolemic shock. *Internal fluid loss* results from internal hemorrhage (such as GI bleeding) and third-space fluid shifting (such as in diabetic ketoacidosis). *External fluid loss* results from severe bleeding or from severe diarrhea, diuresis, or vomiting.

Inadequate vascular volume leads to decreased venous return and cardiac output. The resulting drop in arterial blood pressure activates the body's compensatory mechanisms in an attempt to increase vascular volume. If compensation is unsuccessful, decompensation and death may rapidly ensue.

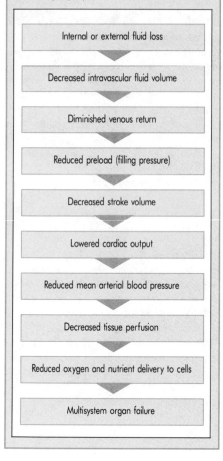

Internal or external fluid loss

⬇

Decreased intravascular fluid volume

⬇

Diminished venous return

⬇

Reduced preload (filling pressure)

⬇

Decreased stroke volume

⬇

Lowered cardiac output

⬇

Reduced mean arterial blood pressure

⬇

Decreased tissue perfusion

⬇

Reduced oxygen and nutrient delivery to cells

⬇

Multisystem organ failure

COMPLICATIONS

Without immediate treatment, hypovolemic shock can cause adult respiratory distress syndrome, acute tubular necrosis and renal failure, disseminated intravascular coagulation (DIC), multisystem organ failure, and death.

ASSESSMENT

The patient's history will include conditions that reduce blood volume, such as GI hemorrhage, trauma, and severe diarrhea and vomiting. A patient with cardiac disease may report anginal pain.

Inspection may reveal pale skin, decreased sensorium, and rapid, shallow respirations. Urine output usually falls below 25 ml/hour. Palpation may disclose rapid, thready peripheral pulses and cold, clammy skin. Auscultation of blood pressure usually detects a mean arterial pressure (MAP) below 60 mm Hg and a narrowing pulse pressure. In chronic hypotension, the MAP may fall below 50 mm Hg before signs of shock appear. (See *Hemodynamic values in hypovolemic shock.*)

Orthostatic vital signs may also detect shock. Such signs include a systolic blood pressure decrease of 10 mm Hg or more between positions (lying, sitting, and standing) or a pulse rate increase of 10 beats/minute. Likewise, in the tilt test, blood pressure that rises significantly while the patient lies supine with his legs raised above heart level indicates volume depletion and impending hypovolemic shock.

DIAGNOSTIC TESTS

Characteristic laboratory findings include:
• low hematocrit and decreased hemoglobin levels and red blood cell and platelet counts
• elevated serum potassium, sodium, lactate dehydrogenase, creatinine, and blood urea nitrogen levels
• increased urine specific gravity (greater than 1.020) and urine osmolality
• decreased urine creatinine levels
• decreased pH and partial pressure of arterial oxygen and increased partial pressure of arterial carbon dioxide.

X-rays, gastroscopy, aspiration of gastric contents through a nasogastric tube, and tests for occult blood identify internal bleeding sites. Coagulation studies may detect coagulopathy from DIC.

TREATMENT

Emergency treatment relies on prompt and adequate blood and fluid replacement to restore intravascular volume and to raise blood pressure and maintain it above 60 mm Hg. Rapid infusion of 0.9% sodium chloride or lactated Ringer's solution and, possibly, albumin or other plasma expanders may expand volume adequately until whole blood can be matched.

Treatment may also include application of a pneumatic antishock garment, oxygen administration, control of bleeding, dopamine or another inotropic drug and, possibly, surgery. To be effective, dopamine or other inotropic drugs require vigorous fluid resuscitation.

KEY NURSING DIAGNOSES AND PATIENT OUTCOMES

Altered tissue perfusion (cardiopulmonary, cerebral, renal) related to decreased cardiac output caused by blood loss. Based on this nursing diagnosis, you'll establish these patient outcomes. The patient will:
• not develop chest pain, cardiac arrhythmias, or shortness of breath
• stay alert and oriented to time, person, and place
• maintain urine output of at least 30 ml/hour
• regain or maintain normal GI function
• regain normal peripheral pulses, color, and temperature.

Decreased cardiac output related to diminished venous return caused by blood loss. Based on this nursing diagnosis, you'll establish these patient outcomes. The patient will:
• regain normal cardiac output, as evidenced by normal blood pressure, central venous pressure (CVP), right atrial pressure (RAP), pulmonary artery pressure (PAP), and pulmonary artery wedge pressure (PAWP) readings
• identify early signs and symptoms of decreased cardiac output (dizziness, syncope, cool or clammy skin, fatigue, and dyspnea), and ex-

---

Hemodynamic values in hypovolemic shock

Hemodynamic monitoring helps you evaluate the patient's cardiovascular status in hypovolemic shock. Look for values below the following normal ranges:
• central venous pressure below the normal range of 4 to 12 cm H_2O
• right atrial pressure below the normal mean of 1 to 6 mm Hg
• pulmonary artery pressure below the normal mean of 10 to 20 mm Hg
• pulmonary artery wedge pressure below the normal mean of 4 to 12 mm Hg
• cardiac output below the normal range of 4 to 6 liters/minute.

---

press the importance of seeking immediate medical attention if they occur.

Fluid volume deficit related to blood loss. Based on this nursing diagnosis, you'll establish these patient outcomes. The patient will:
• recover and maintain normal fluid volume as evidenced by stable vital signs and adequate urine output
• recover normal hemoglobin levels, hematocrit, red blood cell and platelet counts, arterial blood gas (ABG) and electrolyte levels, and urine specific gravity
• identify causes of fluid volume deficit and express the rationale for following a prescribed diet, taking medications, maintaining his activity level, and obtaining follow-up care.

NURSING INTERVENTIONS

• Check for a patent airway and adequate circulation. In cardiac or respiratory arrest, start cardiopulmonary resuscitation.
• Begin an I.V. infusion with 0.9% sodium chloride or lactated Ringer's solution given through a large-bore (14G to 18G) catheter.
• Help insert a central venous line and pulmonary artery catheter for hemodynamic monitoring.
• Insert an indwelling urinary catheter. If output falls below 30 ml/hour in an adult, in-

crease the fluid infusion rate, but watch for fluid overload (signaled by elevated PAWP). Notify the doctor if urine output doesn't increase.

• If the doctor orders an osmotic diuretic to increase renal blood flow and urine output, determine how much fluid to give by checking blood pressure, urine output, and CVP or PAWP.

• Draw an arterial blood sample to measure ABG levels. Give oxygen by face mask or airway to ensure adequate tissue oxygenation. Adjust the oxygen flow rate according to ABG measurements.

• Obtain and record the patient's blood pressure, pulse and respiratory rates, and peripheral pulse rates. When systolic blood pressure drops below 80 mm Hg, increase the oxygen flow rate, and notify the doctor immediately because systolic blood pressure below 80 mm Hg usually results in inadequate coronary artery blood flow, cardiac ischemia, arrhythmias, and further complications of low cardiac output.

• Also notify the doctor, and increase the infusion rate if the patient experiences a progressive drop in blood pressure and a thready pulse. This usually signals inadequate cardiac output from reduced intravascular volume.

• Draw venous blood for a complete blood count, electrolyte measurements, type and cross-matching, and coagulation studies.

Monitoring

• Record blood pressure, pulse and respiratory rates, and peripheral pulse rates every 15 minutes until stable. Monitor cardiac rhythm continuously.

• Monitor the patient's CVP, RAP, PAP, PAWP, and cardiac output hourly or as ordered.

• Measure the patient's urine output hourly.

• Monitor the patient's ABG and electrolyte levels frequently as ordered.

• During therapy, assess skin color and temperature, and note any changes. Cold, clammy skin may signal continuing peripheral vascular constriction, indicating progressive shock.

• Watch for signs of impending coagulopathy (petechiae, bruising, or bleeding or oozing from gums or venipuncture sites).

Patient teaching

• Explain all procedures, and discuss the risks associated with blood transfusions with the patient and his family.

6
Neurologic disorders

As the body's communications network, the nervous system coordinates and directs the functions of all body systems. As a result, any disease or trauma that alters nerve function can impair other organs and quickly become life-threatening. What's more, neurologic disease or trauma may trigger a downward spiral. For example, impaired cardiac output or gas exchange may traumatize the nervous system even more because of its need for adequate tissue oxygenation.

In this section, you'll find information on such acute, life-threatening neurologic disorders as head and spinal cord injury, cerebral aneurysm, status epilepticus, and myasthenic crisis. You'll also learn about infectious disorders that affect the nervous system, such as meningitis, encephalitis, and brain abscess.

As you care for the patient with an acute neurologic disorder, be alert for subtle changes in his condition that may herald an emergency. Perform frequent neurologic assessments, and monitor him closely to detect abnormalities so that you can intervene appropriately. Give supportive care, such as preventing further injury and providing comfort, to help avoid complications and ensure the patient's full recovery.

Initial neurologic care

Check for:
- history of neurologic conditions, especially chronic ones or head or spinal cord trauma
- medication history of drugs that alter neurologic function
- sensory, perceptual, or motor deficits
- airway obstruction, the presence and quality of respirations, and signs of hypoxia
- changes in heart rate, pulses, and blood pressure
- signs of increased intracranial pressure
- presence of spinal cord injury
- level of consciousness or pupillary changes
- paresis or paralysis
- leakage of cerebrospinal fluid from nose and ears
- restlessness or seizure activity
- aphasia, dysphasia, or slurred speech
- incontinence
- abnormal reflexes
- nuchal rigidity
- cranial nerve dysfunction
- temperature alterations.

Intervene by:
- notifying the doctor immediately
- initiating CPR, if needed
- stabilizing the spine
- administering oxygen
- inserting a large-bore needle for an I.V. line
- monitoring vital signs and neurologic status continuously.

Prepare for:
- medication administration
- possible intubation and mechanical ventilation
- emergency diagnostic studies
- emergency measures to correct underlying cause.

HEAD INJURIES

Injury to the head may result in a concussion, a cerebral contusion, or a skull fracture. By far the most common head injury, a *concussion* results from a blow to the head that's hard enough to jostle the brain and make it strike the skull, causing temporary neural dysfunction, but not hard enough to cause a cerebral contusion. Most concussion victims recover completely within 48 hours. Repeated concussions, however, exact a cumulative toll on the brain.

More serious than a concussion, a *cerebral contusion* is an ecchymosis of brain tissue that results from a severe blow to the head. A contusion disrupts normal nerve functions in the bruised area and may cause loss of consciousness, hemorrhage, edema, and even death.

A *skull fracture* is always considered serious and at times may be life-threatening. Because the primary concern isn't the fracture itself but possible damage to the brain, the injury is considered a neurosurgical condition. Signs and symptoms reflect the severity and extent of the head injury.

Skull fractures may be simple (closed) or compound (open) and may or may not displace bone fragments. They're also described as linear, comminuted, or depressed. A linear, or hairline, fracture doesn't displace structures and seldom requires treatment. A comminuted fracture splinters or crushes the bone into several fragments. A depressed fracture pushes the bone toward the brain; it's considered serious only if it compresses underlying structures.

Skull fractures also are classified according to location, such as cranial vault or basilar. A basilar fracture occurs at the base of the skull and involves the cribiform plate and the frontal sinuses. Because of the danger of cranial complications and meningitis, basilar fractures usually are far more serious than cranial vault fractures.

CAUSES

A traumatic blow to the head causes a head injury. The blow is usually sudden and forceful, such as a fall, a motor vehicle accident, or a punch to the head. If the blow causes an acceleration-deceleration or coup-contrecoup injury, then a cerebral contusion results.

Acceleration-deceleration or coup-contrecoup injuries can occur directly beneath the site of impact when the brain rebounds against the skull from the force of a blow (a beating with a blunt instrument, for example), when the force of the blow drives the brain against the opposite side of the skull, or when the head is hurled forward and stopped abruptly (as in a motor vehicle accident when the driver's head forcefully strikes the windshield). The brain continues moving and slaps against the skull (acceleration) and then rebounds (deceleration).

COMPLICATIONS

A *concussion* usually causes no significant anatomic brain injury. Seizures, persistent vomiting, or both may occur. Rarely, a concussion leads to intracranial hemorrhage (subdural, epidural, or parenchymal).

A *cerebral contusion* can cause intracranial hemorrhage or hematoma if the injury causes the brain to strike against bony prominences inside the skull (especially the sphenoidal ridges). Residual headaches and vertigo may complicate recovery. Secondary effects, such as brain swelling, may accompany serious contusions, resulting in increased intracranial pressure (ICP) and herniation. (See *What happens in increased ICP.*)

Skull fractures can lead to infection, intracerebral hemorrhage and hematoma, brain abscess, and increased ICP from edema. Recovery from the injury also can be complicated by residual effects of the injury, such as seizure disorders, hydrocephalus, and organic mental syndrome.

ASSESSMENT

The patient's history (which may be obtained from the patient, his family, eyewitnesses, or emergency personnel) reveals a traumatic in-

What happens in increased ICP

Increased intracranial pressure (ICP) is the force exerted within the intact skull by intracranial volume—about 10% blood, 10% cerebrospinal fluid (CSF), and 80% brain tissue and water. The rigid skull allows little space for expansion of these substances. When ICP increases dramatically, brain damage can result.

The brain compensates for increases by regulating the volume of the three substances by:
• limiting blood flow to the head

• displacing CSF into the spinal canal
• increasing absorption or decreasing production of CSF—withdrawing water from brain tissue into the blood and excreting it through the kidneys. When compensatory mechanisms become overworked, small changes in volume lead to large changes in pressure.

The flowchart will help you understand the pathophysiology of increased ICP.

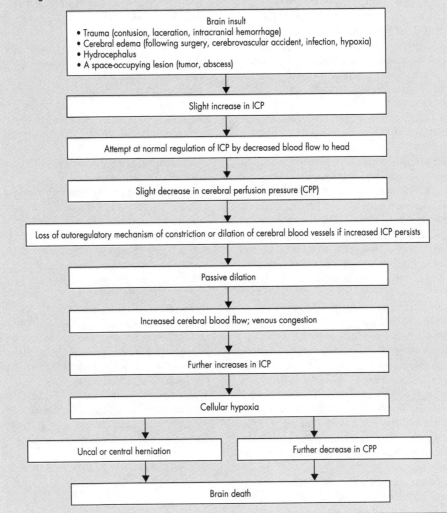

Brain insult
• Trauma (contusion, laceration, intracranial hemorrhage)
• Cerebral edema (following surgery, cerebrovascular accident, infection, hypoxia)
• Hydrocephalus
• A space-occupying lesion (tumor, abscess)

↓

Slight increase in ICP

↓

Attempt at normal regulation of ICP by decreased blood flow to head

↓

Slight decrease in cerebral perfusion pressure (CPP)

↓

Loss of autoregulatory mechanism of constriction or dilation of cerebral blood vessels if increased ICP persists

↓

Passive dilation

↓

Increased cerebral blood flow; venous congestion

↓

Further increases in ICP

↓

Cellular hypoxia

↓

Uncal or central herniation   Further decrease in CPP

↓   ↓

Brain death

jury to the head. A period of unconsciousness may follow the trauma. If unconscious, the patient may appear pale and motionless. If conscious, he may appear drowsy or easily disturbed by any form of stimulation, such as noise or light.

If the patient has a concussion, a family member or friend may report behavioral changes, saying that the patient is behaving out of character. The patient usually complains of dizziness, nausea, and severe headache. He may also exhibit anterograde and retrograde amnesias. The patient not only can't remember what happened immediately after the injury but also has difficulty remembering events that led up to it. Typically, he repeats the same questions. The presence of anterograde amnesia and the duration of retrograde amnesia reliably correlate with the injury's severity.

A conscious patient with a cerebral contusion may become agitated and even violent. If he has a skull fracture, he may complain of a persistent, localized headache. Depending on the type and location of the fracture, he may appear dazed, anxious, or agitated.

Your assessment findings will vary, depending on the type and location of the head injury. Vital signs will be normal in a patient with a concussion. In the conscious patient with a cerebral contusion, vital signs will vary with his emotional status; if he's unconscious, you may find below-normal blood pressure and temperature, a feeble but normal pulse rate, and shallow, labored respirations. In the patient with a skull fracture, you may assess decreased pulse and respiratory rates as well as labored respirations.

Because scalp wounds commonly accompany a cerebral contusion or skull fracture, scalp inspection may reveal abrasions, contusions, lacerations, or avulsions. If the scalp was lacerated or torn away, you may note profuse bleeding, although seldom heavy enough to induce hypovolemic shock. However, the patient may be in shock from other injuries or from medullary failure if the head injury is severe.

Other inspection findings in a patient with a skull fracture may include bleeding in the nose, pharynx, or ears; under the conjunctivae; under the periorbital skin (raccoon eyes); and behind the eardrum. You also may note Battle's sign. Inspection of the ears and nose may reveal cerebrospinal fluid (CSF) and brain tissue leakage. (Leakage may be found on the patient's pillowcase or bed linens.) Basilar fractures of the skull commonly produce hemorrhage from these areas. Red-tinged CSF drainage indicates brain injury.

Palpation of the skull may reveal tenderness or hematomas in a patient with a concussion. It may reveal palpable fractures, areas of swelling and, possibly, hematoma formation in a patient with a skull fracture. A vault fracture commonly causes soft-tissue swelling near the site, making other fractures hard to detect without X-rays.

A neurologic assessment usually produces normal findings in a patient with a concussion and abnormal findings in a patient with a cerebral contusion or skull fracture. A patient with a cerebral contusion may display hemiparesis, decorticate or decerebrate posturing, and unequal pupillary response. With effort, you may be able to rouse an unconscious patient temporarily. If the acute stage has passed, you may find that the patient has returned to a relatively alert state, perhaps with temporary aphasia, slight hemiparesis, or unilateral numbness.

If the patient has a skull fracture, you may note an altered level of consciousness (LOC) along with other classic signs of brain injury. These include agitation and irritability, abnormal deep tendon reflexes, altered pupillary and motor responses, hemiparesis, dizziness, seizures, and projectile vomiting. Loss of consciousness may last for hours, days, weeks, or indefinitely. Many findings, however, will vary with the location and severity of the fracture. For example, a linear fracture associated only with a concussion won't produce loss of consciousness; a sphenoidal fracture may produce vision loss; a temporal fracture may trigger unilateral hearing loss or facial paralysis.

DIAGNOSTIC TESTS

• *Skull X-rays* will locate a fracture, if present, unless the fracture is of the cranial vault. (These fractures aren't visible or palpable.)
• *Cerebral angiography* locates vascular disruptions from internal pressure or injury that result from a cerebral contusion or skull fracture.
• *Computed tomography scan* will disclose intracranial hemorrhage from ruptured blood vessels, ischemic or necrotic tissue, cerebral edema, areas of petechial hemorrhage, a shift in brain tissue, and subdural, epidural, and intracerebral hematomas that may have occurred from the head injury.
• *Magnetic resonance imaging* and a *radioisotope scan* may also disclose intracranial hemorrhage from ruptured blood vessels in a patient with a skull fracture.

TREATMENT

Treatment depends on the type of injury. Most patients with a concussion require no treatment except bed rest, observation, and acetaminophen for headache.

However, a patient with a cerebral contusion may require immediate emergency treatment, including establishment of a patent airway and, if necessary, a tracheotomy or endotracheal intubation. Treatment also may consist of I.V. fluids (dextrose 5% in 0.45% sodium chloride solution), I.V. mannitol to reduce ICP, and restricted fluid intake to decrease intracerebral edema. The patient's ICP may be reduced by maintaining his level of partial pressure of carbon dioxide in arterial blood ($Paco_2$) between 25 and 30 mm Hg, which will constrict cerebral blood vessels. (See *Types of ICP monitoring,* pages 166 and 167.) If necessary, additional treatments for the patient with a cerebral contusion may include blood transfusion and craniotomy.

Specific treatment for a skull fracture depends on the type of fracture. In general, if the patient hasn't lost consciousness, he should be observed in the emergency department for at least 4 hours. After this period, a patient with stable vital signs can be discharged. He should receive an instruction sheet for 24 to 48 hours of observation at home.

Although a simple linear skull fracture can tear an underlying blood vessel or cause a CSF leak, most linear fractures require only supportive treatment. Such treatment includes mild analgesics (acetaminophen) and wound management (local injection of procaine, shaving the scalp around the wound, and cleaning and debriding the wound).

More severe vault fractures, especially depressed fractures, usually require a craniotomy to elevate or remove fragments that have been driven into the brain and to extract foreign bodies and necrotic tissue. This reduces the risk of infection and further brain damage. Cranioplasty follows the use of tantalum mesh or acrylic plates to replace the removed skull section. The patient commonly requires antibiotics and, in profound hemorrhage, blood transfusions.

A basilar fracture calls for immediate prophylactic antibiotics to prevent meningitis from CSF leakage. The patient also needs close observation for secondary hematomas and hemorrhages; surgery may be necessary. Also, a patient with a basilar or vault fracture requires I.V. or I.M. dexamethasone to reduce cerebral edema and minimize brain tissue damage.

For status epilepticus, which may result from head injury, the patient may receive an anticonvulsant; usually, 10 to 15 mg/kg of I.V. phenytoin sodium is given at a rate of not more than 50 mg/minute or according to hospital policy.

KEY NURSING DIAGNOSES AND PATIENT OUTCOMES

Anxiety related to the threat of permanent neurologic injury or death. Based on this nursing diagnosis, you'll establish these patient outcomes. The patient will:
• express his feelings of anxiety
• use available support systems to help cope with his anxiety
• demonstrate that he experiences fewer physical symptoms caused by anxiety.

High risk for injury related to complications of head injury. Based on this nursing di-

Types of ICP monitoring

The four types of intracranial pressure (ICP) monitoring described here have important advantages and disadvantages.

Intraventricular catheter monitoring

In this procedure, which monitors ICP directly, the doctor inserts a catheter into the lateral ventricle through a burr hole.

Although this method measures ICP most accurately, it carries the greatest risk of infection. This is the only type of ICP monitoring that allows evaluation of brain compliance and drainage of significant amounts of cerebrospinal fluid (CSF).

Contraindications usually include stenotic cerebral ventricles, cerebral aneurysms in the path of catheter placement, and suspected vascular lesions.

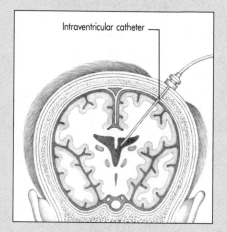

Intraventricular catheter

Subarachnoid screw monitoring

This procedure involves insertion of a special screw with a hollow bolt into the subarachnoid space through a twist-drill burr hole that's positioned in the front of the skull behind the hairline.

Placing the screw is easier than placing an intraventricular catheter, especially if a computed tomography scan reveals that the cerebrum has shifted or the ventricles have collapsed. This type of ICP monitoring also carries less risk of infection and parenchymal damage than intraventricular catheter monitoring because the screw doesn't penetrate the cerebrum.

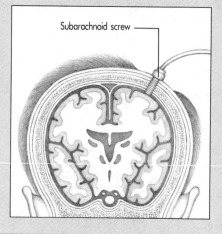

Subarachnoid screw

agnosis, you'll establish these patient outcomes. The patient will:
• avoid permanent neurologic deficit because of the head injury
• exhibit normal neurologic findings after the head injury heals.

Pain related to altered brain or skull tissue. Based on this nursing diagnosis, you'll establish these patient outcomes. The patient will:
• maintain normal ICP
• express pain relief with treatment
• obtain complete pain relief after the head injury heals.

Epidural sensor monitoring

The least invasive method with the lowest incidence of infection, this monitoring system uses a sensor inserted into the epidural space through a bur hole.

Unlike an intraventricular catheter or a subarachnoid screw, the sensor can't become occluded with blood or brain tissue. Accuracy is questionable, however, because the epidural sensor doesn't measure ICP directly from a CSF-filled space. Several types of sensors are available; some can be recalibrated repeatedly. Fiber-optic sensors must be calibrated before they're inserted.

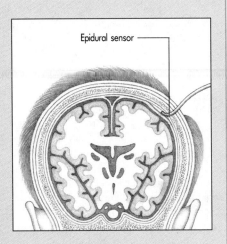

Intraparenchymal monitoring

In this procedure, the doctor inserts a catheter through a small subarachnoid bolt and, after puncturing the dura, advances the catheter a few centimeters into the brain's white matter. There's no need to balance or calibrate the equipment after insertion.

Although this method doesn't provide direct access to CSF, ICP measurements are accurate because brain tissue pressures correlate well with ventricular pressures. Intraparenchymal monitoring may be used to obtain ICP measurements in patients with compressed or dislocated ventricles.

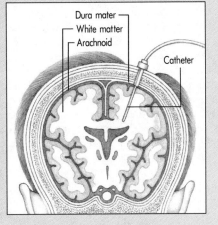

NURSING INTERVENTIONS

• Maintain a patent airway. Assist with endotracheal intubation or tracheotomy, as necessary.

• Administer medications as ordered. Give acetaminophen for pain, as ordered.

◆ NURSING ALERT. However, don't administer narcotics or sedatives because they may depress respirations, raise PaCO$_2$ levels, and lead to increased ICP. They also can mask changes in neurologic status.

• Protect the patient from injury according to his condition. Use side rails, assist the unsteady patient with walking, stay with the patient while he uses the bathroom, and place the confused patient where he can be easily observed.

• Insert an indwelling urinary catheter, if ordered.

• If the patient is unconscious, insert a nasogastric tube to prevent aspiration – but only after a basilar skull fracture has been ruled out. Otherwise, the tube may be inserted into the cranial vault.

• If the patient has CSF leakage or is unconscious, elevate the head of the bed 30 degrees; otherwise, leave it flat. Remember that such a patient is at risk for jugular compression, leading to increased ICP, when he's not positioned on his back. So be sure to keep his head properly aligned. Enforce bed rest.

• Position the patient so that secretions drain properly. If you detect CSF leakage from the nose, place a gauze pad under the nostrils. If CSF leaks from the ear, position the patient so his ear drains naturally; don't pack the ear or nose. If the patient requires suctioning, suction him through the mouth, not the nose, to avoid introducing bacteria into CSF.

• To reduce volume and intracerebral swelling, if indicated, restrict total fluid intake to 1,200 to 1,500 ml/day.

• To decrease the patient's anxiety, speak calmly to him and explain your actions, even if he's unconscious. Don't make any sudden, unexpected moves. Touch the patient gently.

• After the patient is stabilized, clean and dress any superficial scalp wounds. Be sure to wear sterile gloves. (If the skin has been broken, the patient may need tetanus prophylaxis.) Assist with suturing if needed. Carefully cover scalp wounds with a sterile dressing; control any bleeding as necessary.

• If the patient develops temporary aphasia, provide an alternative means of communication.

• Institute seizure precautions, but don't restrain the patient.

• Prepare the patient for a craniotomy, as indicated.

Monitoring

• Initially, monitor vital signs continuously and check for additional injuries. Abnormal respirations could indicate a breakdown in the brain's respiratory center and possibly an impending tentorial herniation – a neurologic emergency.

• Continue to check vital signs and neurologic status, including LOC and pupil size, every 15 minutes. If the patient's condition worsens or fluctuates, arrange for a neurosurgical consultation.

• Monitor the patient's ICP, if indicated.

• Observe the patient for headache, dizziness, irritability, and anxiety. If his condition worsens, perform a complete neurologic evaluation and notify the doctor.

• Monitor fluid and electrolyte levels and replace them as necessary.

• Assess the patient's oxygenation status through serial arterial blood gas studies, as ordered – especially if he's intubated.

• Carefully observe the patient for CSF leakage. Check the bed sheets for a blood-tinged spot surrounded by a lighter ring (halo sign).

• Observe the patient for agitated behavior, which may stem from hypoxia or increased ICP.

• Monitor the older patient especially closely. He may have brain atrophy and therefore more space for cerebral edema; ICP may increase, yet cause no signs.

• If the patient remains stable after 4 or more hours of observation, he can be discharged in the care of a responsible adult.

Patient teaching

• Explain to the patient who is discharged from the emergency department that a responsible adult, such as a family member or friend, should continue to observe his condition at home for the next 24 to 48 hours. If this isn't possible, the patient may be hospitalized briefly. Be sure to provide a head injury instruction sheet.

• Instruct the caregiver to awaken the patient every 2 hours throughout the night and to ask him his name, where he is, and whether he can identify the person. Tell the caregiver to return the patient to the hospital if he is difficult to arouse, is disoriented, or has seizures.

• Advise the caregiver to keep the sleep area quiet so the patient can sleep between the 2-hour intervals.

• Tell the patient to return to the hospital if he experiences a persistent or worsening head-

ache, forceful or constant vomiting, blurred vision, any change in personality, abnormal eye movements, a staggering gait, or twitching.
• Instruct the patient not to take anything stronger than acetaminophen for a headache. Warn him not to take aspirin because it may heighten the risk of bleeding.
• If vomiting occurs, instruct the patient to eat lightly until it stops. (Occasional vomiting is normal after a concussion.)
• Teach the patient to recognize symptoms of postconcussion syndrome—headache, dizziness, vertigo, anxiety, and fatigue. Tell him that the syndrome may persist for several weeks.
• Tell the patient with a cerebral contusion not to cough, sneeze, or blow his nose because these activities can increase ICP.
• Teach the patient and his family how to care for his scalp wound, if applicable. Emphasize the need to return for suture removal and follow-up evaluation.

SPINAL INJURIES

Usually the result of trauma to the head or neck, spinal injuries (other than spinal cord damage) include fractures, contusions, and compressions of the vertebral column. Spinal injuries most commonly occur in the twelfth thoracic, first lumbar, and fifth, sixth, and seventh cervical areas. The real danger from such injuries lies in associated damage to the spinal cord, which is potentially life-threatening.

CAUSES

Most serious spinal injuries result from motor vehicle accidents, falls, diving into shallow water, and gunshot wounds; less serious injuries, from lifting heavy objects and minor falls. Spinal dysfunction also may result from hyperparathyroidism and neoplastic lesions.

COMPLICATIONS

Spinal injury may damage the spinal cord, leading to neurogenic shock, paralysis, and even death. The extent of damage to the spinal cord depends on the level of injury to the spinal column.

ASSESSMENT

The patient's history may reveal trauma, a neoplastic lesion, an infection that could produce a spinal abscess, or an endocrine disorder. The patient typically complains of muscle spasm and back or neck pain that worsens with movement. In cervical fractures, point tenderness may be present; in dorsal and lumbar fractures, pain may radiate to other body areas, such as the legs.

Physical assessment (including a neurologic assessment) helps locate the level of injury and detect any cord damage. (See *Evaluating levels of innervation*, page 170.) General observation of the patient reveals that he limits movement and activities that cause pain. Inspection detects any surface wounds that occurred with the spinal injury. Palpation can identify pain location and loss of sensation.

If the injury damages the spinal cord, you'll note clinical effects that range from mild paresthesia to quadriplegia and shock.

DIAGNOSTIC TESTS

Spinal X-rays, myelography, and computed tomography and magnetic resonance imaging scans locate the fracture or site of the compression.

TREATMENT

The primary treatment after spinal injury is immediate immobilization to stabilize the spine and prevent cord damage; other treatment is supportive.

Cervical injuries require immobilization, using sandbags on both sides of the patient's head, a plaster cast, a hard cervical collar, or skeletal traction with skull tongs (Crutchfield, Barton, Vinke) or a halo device. (See *Skeletal traction devices*, page 171.)

Treatment of stable lumbar and dorsal fractures consists of bed rest on a firm surface (such as a bed board), analgesics, and muscle relaxants until the fracture stabilizes (usually in 10 to 12 weeks). Later treatment includes exercises to strengthen the back muscles and a back brace or corset to provide support while walking.

Evaluating levels of innervation

This chart will help you determine muscle movements to assess your patient's level of innervation. Grade the quality of these movements on a motor strength scale. Using such a scale, 5 is normal; 4 means range of motion (ROM) with resistance; 3 means full ROM against gravity; 2, full ROM with gravity eliminated; and 1, visible or palpable contractions.

LEVEL OF INNERVATION	MUSCLE INVOLVED	PATIENT INSTRUCTIONS
Third or fourth cervical vertebra	Diaphragm Trapezius	• To inhale deeply • To shrug his shoulders
Fourth or fifth cervical vertebra	Deltoid	• To flap his arms • To push his shoulders forward and backward
Fifth cervical vertebra	Biceps	• To bend his arm up and make a muscle
Sixth cervical vertebra	Wrist	• To move his wrist up and down *Note:* Be sure to prevent arm supination and pronation, which the patient may substitute for the actual muscle movement.
Seventh cervical vertebra	Triceps	• To bring his arm across his chest, then straighten his arm with his thumb pointing to his chest and his supporting elbow up *Note:* The patient can substitute the deltoid and extensor biceps to perform this movement.
Eighth cervical vertebra	Hand	• To squeeze your hand • To open his hand and spread his fingers
First lumbar vertebra	Iliopsoas Hip rotator	• To lift his leg off the bed • To pull his leg back
Second to fourth lumbar vertebrae	Quadriceps	• To bend his knee and straighten his leg. Tell him to support the knee with his arm if necessary.
Fifth lumbar vertebra	Ankle dorsiflexion muscles	• To pretend he's stepping on the gas pedal
First or second sacral vertebra	Ankle plantarflexion muscles	• To pull his toes toward his head

An unstable dorsal or lumbar fracture requires a plaster cast, a turning frame and, in severe fracture, laminectomy and spinal fusion.

When the damage results in compression of the spinal column, neurosurgery may relieve the pressure. If the cause of compression is a neoplastic lesion, chemotherapy and radiation may relieve the compression by shrinking the lesion. Surface wounds that accompany the spinal injury require wound care and tetanus prophylaxis unless the patient has recently been immunized.

KEY NURSING DIAGNOSES AND PATIENT OUTCOMES

Fear related to potential for permanent neurologic deficits or death. Based on this nursing diagnosis, you'll establish these patient outcomes. The patient will:
• identify and express feelings of fear
• use available support systems to cope with fear

Skeletal traction devices

A halo-vest traction device or skull tongs may be used to immobilize the head and neck of a patient with a cervical vertebrae injury.

Halo-vest traction device

Halo devices consist of a metal ring that fits over the patient's head and metal bars that connect the ring to a plastic vest that distributes the weight of the entire apparatus around the chest. This device allows greater mobility than skull tongs and carries less risk of infection because it doesn't require skin incisions and drill holes to position skull pins.

In the low-profile (standard) device, traction and compression are produced by threaded support rods on either side of the halo ring. Flexion and extension are obtained by moving the swivel arm to an anterior or posterior position, depending on the location of the skull pins.

Skull tongs

Skull (or cervical) tongs consist of a stainless steel body with a pin at the end of each arm. Each pin is about ⅛" (0.3 cm) in diameter with a sharp tip. On Crutchfield tongs, the pins are placed about 5" (13 cm) apart in line with the long axis of the cervical spine.

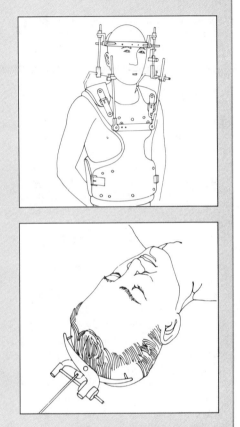

• demonstrate healthy coping behaviors in managing fear.

Decreased cardiac output related to neurogenic shock caused by spinal cord injury. Based on this nursing diagnosis, you'll establish these patient outcomes. The patient will:
• regain and maintain hemodynamic stability exhibited by stable vital signs
• demonstrate no serious adverse effects such as arrhythmias, chest pain, decreased urinary output, or altered mental status
• regain normal cardiac output.

Impaired physical mobility related to neurologic dysfunction. Based on this nursing diagnosis, you'll establish these patient outcomes. The patient will:
• maintain muscle strength and joint range of motion
• show no evidence of complications, such as contractures, venous stasis, or skin breakdown
• achieve the highest level of mobility possible following spinal injury.

NURSING INTERVENTIONS

• As in all spinal injuries, suspect cord damage until proved otherwise.

• During the initial assessment and X-rays, immobilize the patient on a firm surface, with sandbags on both sides of his head. Tell him not to move.

• If possible, avoid moving him because hyperflexion can damage the cord. If you must move him, get at least one other member of the staff to help you logroll him so that you don't disturb his body alignment.

• Offer comfort and reassurance to the patient, talking to him quietly and calmly. Remember, the fear of possible paralysis will be overwhelming. Allow a family member who isn't too distraught to stay with him.

• If the injury necessitates surgery, administer prophylactic antibiotics, as ordered. Catheterize the patient as ordered to avoid urine retention, and monitor defecation patterns to avoid impaction.

• If the patient has a halo or skull tong traction device, clean the pin sites daily, trim his hair short, and provide analgesics for headaches. During traction, turn the patient often to prevent pneumonia, embolism, and skin breakdown. Perform passive range-of-motion exercises to maintain muscle tone. If available, use a CircOlectric bed or Stryker frame to facilitate turning and to avoid spinal cord injury.

• To prevent aspiration, turn the patient on his side during feedings. Create a relaxed atmosphere at mealtimes.

• If necessary, insert a nasogastric tube to prevent gastric distention.

• Suggest appropriate diversionary activities to fill the hours of immobility. Offer prism glasses for reading.

• Help the patient walk as soon as the doctor allows; he'll probably have to wear a back brace.

Monitoring

• Watch closely for neurologic changes. Immediately report changes in skin sensation and loss of muscle strength. Either could point to pressure on the spinal cord, possibly as a result of edema or shifting bone fragments.

• Observe the patient closely for signs and symptoms of complications associated with spinal injuries or prolonged immobility, such as pneumonia, skin breakdown, and renal calculi.

Patient teaching

• Explain traction methods to the patient and his family, and reassure them that a halo traction device or skull tongs don't penetrate the brain.

• Tell the patient about the prescribed regimen for home care.

• Teach the patient exercises to maintain physical mobility.

• Instruct the patient about his medications, including adverse effects and the duration of treatment.

• Stress the importance of follow-up examinations.

CEREBRAL ANEURYSM

This localized dilation of a cerebral artery results from a weakness in the arterial wall. Its most common form is the saccular (berry) aneurysm, a saclike outpouching in a cerebral artery. (See *Comparing cerebral aneurysms.*) Cerebral aneurysms commonly rupture, causing subarachnoid hemorrhage. Sometimes bleeding also spills into the brain tissue and subsequently forms a clot. This may result in potentially fatal increased intracranial pressure (ICP) and brain tissue damage.

Most cerebral aneurysms occur at bifurcations of major arteries in the circle of Willis and its branches. An aneurysm can produce neurologic symptoms by exerting pressure on the surrounding structures, such as the cranial nerves. (See *Common sites of cerebral aneurysm,* page 174.)

Cerebral aneurysms are much more common in adults than in children. Incidence is slightly higher in women than in men, especially women in their late 40s or early to middle 50s, but cerebral aneurysm may occur at

Comparing cerebral aneurysms

Cerebral aneurysms may be classified by their size, shape, cause, and other characteristics. The following lists the various types of aneurysms and their characteristics.

Saccular (berry) aneurysm
• Most common type
• Secondary to congenital weakness of media
• Usually occurs at major vessel bifurcations
• Occurs at the circle of Willis
• Has a neck or stem
• Has a sac that may be partly filled with a blood clot

Fusiform (spindle-shaped) aneurysm
• Occurs with atherosclerotic disease
• Characterized by irregular vessel dilation
• Develops on internal carotid or basilar arteries
• Rarely ruptures
• Produces brain and cranial nerve compression or cerebrospinal fluid obstruction

Mycotic aneurysm
• Rare
• Associated with septic emboli that occur secondary to bacterial endocarditis
• Develops when emboli lodge in the arterial lumen, causing arteritis; the arterial wall weakens and dilates

Dissecting aneurysm
• Caused by arteriosclerosis, head injury, syphilis, or trauma during angiography
• Develops when blood is forced between layers of arterial walls, stripping intima from the underlying muscle layer

Traumatic aneurysm
• Develops in the carotid system
• Associated with fractures and intimal damage
• May thrombose spontaneously

Giant aneurysm
• Similiar to saccular, but larger – 1⅛" (3 cm) or more in diameter
• Behaves like a space-occupying lesion, producing cerebral tissue compression and cranial nerve damage
• Associated with hypertension

Charcot-Bouchard aneurysm
• Microscopic
• Associated with hypertension
• Involves basal ganglia or brain stem

any age. In about 20% of patients, multiple aneurysms occur.

The prognosis is usually guarded but depends on the patient's age and neurologic condition, the presence of other diseases, and the extent and location of the aneurysm. About half the patients who suffer subarachnoid hemorrhages die immediately. With new and better treatment, the prognosis is improving.

CAUSES
Cerebral aneurysm results from a congenital defect of the vessel wall, head trauma, hypertensive vascular disease, advanced age, infection, or atherosclerosis, which can weaken the vessel wall.

COMPLICATIONS
Potentially fatal complications after rupture of an aneurysm include subarachnoid hemorrhage and brain tissue infarction. Cerebral vasospasm, probably the most common cause of death after rupture, occurs in about 40% of all patients after subarachnoid hemorrhage occurs.

Other possible complications include rebleeding, which usually occurs within the first 24 to 48 hours after rupture but can occur any time within the first 6 months; meningeal irritation from blood in the subarachnoid space; and hydrocephalus, which can occur weeks or even months after rupture if blood obstructs the fourth ventricle.

Common sites of cerebral aneurysm

Cerebral aneurysms usually arise at arterial bifurcations in the circle of Willis and its branches. The illustration below shows the most common aneurysm sites around this circle.

ASSESSMENT

Most cerebral aneurysms produce no symptoms until rupture occurs. A history may have to be obtained from a family member if the patient is unconscious or severely neurologically impaired.

Usually, the patient's history reveals the onset of an unusually severe headache that is accompanied by nausea, vomiting and, commonly, loss of consciousness. The patient or family member may report that rupture of the aneurysm was preceded by a period of activity, such as exercise, labor and delivery, or sexual intercourse. The patient also may have a history of hypertension, infection, or head injury.

◆ NURSING ALERT. Although cerebral aneurysms usually rupture without warning, they sometimes leak blood for up to several days, causing premonitory symptoms of rupture. If your patient reports nuchal rigidity, stiff back and legs, and intermittent nausea, notify the doctor immediately. "Warning leaks" can occur a few hours to a few days before severe bleeding, which causes cerebral damage, coma, and death.

Other findings vary with the location of the aneurysm and the extent and severity of hemorrhage. Bleeding causes meningeal irritation, which can result in nuchal rigidity, back and leg pain, fever, restlessness, irritability, occasional seizures, and blurred vision. If the aneurysm is adjacent to the oculomotor nerve, ptosis and vision disturbances such as diplopia and vision loss may occur. If the bleeding extends into the brain tissue, hemiparesis, unilateral sensory deficits, dysphagia, visual defects, and altered consciousness may occur.

To better describe the condition of patients with ruptured cerebral aneurysm, the following grading system has been developed:
• *Grade I (minimal bleeding)*—patient is alert, with no neurologic deficit; he may have a slight headache and nuchal rigidity.
• *Grade II (mild bleeding)*—patient is alert with a mild to severe headache, nuchal rigidity and, possibly, third nerve palsy.
• *Grade III (moderate bleeding)*—patient is confused or drowsy, with nuchal rigidity and, possibly, a mild focal deficit.
• *Grade IV (severe bleeding)*—patient is stuporous, with nuchal rigidity and, possibly, mild to severe hemiparesis.
• *Grade V (moribund [often fatal])*—if nonfatal, patient is in deep coma or decerebrate.

DIAGNOSTIC TESTS

The following tests help establish a diagnosis, which, unfortunately, usually follows aneurysmal rupture:
• *Angiography* confirms an unruptured cerebral aneurysm.
• *Lumbar puncture* can detect blood in the cerebrospinal fluid (CSF), but this procedure is contraindicated if the patient shows signs of increased ICP.
• *Skull X-rays* may show calcification in the walls of a large aneurysm.
• *EEG* commonly shows flattened or depressed T waves.

• *Computed tomography scan* locates the clot and identifies hydrocephalus, areas of infarction, and the extent of blood spillage within the cisterns around the brain.

TREATMENT

Initial emergency treatment includes oxygenation and ventilation. Then, to reduce the risk of rebleeding, the doctor may attempt to repair the aneurysm. Usually, surgical repair (by clipping, ligating, or wrapping the aneurysm neck with muscle) takes place 7 to 10 days after the initial bleed; however, surgery performed within 1 to 2 days after hemorrhage has also shown promise in grades I and II.

After surgical repair, the patient's condition depends on the extent of damage from the initial bleed and the degree of successful treatment of the resulting complications. Surgery can't improve the patient's neurologic condition unless it removes a hematoma or reduces the compression effect.

When surgical correction poses too much risk (for example, in older patients and those with heart, lung, or other serious diseases), when the aneurysm is in a particularly dangerous location, or when vasospasm necessitates a delay in surgery, the patient may receive conservative treatment. This includes:
• bed rest in a quiet, darkened room, with the head of the bed flat or raised less than 30 degrees; if immediate surgery isn't possible, such bed rest may continue for 4 to 6 weeks
• avoidance of coffee, other stimulants, and aspirin
• codeine or another analgesic, as needed
• hydralazine or another antihypertensive agent, if the patient is hypertensive
• a vasoconstrictor to maintain blood pressure at the optimum level (20 to 40 mm Hg above normal), if necessary
• corticosteroids to reduce cerebral edema
• phenobarbital or another sedative to keep the patient relaxed
• aminocaproic acid, a fibrinolytic inhibitor, to minimize the risk of rebleeding by delaying blood clot lysis; however, this drug's effectiveness is controversial.

KEY NURSING DIAGNOSES AND PATIENT OUTCOMES

Altered thought processes related to neurologic impairment caused by a ruptured cerebral aneurysm. Based on this nursing diagnosis, you'll establish these patient outcomes. The patient will:
• remain free from injury
• exhibit normal thought processes.

Altered cerebral tissue perfusion related to inadequate oxygenation of cerebral tissue caused by bleeding from a ruptured cerebral aneurysm. Based on this nursing diagnosis, you'll establish these patient outcomes. The patient will:
• regain adequate cerebral tissue perfusion as exhibited by being oriented to time, person, and place
• demonstrate normal neurologic function.

High risk for injury related to increased ICP caused by a ruptured cerebral aneurysm. Based on this nursing diagnosis, you'll establish these patient outcomes. The patient will:
• have a normal ICP
• experience no signs of permanent neurologic injury, such as paralysis, speech impairment, or memory loss.

NURSING INTERVENTIONS

• Establish and maintain a patent airway because the patient may need supplemental oxygen. Position the patient to promote pulmonary drainage and prevent upper airway obstruction. Following hospital policy, suction secretions from the airway as necessary to prevent hypoxia and vasodilation from carbon dioxide accumulation. Suction for fewer than 20 seconds to avoid increased ICP.
• Prepare the patient for an emergency craniotomy, if indicated.
• If surgery can't be performed immediately, institute aneurysm precautions to minimize the risk of rebleeding and to avoid increasing the patient's ICP. Limit the patient's visitors, restrict his fluid intake, and tell the patient to avoid performing Valsalva's maneuver.
• Administer hydralazine or another antihypertensive agent, as ordered.

• Administer aminocaproic acid I.V. in dextrose 5% in water, as ordered. Administer the drug at least every 2 hours to maintain therapeutic serum drug levels. (If the patient has renal insufficiency, he may require a dosage adjustment.)

• Turn the patient often. Encourage deep breathing and leg movement. Assist with active range-of-motion (ROM) exercises; if the patient is paralyzed, perform passive ROM exercises.

• Apply elastic stockings to the patient's legs to reduce the risk of deep vein thrombosis.

• Provide frequent nose and mouth care.

• Give fluids, as ordered, and monitor I.V. infusions to avoid overhydration, which may increase ICP.

• If the patient has facial weakness, assist him during meals; assess his gag reflex, and place the food in the unaffected side of his mouth.

• If the patient can't swallow, insert a nasogastric tube, as ordered, and give all tube feedings slowly. Prevent skin breakdown by taping the tube so it doesn't press against the nostril.

• If the patient can eat, provide a high-bulk diet (bran, salads, and fruit) to prevent straining during defecation, which can increase ICP. Get an order for a stool softener, such as dioctyl sodium sulfosuccinate, or a mild laxative, and administer as ordered. Don't force fluids. Implement a bowel elimination program based on previous habits. If the patient is receiving steroids, check the stool for blood.

• If the patient has third or facial nerve palsy, administer artificial tears to the affected eye, and tape the eye shut at night to prevent corneal damage.

• Raise the bed's side rails to protect the patient from injury. If possible, avoid using restraints because these can cause agitation and raise ICP.

• Provide emotional support to the patient and his family. To minimize stress, encourage the patient to use relaxation techniques. Encourage him to express his concerns if he's able.

Monitoring

• Closely observe the patient for signs of increasing ICP, such as restlessness, weakness, or a changed speech pattern. Also watch for decreased level of consciousness (LOC), a unilaterally enlarged pupil, onset or worsening of hemiparesis or motor deficit, increased blood pressure, decreased heart rate, worsened or sudden headache, renewed or persistent vomiting, and renewed or worsened nuchal rigidity. These signs and symptoms may indicate an enlarging aneurysm, rebleeding, an intracranial clot, vasospasm, or another complication; report them immediately.

• Carefully monitor the patient's blood pressure. Report any significant changes, particularly a rise in systolic pressure.

• If the patient is receiving aminocaproic acid, watch for adverse reactions. Common adverse reactions include nausea and diarrhea with oral administration and phlebitis with I.V. administration.

• Frequently check the patient's arterial blood gas values, intake and output, and vital signs. Don't take the patient's temperature rectally. Doing so could stimulate the vagus nerve and lead to cardiac arrest.

Patient teaching

• Teach the patient, if possible, and his family about his condition. Encourage family members to adopt a realistic attitude, but don't discourage hope. Answer questions honestly.

• Explain all tests, neurologic examinations, treatments, and procedures to the patient even if he's unconscious.

• Warn the patient who will be treated conservatively to avoid all unnecessary physical activity.

• If surgery will be performed, provide preoperative teaching if the patient's condition permits. Make sure the patient, if possible, and the family understand the surgery and its possible complications. Reinforce the doctor's explanations as necessary.

• Before discharge, make a referral to a home health care nurse, or a rehabilitation center when necessary.

• Teach family members to recognize and immediately report signs of rebleeding, such as headache, nausea, vomiting, and changes in LOC.

STATUS EPILEPTICUS

In this disorder, the patient suffers a series of rapidly repeated seizures without recovering neurologic function between attacks. Although status epilepticus may involve any type of seizure, generalized tonic-clonic seizures are the most common type; they're also the most dangerous and life-threathening because they increase the risk of anoxia, arrhythmias, and systemic lactic acidosis.

CAUSES

In most patients, the cause of status epilepticus remains unknown. However, factors that may precipitate it include abrupt withdrawal of anticonvulsant drugs or alcohol, inadequate blood glucose levels, a brain tumor, a head injury, a high fever, central nervous system infections, and poisoning.

COMPLICATIONS

Status epilepticus may cause traumatic injury from a fall as well as various life-threatening complications, such as aspiration (from an altered level of consciousness [LOC] and a compromised airway); hypoxia (from altered respiratory processes and airway occlusion); and anoxia (from altered respiratory processes and airway occlusion). These conditions may lead to brain cell death and cytotoxic cerebral edema, which in turn may cause brain herniation and metabolic disturbances. Rhabdomyolysis—muscle disintegration or dissolution resulting from increased energy consumption due to rapid, repetitive contraction—also may occur and poses a grave risk. Death may ensue from multisystem collapse or from brain cell death.

ASSESSMENT

The history may reveal a known precipitating factor and a preexisting seizure disorder.

Inspection reveals a continuous seizure state. One of three types of status epilepticus may be evident. Patients with generalized tonic-clonic status epilepticus, the most life-threatening form, exhibit continuous generalized tonic-clonic seizures with no intervening return of consciousness. Respiratory distress is also evident. In the second type, absence status, the patient may exhibit 200 to 300 "absences" per day. In the third type, partial or focal status (also known as epilepsia continua), focal seizures occur continuously or regularly, and the patient usually remains conscious unless generalization occurs.

DIAGNOSTIC TESTS

The immediate diagnosis of status epilepticus is based on the patient's presentation in a continuous seizure state. In addition, the doctor may order the following tests to try to determine the underlying cause:
• *Complete blood count* may reveal an elevated white blood cell count, which may indicate infection.
• *Electrolyte analysis* may disclose hyponatremia, hypomagnesemia, or acid-base imbalance.
• *Renal studies* may reveal uremia, whereas *liver function studies* may disclose metabolic disturbances.
• *Computed tomography scan* may be ordered, once the patient is stabilized, to rule out traumatic injury or brain tumor.
• *Magnetic resonance imaging scan* and *cerebral arteriography* may be ordered to reveal any cerebral or vascular abnormalities.
• *Lumbar puncture* may be performed if the doctor suspects an infectious cause, such as meningitis, encephalitis, or a brain abscess.

In addition, an *EEG* supports the diagnosis, helps determine the type of seizure, and may help establish the prognosis.

TREATMENT

The first priority is to maintain adequate oxygenation and an open airway. Status epilepticus is then treated with aggressive intravenous anticonvulsant therapy to halt the seizures. The most commonly used I.V. drugs are diazepam, phenobarbital, and phenytoin. (See *Identifying drug dosages in status epilepticus,* page 178.) Other I.V. drugs that may be ordered are dextrose 50% (when seizures are secondary to hypoglycemia) and thiamine (in the presence of chronic alcoholism or withdrawal).

Identifying drug dosages in status epilepticus

The following drugs are used to halt status epilepticus.

Diazepam
To treat status epilepticus and recurrent seizures, give an adult 5 to 10 mg by slow I.V. push at 2 to 5 mg/minute. If necessary, repeat the dose every 10 to 15 minutes. The maximum dose is 30 mg. For older or debilitated patients, give 2 to 5 mg I.M. or I.V.
For recurrent seizures, the dose may be repeated in 20 to 30 minutes.

Phenobarbital
To treat status epilepticus and other acute seizure disorders not controlled by diazepam, give an adult 200 to 600 mg by slow injection at a rate not exceeding 60 mg/minute. Don't exceed a total dose of 20 mg/kg or 600 mg.

Phenytoin
To treat status epilepticus, give an adult 150 to 250 mg by direct injection. If necessary after 30 minutes, give 100 to 150 mg, or give 8 to 18 mg/kg at a rate not to exceed 50 mg/minute. The maximum daily dose is 1.5 g.

If these drugs don't halt seizure activity quickly, the doctor may induce pharmacologic paralysis to ease intubation and ensure respiratory support.

◆ NURSING ALERT. Be aware that stopping the visible seizure activity with a paralytic agent doesn't necessarily abolish the seizure. To avoid clinical confusion about halting the seizure versus masking the motor responses, some doctors use a short-acting nondepolarizing muscle relaxant, such as vecuronium.

KEY NURSING DIAGNOSES AND PATIENT OUTCOMES

Inability to sustain spontaneous ventilation related to continuous muscle contraction caused by seizures. Based on this nursing diagnosis, you'll establish these patient outcomes. The patient will:

• be intubated immediately and placed on mechanical ventilation
• regain and maintain normal arterial blood gas (ABG) and oxygen saturation values
• be able to breathe spontaneously after ventilator support is withdrawn.

High risk for injury related to hypoxia and anoxia caused by seizure activity. Based on this nursing diagnosis, you'll establish these patient outcomes. The patient will:
• have his altered state detected quickly and promptly treated
• show no residual neurologic deficits after seizure activity has ceased.

Ineffective airway clearance related to involuntary muscle contraction caused by seizure activity. Based on this nursing diagnosis, you'll establish these patient outcomes. The patient will:
• maintain a patent airway
• exhibit no adventitious breath sounds.

NURSING INTERVENTIONS

• Notify the doctor immediately but don't leave the patient unattended.
• Ensure a patent airway.

◆ NURSING ALERT. Don't attempt to insert an artificial airway until the patient's muscles have relaxed. Otherwise, his tongue may occlude the airway or his teeth may break, creating a partial occlusion.
• Establish an I.V. line and be prepared to administer I.V. medication to stop seizure activity. Maintain I.V. access until seizure activity has stopped and an effective therapeutic regimen has been established.
• Draw blood for glucose, electrolyte, blood urea nitrogen, ABG, and creatine kinase levels to determine possible causes.
• Ongoing care focuses on ensuring overall patient well-being, avoiding more seizures, and preventing complications such as injury.
• Arrange for a nutritional consultation to counter the effects of the catabolism caused by status epilepticus. During seizures, muscles consume oxygen and nutrients create an oxygen debt, depriving other body tissues of oxygen and nutrients. Make sure you're familiar with the effects of food on the absorption rates of prescribed anticonvulsants to ensure opti-

mal absorption and maintenance of serum levels.

• To avoid injury and minimize the risk of inducing seizures, maintain seizure precautions at all times: Enforce bed rest or supervise the patient's activities. Keep the bed's side rails up and padded, and keep airway and suction equipment at the bedside. Make sure the patient wears only loose-fitting clothes.

Monitoring

• Continuously monitor the patient during status epilepticus.

• Frequently check ABG values during status epilepticus and for 24 hours afterward to help detect hypoxia and acid-base imbalances. Also evaluate the patient's glucose, electrolytes, and renal function studies for abnormalities.

• Monitor the patient's vital signs closely to ensure adequate blood pressure and heart rate.

• Perform a neurologic assessment every hour. Watch for desired and adverse effects of anticonvulsant drugs, and monitor blood drug levels closely.

Patient teaching

• Teach the patient and family about seizures, and emphasize the need to get emergency care when one occurs. Instruct the patient to stay alert for prodromal (warning) signs: mood or behavioral changes and an aura, such as a metallic taste, a flash of light, or an unusual smell or sound.

• As appropriate, refer the patient to the Epilepsy Foundation of America for support.

MENINGITIS

In this disorder, the brain and the spinal cord meninges become inflamed. Such inflammation may involve all three meningeal membranes — the dura mater, the arachnoid membrane, and the pia mater.

For most patients, meningitis follows onset of respiratory symptoms. In about 50% of patients, it develops over 1 to 7 days; in just under 20% of patients, it occurs 1 to 3 weeks after respiratory symptoms appear. Unheralded by respiratory symptoms, meningitis has a sudden onset in about 25% of patients, who become seriously ill within 24 hours.

The prognosis is good and complications are rare, especially if the disease is recognized early and the infecting organism responds to antibiotics. However, mortality in untreated meningitis is 70% to 100%. The prognosis is poorer for older people.

CAUSES

Meningitis can be caused by bacteria, viruses, protozoa, or fungi. It most commonly results from bacterial infection, usually caused by *Neisseria meningitidis, Haemophilus influenzae, Streptococcus pneumoniae,* and *Escherichia coli.* In some patients, no causative organism can be found.

In most patients, the infection that causes meningitis is secondary to another bacterial infection, such as bacteremia (especially from pneumonia, empyema, osteomyelitis, and endocarditis), sinusitis, otitis media, encephalitis, myelitis, and brain abscess. Meningitis may also follow skull fracture, a penetrating head wound, lumbar puncture, or ventricular shunting procedures.

When meningitis is caused by a virus, it's known as aseptic viral meningitis. (See *What you should know about aseptic viral meningitis,* page 180.)

Older people have the highest risk of developing meningitis. In addition to age, other risk factors include malnourishment, immunosuppression (as from radiation therapy, chemotherapy, or long-term steroid therapy), and central nervous system trauma.

COMPLICATIONS

Depending on the cause and severity of the illness, potential complications of meningitis include visual impairment, optic neuritis, cranial nerve palsies, deafness, personality change, headache, paresis or paralysis, endocarditis, coma, vasculitis, and cerebral infarction.

What you should know about aseptic viral meningitis

A benign syndrome, aseptic viral meningitis is characterized by headache, fever, vomiting, and meningeal symptoms. It results from some form of viral infection, such as from an enterovirus (most common), arbovirus, herpes simplex virus, mumps virus, or lymphocytic choriomeningitis virus.

Assessment

The history of a patient with aseptic viral meningitis usually shows that the disease began suddenly with a fever up to 104° F (40° C), alterations in level of consciousness (drowsiness, confusion, stupor), and neck or spinal stiffness that is slight at first. The patient experiences such stiffness when bending forward. The history also may reveal a recent illness.

Other signs and symptoms may include headache, nausea, vomiting, abdominal pain, poorly defined chest pain, and sore throat.

The patient history and your knowledge of seasonal epidemics are essential in differentiating among the many forms of aseptic viral meningitis. Negative bacteriologic cultures and cerebrospinal fluid (CSF) analysis showing pleocytosis and increased protein suggest the diagnosis. Isolation of the virus from CSF confirms it.

Supportive treatment

Management of aseptic meningitis includes bed rest, maintenance of fluid and electrolyte balance, analgesics for pain, and exercises to combat residual weakness. Isolation isn't necessary. Careful handling of excretions and good handwashing technique prevent the spread of the disease.

ASSESSMENT

Signs and symptoms of infection and increased intracranial pressure (ICP) are the cardinal signs of meningitis. (See *Nursing care in meningitis*, pages 182 and 183.)

The patient's history may detail headache, stiff neck and back, malaise, photophobia, chills and, in some patients, vomiting, twitching, and seizures. The patient or a family member may also report altered level of consciousness (LOC), such as confusion and delirium. Vital signs may reveal fever.

In pneumococcal meningitis, the patient's history may uncover a recent lung, ear, or sinus infection or endocarditis. It may also reveal the presence of other conditions, such as alcoholism, sickle cell disease, basal skull fracture, recent splenectomy, or organ transplant.

In *H. influenzae* meningitis, patient history may reveal recent respiratory tract or ear infection.

Physical findings vary, depending on the severity of the meningitis. You may note opisthotonos (a spasm in which the back and extremities of a supine patient arch backward so that the body rests on the head and heels), a sign of meningeal irritation. In meningococcal meningitis, you may also see a petechial, purpuric, or ecchymotic rash on the lower part of the body.

Neurologic examination may uncover other indications of meningeal irritation, including positive Brudzinski's and Kernig's signs and exaggerated and symmetrical deep tendon reflexes. Neurologic examination may also reveal altered LOC, ranging from confusion or delirium to deep stupor or coma.

Vision testing may demonstrate diplopia and other visual problems. Ophthalmoscopic examination may show papilledema (another sign of increased ICP), although this is rare.

DIAGNOSTIC TESTS

• *Lumbar puncture* shows typical cerebrospinal fluid (CSF) findings associated with meningitis (elevated CSF pressure, cloudy or milky white CSF, high protein level, positive Gram stain and culture that usually identifies the infecting organism [unless it's a virus], and depressed CSF glucose concentration).

• *Chest X-rays* are especially important because they may reveal pneumonitis or lung abscess, tubercular lesions, or granulomas secondary to fungal infection. *Sinus* and *skull films* may help identify the presence of cranial osteomyelitis, paranasal sinusitis, or skull fracture.

• *White blood cell count* usually indicates leukocytosis, and *serum electrolyte levels* often are abnormal.

• *Computed tomography scan* can rule out cerebral hematoma, hemorrhage, or tumor.

TREATMENT

Medical management of meningitis includes appropriate antibiotic therapy and vigorous supportive care.

Usually, I.V. antibiotics are given for at least 2 weeks, followed by oral antibiotics. Such antibiotics include penicillin G, ampicillin, or nafcillin. However, if the patient is allergic to penicillin, anti-infective therapy includes tetracycline, chloramphenicol, or kanamycin. Other drugs include a digitalis glycoside (such as digoxin) to control arrhythmias, mannitol to decrease cerebral edema, an anticonvulsant (usually given I.V.) or a sedative to reduce restlessness, and aspirin or acetaminophen to relieve headache and fever.

Supportive measures consist of bed rest, hypothermia, and fluid therapy to prevent dehydration. Isolation is necessary if nasal cultures are positive. Treatment includes appropriate therapy for any coexisting conditions, such as endocarditis or pneumonia.

To prevent meningitis, prophylactic antibiotics are sometimes used after ventricular shunting procedures, skull fracture, or penetrating head wounds, but this use is controversial.

KEY NURSING DIAGNOSES AND PATIENT OUTCOMES

High risk for injury related to increased intracranial pressure (ICP). Based on this nursing diagnosis, you'll establish these patient outcomes. The patient will:

• avoid permanent neurologic deficits caused by increased ICP

• regain and maintain normal intracranial pressure.

Hyperthermia related to infection caused by the organism responsible for meningitis. Based on this nursing diagnosis, you'll establish these patient outcomes. The patient will:

• exhibit a reduced temperature after antipyretic measures

• avoid complications associated with hyperthermia, such as dehydration and seizures

• regain and maintain a temperature within the normal range.

Pain related to meningeal irritation. Based on this nursing diagnosis, you'll establish these patient outcomes. The patient will:

• express relief of pain after analgesic administration

• become pain-free with eradication of meningitis.

NURSING INTERVENTIONS

• Maintain respiratory isolation for 24 hours after the start of antibiotic therapy. Discharges from the nose and the mouth are considered infectious. Follow strict aseptic technique when treating patients with head wounds or skull fractures.

• Administer prescribed medications.

• Administer oxygen as required to maintain partial pressure of oxygen at desired levels. If necessary, maintain the patient on mechanical ventilation and care for his endotracheal tube or tracheostomy.

• Maintain adequate fluid intake to avoid dehydration, but avoid fluid overload because of the danger of cerebral edema.

• Position the patient carefully to prevent joint stiffness and neck pain. Turn him often, according to a planned positioning schedule. Assist with range-of-motion exercises.

• Maintain adequate nutrition. You may need to provide small, frequent meals or to supplement these meals with nasogastric tube or parenteral feedings.

• To prevent constipation and minimize the risk of increased ICP resulting from straining during defecation, give the patient a mild laxative or stool softener, as ordered.

• Provide mouth care regularly.

• Ensure the patient's comfort, and maintain a quiet environment. Darkening the room may decrease photophobia. Relieve headache with a nonnarcotic analgesic, such as aspirin or acetaminophen, as ordered. (Narcotics interfere with accurate neurologic assessment.)

• Provide reassurance and support. The patient may be frightened by his illness and frequent lumbar punctures. If he's delirious or

PRIORITY FLOWCHART

Nursing care in meningitis

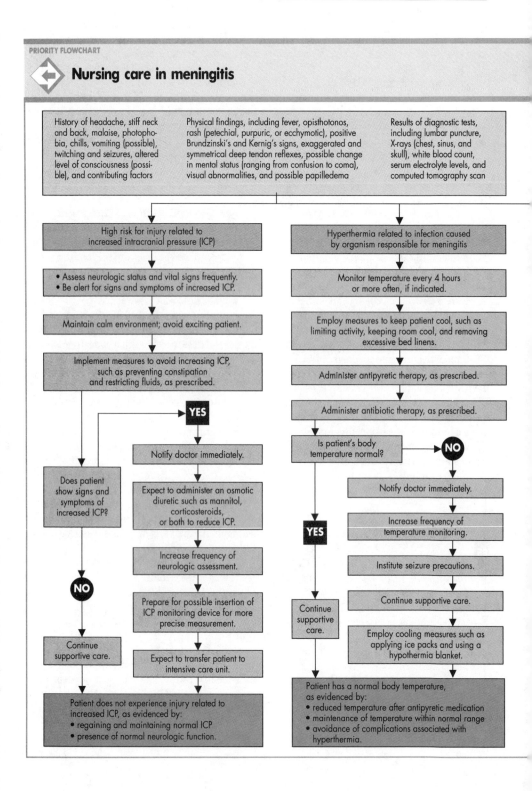

History of headache, stiff neck and back, malaise, photophobia, chills, vomiting (possible), twitching and seizures, altered level of consciousness (possible), and contributing factors

Physical findings, including fever, opisthotonos, rash (petechial, purpuric, or ecchymotic), positive Brundzinski's and Kernig's signs, exaggerated and symmetrical deep tendon reflexes, possible change in mental status (ranging from confusion to coma), visual abnormalities, and possible papilledema

Results of diagnostic tests, including lumbar puncture, X-rays (chest, sinus, and skull), white blood count, serum electrolyte levels, and computed tomography scan

High risk for injury related to increased intracranial pressure (ICP)

- Assess neurologic status and vital signs frequently.
- Be alert for signs and symptoms of increased ICP.

Maintain calm environment; avoid exciting patient.

Implement measures to avoid increasing ICP, such as preventing constipation and restricting fluids, as prescribed.

YES

Does patient show signs and symptoms of increased ICP?

Notify doctor immediately.

Expect to administer an osmotic diuretic such as mannitol, corticosteroids, or both to reduce ICP.

Increase frequency of neurologic assessment.

NO

Continue supportive care.

Prepare for possible insertion of ICP monitoring device for more precise measurement.

Expect to transfer patient to intensive care unit.

Patient does not experience injury related to increased ICP, as evidenced by:
- regaining and maintaining normal ICP
- presence of normal neurologic function.

Hyperthermia related to infection caused by organism responsible for meningitis

Monitor temperature every 4 hours or more often, if indicated.

Employ measures to keep patient cool, such as limiting activity, keeping room cool, and removing excessive bed linens.

Administer antipyretic therapy, as prescribed.

Administer antibiotic therapy, as prescribed.

Is patient's body temperature normal?

NO

Notify doctor immediately.

Increase frequency of temperature monitoring.

Institute seizure precautions.

Continue supportive care.

YES

Continue supportive care.

Employ cooling measures such as applying ice packs and using a hypothermia blanket.

Patient has a normal body temperature, as evidenced by:
- reduced temperature after antipyretic medication
- maintenance of temperature within normal range
- avoidance of complications associated with hyperthermia.

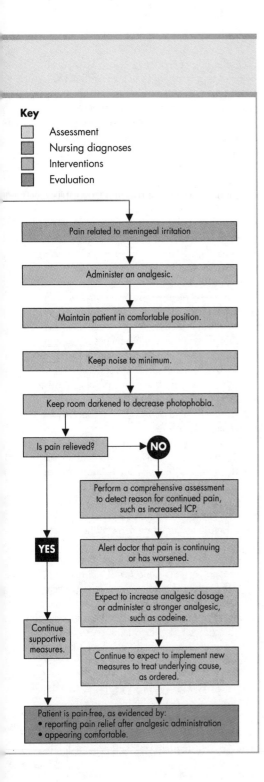

Key

- ☐ Assessment
- ☐ Nursing diagnoses
- ☐ Interventions
- ■ Evaluation

Pain related to meningeal irritation

↓

Administer an analgesic.

↓

Maintain patient in comfortable position.

↓

Keep noise to minimum.

↓

Keep room darkened to decrease photophobia.

↓

Is pain relieved? → **NO**

Is pain relieved? → **YES**

Perform a comprehensive assessment to detect reason for continued pain, such as increased ICP.

↓

Alert doctor that pain is continuing or has worsened.

↓

Expect to increase analgesic dosage or administer a stronger analgesic, such as codeine.

↓

Continue to expect to implement new measures to treat underlying cause, as ordered.

Continue supportive measures.

Patient is pain-free, as evidenced by:
- reporting pain relief after analgesic administration
- appearing comfortable.

confused, attempt to reorient him often. Reassure the family that the delirium and behavior changes caused by meningitis usually disappear. However, if a severe neurologic deficit appears permanent, refer the patient to a rehabilitation program as soon as the acute phase of this illness has passed.

Monitoring

- Continually assess the patient's clinical status, including neurologic function and vital signs. Monitor for changes in LOC and signs of increased ICP (plucking at the bedcovers, vomiting, seizures, and changes in motor function and vital signs). Also watch for signs of cranial nerve involvement (ptosis, strabismus, and diplopia).
- Regularly observe the patient for signs of deterioration. Be especially alert for a temperature increase, deteriorating LOC, seizures, and altered respirations. All of these signs may herald an impending crisis.
- Monitor arterial blood gas measurements as ordered.
- Assess the patient's fluid volume. Measure and record central venous pressure, and document intake and output accurately.
- Monitor for desired and adverse effects of prescribed medications.

Patient teaching

- Inform the patient and his family of the contagion risks, and tell them to notify anyone who comes into close contact with the patient. Such people require antimicrobial prophylaxis and immediate medical attention if fever or other signs of meningitis develop.
- To help prevent the development of meningitis, teach patients with chronic sinusitis or other chronic infections the importance of proper medical treatment.

ENCEPHALITIS

A severe inflammation of the brain, encephalitis is characterized by intense lymphocytic infiltration of brain tissues and the leptomeninges. This causes cerebral edema, degenera-

Types of encephalitis

Eastern equine encephalitis may produce permanent neurologic damage and is often fatal. It occurs in the eastern regions of North, Central, and South America. *Western equine encephalitis* occurs throughout the western hemisphere; *California encephalitis,* throughout the United States; *St. Louis encephalitis,* in Florida and in the western and southern United States; and *Venezuelan equine encephalitis,* in South America.

Between World War I and the depression, a type of encephalitis known as *lethargic encephalitis, von Economo's disease,* or *sleeping sickness* occurred with some regularity. The causative virus was never clearly identified, and the disease is rare today. Even so, the term sleeping sickness persists and is often mistakenly used to describe other types of encephalitis as well.

tion of the brain's ganglion cells, and diffuse nerve cell destruction.

Encephalitis is usually caused by a mosquito-borne or, in some areas, a tick-borne virus. However, transmission by other means may occur through ingestion of infected goat's milk and accidental injection or inhalation of the virus. (See *Types of encephalitis.*)

CAUSES

Encephalitis usually results from infection with arboviruses specific to rural areas. In urban areas, encephalitis is usually caused by enteroviruses (coxsackievirus, poliovirus, and echovirus). Other causes include herpesvirus, mumps virus, adenoviruses, and demyelinating diseases after measles, varicella, rubella, or vaccination.

COMPLICATIONS

Potential complications associated with viral encephalitis include bronchial pneumonia, urine retention, urinary tract infection, pressure ulcers, and coma. Seizure disorder, parkinsonism, and mental deterioration may also occur.

ASSESSMENT

Depending on the severity of the disease, all forms of viral encephalitis have similar clinical features. The severity of arbovirus encephalitis may range from subclinical to rapidly fatal necrotizing disease. Herpes encephalitis also produces signs and symptoms that vary from subclinical to acute and usually fatal fulminating disease.

If encephalitis is the primary illness, the patient may be acutely ill when he seeks treatment because the nonspecific symptoms that occur before the onset of acute neurologic symptoms aren't recognized as signs of encephalitis. Thus, patient history may include reports of systemic symptoms, such as headache, muscle stiffness, malaise, sore throat, and upper respiratory tract symptoms, that existed for several days before the onset of neurologic symptoms.

After neurologic symptoms occur, patient history may reveal the sudden onset of altered levels of consciousness, from lethargy or drowsiness to stupor. The patient or a family member may also report the occurrence of seizures, which may be the only presenting sign of encephalitis.

On neurologic examination, the patient may be confused, disoriented, or hallucinating. He may also demonstrate tremor, cranial nerve palsies, exaggerated deep tendon reflexes, absent superficial reflexes, and paresis or paralysis of the extremities. Additionally, the patient may complain of a stiff neck when his head is bent forward.

Vital signs usually reveal fever. The patient may also experience nausea and vomiting.

If the cerebral hemispheres are involved, assessment findings may include aphasia; involuntary movements identified on inspection; ataxia; sensory defects, such as disturbances of taste and smell; and poor memory retention.

DIAGNOSTIC TESTS

During an encephalitis epidemic, diagnosis is readily made from clinical findings and patient history. However, sporadic cases are difficult to distinguish from other febrile illnesses, such as gastroenteritis or meningitis. The following tests help establish a diagnosis:

• *Blood analysis* or, rarely, *cerebrospinal fluid (CSF) analysis* identifies the virus and confirms the diagnosis. The common viruses that also cause herpes, measles, and mumps are easier to identify than arboviruses. Arboviruses and herpesviruses can be isolated by inoculating young mice with a specimen taken from the patient.

• *Serologic studies* in herpes encephalitis may show rising titers of complement-fixing antibodies.

• *Lumbar puncture* discloses CSF pressure elevated in all forms of encephalitis. Despite inflammation, *CSF analysis* often reveals clear fluid. White blood cell count and protein levels in CSF are slightly elevated, but the glucose level remains normal.

• *EEG* reveals abnormalities, such as generalized slowing of waveforms.

• *Computed tomography scan* may be ordered to check for temporal lobe lesions that indicate herpesvirus and to rule out cerebral hematoma.

TREATMENT

The antiviral agent vidarabine monohydrate is effective only against herpes encephalitis and only if it's administered before the onset of coma.

Treatment of all other forms of encephalitis is supportive. Drug therapy includes reduction of intracranial pressure (ICP) with I.V. mannitol and corticosteroids (to reduce cerebral inflammation and resulting edema); phenytoin or another anticonvulsant, usually given I.V.; sedatives for restlessness; and aspirin or acetaminophen to relieve headache and reduce fever.

Other supportive measures include adequate fluid and electrolyte intake to prevent dehydration; appropriate antibiotics for associated infections, such as pneumonia or sinusitis; maintenance of the patient's airway; administration of oxygen to maintain arterial blood gas levels; and maintenance of nutrition, especially during coma. Isolation is unnecessary.

KEY NURSING DIAGNOSES AND PATIENT OUTCOMES

Altered thought processes related to brain cell dysfunction. Based on this nursing diagnosis, you'll establish these patient outcomes. The patient will:

• remain safe from injury

• regain orientation to time, person, and place and remain oriented after the infection is eradicated.

Hyperthermia related to infection. Based on this nursing diagnosis, you'll establish these patient outcomes. The patient will:

• regain a normal temperature with antipyretic agents and maintain a normal temperature when the infection is eradicated

• sustain no brain damage because of hyperthermia.

Impaired physical mobility related to neurologic dysfunction. Based on this nursing diagnosis, you'll establish these patient outcomes. The patient will:

• develop no complications while mobility is impaired

• skillfully perform the prescribed mobility regimen to prevent complications

• regain normal physical mobility when encephalitis is eliminated.

NURSING INTERVENTIONS

• Maintain adequate fluid intake to prevent dehydration, but avoid fluid overload, which may increase cerebral edema.

• Maintain adequate nutrition. Give small, frequent meals, or supplement meals with nasogastric tube or parenteral feedings.

• As ordered, give vidarabine by slow I.V. infusion only.

• To prevent constipation and minimize the risk of increased ICP resulting from straining during defecation, provide a mild laxative or stool softener.

• Carefully position the patient to prevent joint stiffness and neck pain, and turn him often. Assist with range-of-motion exercises.

• Provide thorough mouth care.

• Maintain a quiet environment. Darkening the room may decrease headache. If the patient naps during the day and is restless at night,

plan daytime activities to minimize napping and promote nighttime sleep.
• If the patient has seizures, take precautions to protect him from injury.
• Because the illness and frequent diagnostic tests can be frightening, provide emotional support and reassurance to the patient and family.
• If the patient becomes delirious or confused, try to reorient him often. Putting a calendar or a clock in his room may help.

Monitoring
• During the acute phase of the illness, assess the patient's neurologic function often. Observe his level of consciousness and signs of increased ICP (increasing restlessness, plucking at the bedcovers, vomiting, seizures, and changes in pupil size, motor function, and vital signs). Also watch for cranial nerve involvement (ptosis, strabismus, diplopia), abnormal sleep patterns, and behavioral changes.
• Measure and record intake and output; monitor for fluid and electrolyte imbalance.
• When administering vidarabine, watch for adverse reactions, such as tremor, dizziness, hallucinations, anorexia, nausea, vomiting, diarrhea, pruritus, rash, and anemia. Also watch for adverse effects from other drugs. Check infusion sites often to prevent problems such as infiltration and phlebitis.
• Watch for complications associated with bed rest, such as skin breakdown, constipation, and muscle weakness.

Patient teaching
• Teach the patient and his family about the disease and its effects. Explain diagnostic tests and treatments. Be sure to explain procedures to the patient even if he's comatose.
• Explain that behavior changes caused by encephalitis are usually transitory, but permanent problems sometimes occur. If a neurologic deficit is severe and appears permanent, refer the patient to a rehabilitation program as soon as the acute phase passes.

BRAIN ABSCESS

Intracranial, or brain, abscess is a free or encapsulated collection of pus typically found in the frontal, parietal, temporal, or occipital lobes. Less commonly, it occurs in the cerebellum or basal ganglia. Brain abscesses can vary in size and may occur singly or in multiple areas. Their incidence is relatively low. Although abscesses can occur at any age, they're most common in people between ages 10 and 35 and rare in older people.

Untreated brain abscess is usually fatal; with treatment, the prognosis is only fair, and about 30% of patients develop focal seizures. Multiple metastatic abscesses secondary to systemic or other infections have the poorest prognosis.

CAUSES
Brain abscess is usually secondary to some other infection, most commonly otitis media, sinusitis, dental abscess, and mastoiditis. It may result from pyogenic bacteria, such as *Staphylococcus aureus, Streptococcus viridans,* and *Streptococcus hemolyticus.* (At least 50% of brain abscesses result from mastoid or ear infections.)

An abscess may also occur secondary to subdural empyema; bacterial endocarditis; bacteremia; pulmonary or pleural infection; pelvic, abdominal, and skin infections; and cranial trauma, such as a penetrating head wound or compound skull fracture. Penetrating head trauma or bacteremia usually leads to staphylococcal infection; pulmonary disease, to streptococcal infection.

Brain abscesses develop on the same side of the brain as the primary infection. Pus may be free at first, causing inflammatory necrosis and edema; but, over several weeks, the brain tissue surrounds the abscess with a thick capsule. The resulting mass produces clinical effects similar to those of a brain tumor.

COMPLICATIONS
Without treatment, the encapsulated abscess breaks, spreading satellite abscesses to white brain matter and ventricles and producing

empyema and meningitis. Even with treatment, hemiparesis, focal seizures, cranial nerve palsies, and visual defects may occur.

ASSESSMENT

Signs and symptoms depend on the location of the abscess; alterations in intracranial dynamics, such as edema and brain shift; and the presence of infection. Most patients have symptoms for 2 weeks or less before seeking treatment.

Typically, the patient reports a recent, current, or recurrent infection – especially of the middle ear, mastoid, nasal sinuses, heart, or lungs – or a history of congenital heart disease. The patient also may complain of nausea, vomiting, and a constant, intractable headache that is worse in the morning. In addition, the patient or his family may report a change in the patient's level of consciousness (LOC), such as increased irritability or decreased alertness. Some patients may be drowsy; others may be stuporous.

Neurologic examination confirms alteration in LOC. It also may reveal that the patient is confused or disoriented and has signs of a focal neurologic disorder. Focal symptoms may include:
• in temporal lobe abscess – auditory-receptive dysphasia, central facial weakness, and hemiparesis
• in cerebellar abscess – dizziness, coarse nystagmus, gaze weakness on lesion side, tremor, and ataxia
• in frontal lobe abscess – expressive dysphasia, hemiparesis with unilateral motor seizure, drowsiness, inattention, and mental function impairment.

Besides decreased LOC and vomiting, other signs of increased intracranial pressure (ICP) may be seen, including abnormal pupillary response and depressed respirations. Additional assessment findings may include signs of an infection, such as fever, bradycardia, and pallor. (If the abscess is encapsulated, these signs may not appear.)

DIAGNOSTIC TESTS

EEG, computed tomography (CT) scan and, occasionally, arteriography (which highlights abscess with a halo) help locate the site.

Cerebrospinal fluid analysis can help confirm infection, but most doctors agree that lumbar puncture is usually too risky because it can release the increased ICP and provoke cerebral herniation.

Other tests include culture and sensitivity of drainage to identify the causative organism, skull X-rays, radioisotope scan and, rarely, ventriculography to further help identify the location of the lesion and its effects on brain tissue.

TREATMENT

Therapy consists of antibiotics to combat the underlying infection and surgical aspiration, drainage, or removal of the abscess after craniotomy. However, surgery is delayed until the abscess becomes encapsulated (CT scan helps determine this) and is contraindicated in patients with congenital heart disease or another debilitating cardiac condition.

After surgery, serial CT scans are performed to ensure that the infection has been eradicated. Administration of a penicillinase-resistant antibiotic, such as nafcillin or methicillin, for at least 2 to 3 weeks before surgery can reduce the risk of spreading infection.

Other treatment during the acute phase is palliative and supportive and includes mechanical ventilation, administration of I.V. fluids with diuretics (urea, mannitol), and glucocorticoids (dexamethasone) to combat increased ICP and cerebral edema. Anticonvulsants, such as phenytoin and phenobarbital, help prevent seizures.

If multiple abscesses are present, treatment usually consists of antimicrobial therapy alone.

KEY NURSING DIAGNOSES AND PATIENT OUTCOMES

Anxiety related to potential threat of death or permanent neurologic deficits. Based on this nursing diagnosis, you'll establish these patient outcomes. The patient will:

• express his fears and concerns about having a brain abscess
• use available support systems to cope with anxiety
• demonstrate decreased physical signs and symptoms of anxiety.

   High risk for injury related to potential for increased ICP and seizures caused by infectious process. Based on this nursing diagnosis, you'll establish these patient outcomes. The patient will:
• remain safe and protected from injury during seizure activity
• exhibit normal neurologic findings after brain abscess is eradicated.

   Pain related to increased ICP caused by presence of thick capsule around abscess. Based on this nursing diagnosis, you'll establish these patient outcomes. The patient will:
• regain and maintain normal ICP
• express pain relief with effective treatment
• obtain complete pain relief after the brain abscess is eradicated.

NURSING INTERVENTIONS

• Administer antibiotic therapy as ordered. Also expect to administer other prescribed drug therapy, such as diuretics, glucocorticoids, and anticonvulsants.
• Depending on the patient's condition, provide supportive care and implement treatment measures, such as mechanical ventilation.
• Maintain seizure precautions at all times.
• If surgery is scheduled, prepare the patient as required.
• After surgery, be sure to change the dressing when it becomes damp, using aseptic technique and noting the amount of drainage. Never allow bandages to remain damp.
• To promote drainage and prevent reaccumulation of the abscess, position the patient on the operative side.
• If the patient remains stuporous or comatose for an extended period, give meticulous skin care to prevent pressure ulcers, and position him to preserve joint function and prevent contractures.

• Ambulate the patient as soon as possible after surgery to prevent complications of immobility.
• Encourage the patient to be as independent as possible. Point out actions that he can perform successfully.
• Provide emotional support. Encourage the patient and family to express their concerns, and answer their questions honestly.

Monitoring

• Frequently assess neurologic status, especially LOC, speech, and motor, sensory, and cranial nerve functions.
• Watch for signs of increased ICP (including decreased LOC, vomiting, abnormal pupil response, and depressed respirations), which may lead to cerebral herniation with such signs as fixed and dilated pupils, widened pulse pressure, tachycardia, and abnormal respirations.
• Monitor vital signs continuously.
• Assess fluid intake and output carefully because fluid overload can contribute to cerebral edema.
• Observe the patient closely for response and adverse reactions to prescribed drug therapy.
• After surgery, monitor the patient's neurologic status continuously as well as vital signs and intake and output.
• Watch the patient for increasing ICP (altered LOC and abnormal respiratory and vasomotor responses) and meningitis (nuchal rigidity, headaches, chills, and sweats).

Patient teaching

• Explain the disorder to the patient and his family. Make sure they understand the diagnostic tests and treatments that will be performed. Explain all procedures to the patient even if he's comatose.
• If surgery is necessary, explain the procedure to the patient and answer his questions.
• If the patient requires isolation because of postoperative drainage, make sure he and his family understand this precaution.
• Inform the family that the residual infection may occur again even after seemingly successful treatment.

• Teach the patient and his family about prescribed medications. Explain that antimicrobial therapy may be necessary for several weeks after the patient is discharged from the hospital. Anticonvulsant therapy is also usually prescribed for an indefinite length of time because epilepsy is a complication of brain abscess. Make sure the patient and his family understand the importance of taking the medication as prescribed and not skipping doses.

• To prevent brain abscess, stress the need for treatment of otitis media, mastoiditis, dental abscess, and other infections. Administer prophylactic antibiotics, as ordered, after a compound skull fracture or penetrating head wound.

MYASTHENIC CRISIS

This medical emergency is an acute exacerbation of myasthenia gravis, a chronic autoimmune disease characterized by abnormal muscle weakness and fatigability. In myasthenia gravis, an autoimmune response presumably reduces the number of acetylcholine-receptor sites on motor end plates. This leads to reduced amplitude of end-plate potentials, which impairs muscle contraction by interfering with impulse transmission and muscle action potentials. Impaired muscle contraction, in turn, produces characteristic muscle weakness.

In myasthenic crisis, extreme muscle weakness may progress to respiratory paralysis and failure. The patient needs immediate intervention to ensure adequate ventilation. (See *What happens in myasthenic crisis,* page 190.)

CAUSES

Conditions that may precipitate myasthenic crisis include insufficient anticholinesterase medication, fatigue, illness, emotional stress, surgery, trauma, and infection (the most common cause). Use of certain drugs also may trigger myasthenic crisis. These include neuromuscular blocking agents, drugs with local anesthetic properties (such as quinidine, pro-

pranolol, and lidocaine), antibiotics (especially neomycin, kanamycin, and gentamicin), barbiturates (such as pentobarbital and secobarbital), and narcotics (such as morphine). In women, myasthenic crisis has been linked to pregnancy and the initiation of menstruation.

COMPLICATIONS

Myasthenic crisis may progress to a life-threatening state within an hour. Difficulty swallowing may precipitate aspiration. Respiratory muscle paralysis may lead to rapid respiratory failure and death. The patient also may develop cholinergic crisis from overmedication with cholinergic drugs used to treat the crisis.

ASSESSMENT

The patient's history may reveal a precipitating factor. The patient may report a sudden onset of extreme weakness, fatigue, difficulty swallowing, anxiety, and shortness of breath. He may also report having ptosis.

Inspection usually reveals the patient to be in acute respiratory distress with exaggerated manifestations of myasthenia gravis – muscle weakness, fatigue, ptosis, dysphagia, increased salivation, a decreased gag reflex, slurred or nasal speech, and absent facial expression. Typically, the patient seems irritable, extremely restless, and anxious. Tachycardia and hypertension may also be present.

DIAGNOSTIC TESTS

In most cases of myasthenic crisis, the patient already has a history of myasthenia gravis and is taking anticholinesterase agents. With this history in mind, the doctor may perform the Tensilon test (using edrophonium chloride) to distinguish myasthenic crisis from cholinergic crisis. In this test, the doctor injects 1 mg of edrophonium I.V. and then assesses the patient's motor responses by having him perform a series of muscle group movements. If signs and symptoms subside quickly after injection of edrophonium I.V., the crisis is myasthenic; if they worsen, the crisis is cholinergic. (See *Differentiating myasthenic crisis from cholinergic crisis,* page 191.)

What happens in myasthenic crisis

These illustrations compare the normal physiology at the neuromuscular junction with the alterations that occur during myasthenic crisis.

Normal motor cell and synapse
Vesicles release acetylcholine (ACh) at special release sites. ACh then crosses the synaptic space, reaching ACh receptors. Acetylcholinesterase in the clefts rapidly hydrolyzes ACh.

During myasthenic crisis
Antibodies attack and destroy ACh-receptor sites, limiting the number of available receptor sites. This decreases motor end-plate action potentials, leading to extreme muscle weakness.

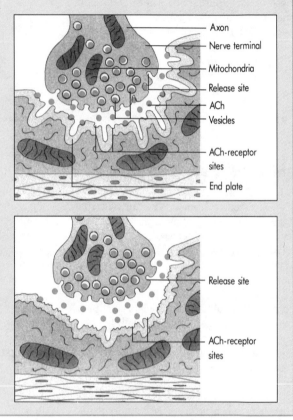

The doctor may then order serum triiodothyronine and thyroxine levels and a thymus scan to determine the cause of myasthenic crisis. Because infection is the most common cause of crisis, the doctor may also order a complete blood count.

If the patient doesn't have a history of myasthenia gravis, the diagnostic tests will include antiacetylcholinesterase-receptor antibody titers and electromyography to confirm myasthenia gravis.

TREATMENT

Therapeutic measures are aimed to halt the crisis while maintaining ventilatory support and preventing complications.

Supplemental oxygen therapy is provided. The patient nearing respiratory failure will be intubated for mechanical ventilation. A tracheotomy may be required if intubation is unsuccessful. Ventilatory augmentation, such as assist-control ventilation or synchronized intermittent mandatory ventilation with pressure support, may be required to promote full

Differentiating myasthenic crisis from cholinergic crisis

Myasthenic crisis is sometimes difficult to differentiate from cholinergic crisis. Use this chart to quickly determine if your patient is experiencing myasthenic crisis or cholinergic crisis. Withdrawal of anticholinesterase drugs for 24 to 72 hours will worsen the signs and symptoms of myasthenic crisis, but those of cholinergic crisis will subside. However, you're unlikely to have 3 days to make a diagnosis.

FEATURE	MYASTHENIC CRISIS	CHOLINERGIC CRISIS
Heart rate	Above normal	Below normal
Blood pressure	Increased	Decreased
Demeanor	Restless	Restless
Secretions	Increased	Increased
Respiratory pattern	Dyspnea	Dyspnea
Muscle strength	Weakened	Weakened, with fasciculations
Swallowing	Impaired	Impaired
Speech	Nasal	Slurred
Bowel sounds	Hypoactive	Hyperactive
Vision	Blurred	Blurred
Ptosis	Present	Present
Results of Tensilon test	Improved strength	No change or increased weakness

ventilation despite weakened respiratory muscles.

Antibiotic therapy is usually prescribed to combat infection. Also, because myasthenia gravis is believed to be an autoimmune disorder, treatment may be targeted to reduce the immune response. This treatment may include steroids, immunosuppressants (such as azathioprine or cyclophosphamide), plasmapheresis or, in some cases, a thymectomy.

KEY NURSING DIAGNOSES AND PATIENT OUTCOMES

Impaired gas exchange related to impaired ventilation. Based on this nursing diagnosis, you'll establish these patient outcomes. The patient will:
• regain and maintain normal arterial blood gas (ABG) and oxygen saturation values

• exhibit no signs or symptoms of profound central nervous system and cardiovascular deterioration.

Inability to sustain spontaneous ventilation related to extreme respiratory muscle weakness. Based on this nursing diagnosis, you'll establish these patient outcomes. The patient will:
• recover muscle strength in respiratory muscles
• resume spontaneous ventilation with treatment
• have ABG values return to and remain normal.

Ineffective breathing pattern related to extreme respiratory muscle weakness. Based on this nursing diagnosis, you'll establish these patient outcomes. The patient will:

• reestablish his respiratory pattern and rate within normal limits

• express a feeling of comfort with his breathing pattern

• have normal breath sounds on auscultation.

NURSING INTERVENTIONS

• Notify the doctor immediately if myasthenic crisis is suspected.

♦ NURSING ALERT. Remember, the patient's condition can deteriorate rapidly within an hour.

• Administer supplemental oxygen, as ordered. To avert respiratory failure, expect the doctor to order intubation and supportive mechanical ventilation.

• Insert a large-bore I.V. line to provide access for volume expanders and other emergency drugs. To avert cholinergic crisis, expect to give atropine I.V., as ordered, as an antidote for anticholinesterase medications, such as neostigmine or pyridostigmine.

• Until the myasthenic crisis passes, withhold all oral intake to prevent aspiration. Perform postural drainage, turning, and suctioning every 2 to 4 hours to avoid pooling of secretions.

• Maintain nutritional support to ensure a smooth recovery after the crisis. Provide a soft diet to reduce the effort of eating. If the patient can't tolerate oral intake, provide feedings through a duodenal tube, as ordered. Many myasthenic patients can't tolerate enteral feedings and require total parenteral nutrition.

• Develop a schedule of alternating rest and activity periods. Schedule activities requiring the greatest muscle strength early in the day, after drug administration.

• Perform range-of-motion exercises and schedule short, assisted exercise periods to reduce muscle atrophy and prevent deep vein thrombosis. To further minimize risk of thrombosis, apply pneumonic compression sleeves and give subcutaneous heparin, as ordered.

Monitoring

• Evaluate the patient's neurologic status every hour and check his muscle strength, ocular motion, speech quality, and swallowing ability. Check for diplopia and ptosis. Repeat this assessment 1 hour after medication administration, and document any changes.

• Every hour, assess the patient's respiratory rate and pattern, accessory muscle use, breath sounds, skin color, tidal volume, and vital capacity. Report any abnormalities or findings outside these desirable ranges: respiratory rate, 35 breaths/minute or less; negative inspiratory force, -20 cm H_2O or more; tidal volume, between 400 and 700 ml, depending on the patient's age, sex, height, and weight; and vital capacity, 1.65 to 4.85 liters in a female and 2.79 to 6.65 liters in a male.

• Use an arterial oxygen saturation monitor or a pulse oximeter to obtain continuous oxygenation data. Evaluate monitor readings in conjunction with periodic ABG values.

• Monitor laboratory studies, such as serum albumin and serum transferrin levels, to help determine the patient's nutritional needs.

Patient teaching

• Teach the patient and his family about myasthenia gravis and factors that may precipitate a crisis. Make sure they know how to identify signs and symptoms of myasthenic crisis. Verify that the patient understands his prescribed medication regimen and the importance of compliance, and teach him about potential adverse drug reactions.

• To help the patient resume his normal roles and responsibilities, urge him to establish a daily routine that includes frequent rest periods. Refer him to the Myasthenia Gravis Foundation for information and emotional support.

7
Musculoskeletal disorders

A complex of muscles, tendons, ligaments, bones, and other connective tissue, the musculoskeletal system gives the body form and shape. Typically, musculoskeletal disorders limit mobility and cause discomfort only temporarily. However, two acute disorders—compartment syndrome and traumatic amputation—can quickly become life-threatening if major complications occur. For example, compartment syndrome can lead to myoglobinuric renal failure and crush syndrome if multiple compartments are involved, and traumatic amputation can rapidly lead to hemorrhage and hypovolemic shock.

If your patient has one of these acute musculoskeletal injuries, you'll need to monitor him closely for life-threatening complications. In this section, you'll find the early warning signs of serious complications. You'll also become familiar with emergency actions required to save not only your patient's traumatized limb but, even more importantly, his life.

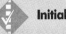

Initial musculoskeletal care

Check for:
- history of trauma
- evidence of blunt or penetrating trauma
- presence of crush injuries
- loss of body part, condition of stump, presence of amputated part, and preservation of amputated part, if saved
- bleeding and swelling at injured site
- deformity, diminished range of motion, immobility or bruises, indicating fracture or dislocation
- poor capillary refill time, absent or diminished pulses, pallor or cool skin
- paralysis, numbness, or impaired sensation at or below injured site
- progressive, intense pain in the injured limb, unaffected by immobilization, elevation, or analgesic administration
- alterations in vital signs suggestive of shock (tachycardia, tachypnea, and hypotension).

Intervene by:
- notifying the doctor immediately
- taking care to prevent further injury to the affected limb
- controlling bleeding
- elevating the patient's affected limb
- monitoring vital signs closely
- starting a peripheral I.V. line
- properly preserving the amputated part, if available and applicable
- removing anything constricting the limb and applying ice packs if compartment syndrome is suspected.

Prepare for:
- emergency surgery or fasciotomy
- fluid and blood replacement
- compartment pressure measurement, if applicable.

COMPARTMENT SYNDROME

An extremely serious neurovascular complication, compartment syndrome can occur following an injury to an extremity. This disorder may arise suddenly, right after a patient's injury, or gradually, over several days. If not detected early, it can lead to permanent dysfunction and deformity. Without treatment, nerves, blood vessels, and muscles at the injury site suffer damage within 6 hours. Within 24 to 48 hours, contracture, paralysis, and sensation loss cause permanent damage.

Compartment syndrome may become life-threatening if multiple compartments are injured. When this occurs, massive or prolonged muscle ischemia may lead to crush syndrome. An acute clinical condition, crush syndrome leads to acidosis (caused by increased lactic acid production), hyperkalemia (caused by increased release of potassium into the blood by injured cells), shock (as a result of fluid imbalance), myoglobulinuria (caused by release of myoglobulin, a muscle protein toxic to the renal system) and, subsequently, renal failure (as a result of myoglobulinuria, shock, and acidosis). If treatment is not given immediately, the patient will die.

CAUSES

Primary causes of compartment syndrome include elbow, forearm and lower leg fractures; crush injuries; and soft tissue injuries with hemorrhage and edema. Other traumatic injuries, such as animal bites, burns with edema, and missile injuries, as well as tight bandages, sutures, casts, poor positioning, and massive intravenous fluid infiltration may also cause compartment syndrome.

Muscle groups enveloped by tough, inelastic fascial tissue form compartments with entry and exit points just large enough for major arteries, nerves, and tendons. Tissue swelling, which occurs after an injury, rapidly compresses these arteries and nerves, causing muscle ischemia.

Initially, ischemia induces histamine release, causing capillary dilation and edema. Edematous tissue compresses the compartment's larger arteries, intensifying muscle ischemia and leading to release of more histamine—a vicious circle that rapidly compounds damage from the initial ischemia. Because the distal portions of the upper and lower extremities have more compartments, injuries to these areas are more likely to cause compartment syndrome.

COMPLICATIONS

Compartment syndrome may cause complications of its own, including infection and subsequent need for amputation of the affected limb. Compartment syndrome also may lead to Volkmann's contracture, which results from shortened ischemic muscles and nerve involvement, or from irreversible motor weakness, stemming from injured nerves in the affected limb. If multiple compartments are involved, such life-threatening complications as myoglobinuric renal failure and crush syndrome may occur.

ASSESSMENT

The patient's history includes a fracture, crush, or soft-tissue or other traumatic injury. He may complain of progressive, intense pain in the injured limb, unaffected by immobilization, elevation, or analgesia administration. Traction may increase the pain. With leg muscle compartment swelling, he may complain of increased pain on passive motion. He also may report numbness, tingling, or loss of sensation in the web space between the first and second toes. If the patient has forearm superficial flexor compartment swelling, he may complain of paresthesia on the hand's medial and ulnar surfaces.

Inspection of the affected limb may or may not show pallid or dusky skin color changes. Increased edema and taut skin also are evident.

Palpation of the peripheral pulses may reveal that they are present, weak, or absent. Capillary refill time may be increased.

DIAGNOSTIC TESTS

Bedside measurement of compartment pressure in the affected extremity is the chief diagnostic tool. An elevated compartment pressure confirms the diagnosis.

TREATMENT

The goal of therapy is to relieve excess pressure within the affected compartment. This may be accomplished through removal of any obvious constriction, such as a dressing or wrap, or having a cast cut to relieve pressure. If these measures are ineffective or the patient's compartment pressure rises to 41 mm Hg or above, an emergency fasciotomy is required.

KEY NURSING DIAGNOSES AND PATIENT OUTCOMES

Altered peripheral tissue perfusion related to increased compartment pressure. Based on this nursing diagnosis, you'll establish these patient outcomes. The patient will:
• regain adequate tissue perfusion to the affected limb, as evidenced by the presence of peripheral pulses, normal capillary refill time, decreased edema at the injured site, and absence of worsening pain
• state his ability to feel sensations in the affected limb.

Altered protection to renal system related to myoglobulin release. Based on this nursing diagnosis, you'll establish these patient outcomes. The patient will:
• maintain normal renal function, as evidenced by a urine output of at least 30 ml/hour and a normal urinalysis
• maintain normal serum creatinine, blood urea nitrogen, and serum electrolyte levels.

High risk for injury related to increased compartment pressure in the affected extremity. Based on this nursing diagnosis, you'll establish these patient outcomes. The patient will:
• regain normal compartment pressure in the affected extremity
• maintain normal function of affected extremity.

NURSING INTERVENTIONS

• Keep the affected limb elevated above the patient's heart level to decrease the edema-ischemic cycle.
• Administer analgesics for pain, as ordered.
• Help the doctor measure compartment pressure frequently.
• Notify the doctor if adverse changes develop in the patient's condition or compartment pressure increases. If compartment pressure starts to rise, loosen any obvious constriction, such as a dressing or wrap, and have a cast cut to relieve pressure, as necessary.
• Anticipate that the doctor may perform an emergency fasciotomy if initial interventions don't provide relief within 30 minutes.

Monitoring

• Frequently assess and record the status of the patient's peripheral pulses and capillary refill time.
• Perform frequent neurovascular assessments on the affected extremity to detect signs or symptoms of worsening compartment pressure, such as a sensory or motor change.
• Frequently ask the patient about any increased pain in the limb.
• Monitor tissue pressure directly with a tissue-pressure monitoring device.

Patient teaching

• If the patient is not acutely ill, briefly teach him about his condition and explain why it is occurring. Tell him how the condition will be treated and explain each new procedure before beginning.
• Stress the importance of alerting the nurse if symptoms worsen.

TRAUMATIC AMPUTATION

The accidental loss of a body part, traumatic amputation usually involves a finger, a toe, an arm, or a leg. In complete amputation, the member is totally severed; in partial amputation, some soft-tissue connection remains.

Although potentially life-threatening because of possible complications, the prog-

Assessing types of amputation

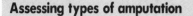

Inspection findings vary in amputation.
• *In a cut amputation,* the wound has well-defined edges and the damage is local.
• *In a crush amputation,* damage involves the tissue and arterial intima.
• *In an avulsive amputation,* the tissue is torn and vascular and neural structures may become separated near the damaged bone or cartilage.
• *In a partial amputation,* palpation detects the status of pulses distal to the amputation.

nosis has improved because of early, improved emergency and critical care management, new surgical techniques, early rehabilitation, prosthesis fitting, and new prosthesis designs. New limb reimplantation techniques have been moderately successful, but incomplete nerve regeneration remains a major limiting factor.

CAUSES
A traumatic amputation may result from a cutting, tearing, or crushing insult involving the use of factory, farm, or power tools, or from a motor vehicle accident.

COMPLICATIONS
Hypovolemic shock and sepsis are possible complications in traumatic amputation. If reimplantation is attempted, residual paralysis may occur.

ASSESSMENT
The patient history reveals the type of accident that caused the amputation. Inspection typically reveals a partially or completely severed body part with hemorrhage and soft-tissue damage. Inspection also discloses the type of amputation. (See *Assessing types of amputation.*)

DIAGNOSTIC TESTS
Ultrasonography is used to monitor the patient's pulses.

X-rays of both the amputated part and the stump can help determine the extent of fractures, and arteriography can help evaluate arterial injury.

TREATMENT
The greatest immediate threat after traumatic amputation is blood loss and hypovolemic shock. Therefore, emergency treatment consists of local measures to control bleeding, fluid replacement with sterile 0.9% sodium chloride solution and colloids, and blood replacement as needed.

Although controversial, reimplantation is becoming more common and successful because of advances in microsurgery. If reconstruction or reimplantation is possible, surgery attempts to preserve the patient's usable joints. When arm or leg amputations are performed, the surgeon creates a stump to be fitted with a prosthesis. A rigid dressing permits early prosthesis fitting and rehabilitation.

KEY NURSING DIAGNOSES AND PATIENT OUTCOMES
• *Decreased cardiac output related to hypovolemic shock.* Based on this nursing diagnosis, you'll establish these patient outcomes. The patient will:
• have hypovolemic shock detected promptly and treated
• demonstrate no significant adverse effects related to decreased cardiac output, such as arrhythmias, chest pain, or altered mental status
• regain and maintain normal cardiac output.
Fluid volume deficit related to fluid and blood loss. Based on this nursing diagnosis, you'll establish these patient outcomes. The patient will:
• recover and maintain normal fluid volume, as evidenced by stable vital signs and adequate urine output
• recover normal hemoglobin levels, hematocrit, red blood cell and platelet counts, arte-

rial blood gas and electrolyte levels, and urine specific gravity.

High risk for infection related to potential for sepsis. Based on this nursing diagnosis, you'll establish these patient outcomes. The patient will:
• maintain a normal body temperature and white blood cell count
• exhibit no signs of infection at the wound site, such as increased redness, swelling, purulent drainage, or worsening pain.

NURSING INTERVENTIONS

• If amputation involved an extremity, ensure I.V. access with at least two large-bore catheters (probably unnecessary with single-digit involvement). Clean the wound and give tetanus prophylaxis, analgesics, and antibiotics, as ordered.
• After a complete amputation, wrap the amputated part in wet dressings soaked with sterile 0.9% sodium chloride solution.

▲ NURSING ALERT. Don't place the part directly in formalin, water, or sterile 0.9% sodium chloride solution, and don't put a tag on the part. Place the amputated part in a dry, clean plastic bag, seal the bag tightly, and label it. Then place the bag on ice (not dry ice). Flush the wound with sterile 0.9% sodium chloride solution, apply a sterile pressure dressing, and elevate the limb (don't use a tourniquet). Notify the reimplantation team.
• After a partial amputation, position the limb in normal alignment, and drape it with towels or dressings soaked in sterile 0.9% sodium chloride solution.
• Preoperative care includes thorough wound irrigation and debridement (using local anesthesia). Postoperative dressing changes require sterile technique to help prevent skin infection and ensure skin graft viability.
• Encourage the patient to verbalize his feelings about his altered body image.
• Allow the patient to verbalize his concerns and fear about his future after the amputation. If necessary, consult with a rehabilitation counselor to help the patient learn a new skill.

• If reimplantation is not viable, inform the patient about community support services and rehabilitation programs.

Monitoring

• Assess and record vital signs frequently to detect hypovolemic shock and sepsis.
• Inspect the wound frequently for signs of bleeding initially; after the wound has been attended to or the amputated part reimplanted, regularly assess the site for signs and symptoms of infection.
• If the amputated part is available, monitor it carefully to ensure it is being properly preserved until reimplantation can occur.
• Assess the patient's pain level and response to administered analgesics. If the amputated part cannot be reattached, evaluate the patient for phantom pain.

Patient teaching

• Reinforce the doctor's explanation of the surgery, as necessary, and clear up any misconceptions the patient or his family may have.
• After surgery, tell the patient to report any drainage through the cast and any warmth, tenderness, or foul odor.
• Teach the patient to immediately wrap the stump with elastic bandages if the cast slips off. Show him how to apply the bandages with even, moderate pressure, avoiding overtightness that could impair circulation. Suggest that he apply the bandages when he awakens in the morning and rewrap the stump at least twice a day to maintain proper compression.
• If the patient is using a custom-fitted, elastic stump shrinker, suggest that he have two available: one to wear while the other is being washed. Explain that he'll need to use elastic bandages or a stump shrinker at all times (except when bathing or exercising) until postoperative edema completely subsides and the prosthesis is properly fitted. Even after adjustment to the prosthesis, he may need to continue nighttime bandaging for many years.
• Teach the patient how to care for his stump. Explain that good stump hygiene will prevent irritation, skin breakdown, and infection. Tell the patient to wash the stump daily with mild soap and water and then rinse and gently dry

it. Suggest that he wash the stump at night and bandage it when dry; advise against bandaging a wet stump because this may lead to skin maceration or infection. Also advise against applying body oil or lotion to the stump because this can interfere with proper fit of the prosthesis.

• Instruct the patient to call the doctor if the incision appears to be opening, looks red or swollen, feels warm, is painful to touch, or is seeping drainage.

• Reinforce the need to follow the prescribed exercise program to minimize complications, maintain muscle tone and strength, and prevent contractures. Also stress the importance of correct positioning to prevent contractures.

• Caution the patient to protect the stump from additional trauma.

8
Gastrointestinal disorders

As the site of digestion, the GI system supplies essential nutrients to the brain, heart, lungs, and other tissues. GI function also profoundly affects the quality of life by its impact on overall health. A malfunction along the GI tract or in one of the accessory GI organs can produce far-reaching metabolic effects, eventually threatening life itself.

This section presents a variety of acute GI disorders, including gastrointestinal hemorrhage, intestinal obstruction, intussusception, volvulus, peritonitis, pancreatitis, liver abscess, pseudomembranous enterocolitis, and blunt and penetrating abdominal injury.

Caring for a patient with a potentially life-threatening GI disorder can be challenging. For example, if your patient has a blunt abdominal injury or liver abscess, acute signs and symptoms warning of an impending crisis may be absent. In other conditions, such as gastrointestinal hemorrhage, intestinal obstruction, intussusception, and volvulus, acute signs and symptoms may occur so rapidly that death may quickly follow if the condition is not detected and treated immediately. Still other acute GI conditions, such as peritonitis, pancreatitis, and pseudomembranous enterocolitis, may initially appear mild but may potentially erupt into a life-threatening crisis at any time.

As a primary caregiver, be alert for any change in the patient's condition, no matter how slight it initially appears, and be ready to provide emergent care.

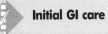
Check for:
- □ history of chronic GI disorders
- □ history of chest or abdominal surgery or trauma
- □ history of drug and alcohol use
- □ recent history of weight loss and nutritional deficiencies
- □ change in eating habits or bowel patterns
- □ nausea, vomiting, or abdominal distention
- □ frank or occult blood in vomitus or feces
- □ abdominal pain, guarding, or rigidity
- □ jaundice
- □ signs of hypovolemic shock (tachycardia, tachypnea, hypotension, diaphoresis, pallor)
- □ fever and chills
- □ change in mental status, restlessness, severe anxiety
- □ absence of, or abnormal, bowel sounds
- □ signs of fluid and electrolyte imbalance.

Intervene by:
- □ notifying the doctor
- □ initiating CPR, if indicated
- □ inserting a large-bore needle for a peripheral I.V. line
- □ administering supplemental oxygen therapy
- □ placing the patient in shock in Trendelenburg's position, unless contraindicated
- □ inserting a nasogastric tube
- □ stabilizing and leaving in place any penetrating object
- □ drawing blood for diagnostic studies and blood typing and crossmatching
- □ monitoring vital signs continuously.

Prepare for:
- □ fluid, blood, and electrolyte replacement
- □ emergency diagnostic studies
- □ medication administration.

GASTROINTESTINAL HEMORRHAGE

Patients with GI hemorrhage require immediate treatment to avoid hypovolemic shock from massive fluid loss. Although acute bleeding can occur at any place along the GI tract, it most often occurs in the upper GI tract.

CAUSES

Hemorrhage of the lower GI tract may result from such GI traumas as ulcerative colitis, diverticulosis, fistulas, cecal ulcers, tumors, angiodysplasia, and bowel infarction.

Upper GI tract hemorrhage may result from esophageal varices, peptic ulcer, and prolapsed gastric mucosa. A stress ulcer may cause massive GI bleeding several days after the initial injury. Typically arising in the esophagus, stomach, or duodenum, stress ulcers result from increased gastric acid secretion—usually in the proximal portion of the stomach. They tend to be deep and of full thickness and, thus, are more likely to perforate. Stress ulcers may occur in patients with central nervous system trauma or in those who chronically ingest drugs toxic to the gastric mucosa. Such drugs fall into three categories:
• those that alter the mucosal barrier, such as nonsteroidal anti-inflammatory drugs and alcohol
• those that decrease gastric mucosal regeneration, such as corticosteroids and phenylbutazone
• those that stimulate acid secretion, such as caffeine, reserpine, and nicotine.

COMPLICATIONS

GI hemorrhage may progress to hypovolemic shock and death.

ASSESSMENT

The patient's history may reveal the source of bleeding. The patient may report abdominal pain, tenderness, or pressure; nausea or bright red or coffee-ground vomitus; changes in taste; swallowing problems; pain after eating; weight loss; and change in bowel habits or color or consistency of stool.

Physical findings vary with the underlying cause of hemorrhage and the amount of blood lost. (See *Four stages of hemorrhage*.)

DIAGNOSTIC TESTS

• *GI X-rays* with a radiopaque contrast medium determine the source of bleeding.
• *GI endoscopy,* such as gastroscopy, also may be performed to directly visualize the gastric mucosa.
• *Laboratory studies,* such as hematocrit, hemoglobin level, blood urea nitrogen (BUN) level, platelet count, mean corpuscular volume, prothrombin time, and partial thromboplastin time, help to evaluate the patient's condition. Some of the values may be abnormal, reflecting the underlying disorder—or may result directly from the bleeding. Abnormal BUN values, for example, may indicate an increase in upper GI bleeding. And a decreased platelet count may contribute to GI bleeding.

TREATMENT

Once the source of the hemorrhage is identified, fluids and oxygen must be administered to maintain adequate perfusion and oxygenation. The doctor may order infusion of blood products to restore lost volume. (See *A closer look at blood products, colloids, and crystalloids,* page 202.)

Patients also may require gastric lavage to arrest active bleeding and vasopressin to inhibit gastric secretion (as well as nitroglycerin or nitroprusside to counteract the adverse effects of vasopressin, if needed). Lavage may be ongoing until bleeding stops or slows. Once the patient has been stabilized and the bleeding site has been identified, he may undergo surgery to remove the cause of bleeding. A rectal tube may be inserted to relieve pressure and bleeding from the lower GI tract.

KEY NURSING DIAGNOSES AND PATIENT OUTCOMES

Altered renal, cerebral, cardiopulmonary, GI, and peripheral tissue perfusion related to active blood loss from GI hemorrhage. Based on

Four stages of hemorrhage

STAGE	COMPENSATORY RESPONSE	EFFECT ON PATIENT
Stage I Up to 15% blood loss	• Compensatory mechanisms (essentially sympathetic nervous system [SNS] responses, such as vasoconstriction) maintain homeostasis.	• Patient remains alert. • Blood pressure stays within normal limits. • Pulse rate stays within normal limits or increases slightly; pulse quality remains strong. • Respiratory rate and depth, skin color and temperature, and urine output all remain normal. • Capillary refill time remains normal.
Stage II 15% to 30% blood loss	• Baroreceptors detect decreased venous return and cardiac output, triggering stronger sympathetic responses. • Vasoconstriction continues to maintain adequate blood pressure, but with some difficulty. • Blood flow shunts to vital organs, with decreased flow to intestines, kidneys, and skin.	• Patient may become confused and restless. • Skin turns pale, cool, and dry from shunting of blood to vital organs. Urine output decreases for the same reason. (Because other signs and symptoms are vague at this stage, decreased urine output may be the first sign of hypovolemia.) • Systolic pressure starts to fall. • Diastolic pressure may rise or fall. It's more likely to rise (from vasoconstriction) or stay the same in otherwise healthy patients with no underlying cardiovascular problems. • Pulse pressure (difference between systolic and diastolic pressures) narrows. • SNS responses also cause tachycardia. Pulse quality weakens. • Respiratory rate increases from SNS stimulation. • Capillary refill time remains normal.
Stage III 30% to 40% blood loss	• Compensatory mechanisms become overtaxed. For example, vasoconstriction can no longer sustain diastolic pressure, which now begins to fall. • Cardiac output and tissue perfusion continue to decrease, becoming potentially life-threatening. (Even at this stage, however, the patient can still recover with prompt treatment.)	• Patient becomes more confused, restless, and anxious. • Classic signs of hypovolemic shock appear—tachycardia, decreased blood pressure, tachypnea, and cool, clammy extremities. • Capillary refill time is delayed. • Urine output continues to decline.
Stage IV More than 40% blood loss	• Compensatory vasoconstriction now becomes a complicating factor in itself, further impairing tissue perfusion and cellular oxygenation.	• Patient becomes lethargic, drowsy, or stuporous. • Signs of shock become more pronounced. Blood pressure continues to fall and pulse pressure narrows further (although if diastolic pressure "drops out," pulse pressure may widen). • Arterial blood gas analysis reveals metabolic acidosis and respiratory alkalosis. • Capillary refill time is very delayed (longer than 3 seconds). • Patient may become severely anuric (output below 20 ml/hour). • Lack of blood flow to the brain and other vital organs ultimately leads to organ failure and death.

A closer look at blood products, colloids, and crystalloids

SUBSTANCE	DESCRIPTION	NURSING CONSIDERATIONS
Whole blood	Blood product: Contains normal components of whole blood; one unit equals 500 ml	• Administer over 2 to 4 hours. • It takes 12 to 24 hours for hemoglobin and hematocrit to equilibrate. • Watch for transfusion reaction and fluid overload.
Packed red blood cells (RBCs)	Blood product: Contains RBCs and 20% plasma (but no clotting factors and less sodium and potassium than whole blood); one unit equals 250 to 300 ml	• Administer at a slower rate than whole blood. • Watch for transfusion reaction.
Fresh frozen plasma	Blood product: Contains liquid portion of whole blood separated from cells, then frozen; one unit equals 200 to 250 ml	• Laboratory should allow 20 minutes to thaw. Use within 2 hours after thawing. • Administer one unit over 1 hour.
Plasmanate	Blood product or colloid: Contains 5% plasma protein fraction solution but no clotting factors; one unit may range from 50 to 500 ml	• Infuse no faster than 10 ml/minute. (Hypotension may occur if infused too rapidly.) • Watch for hypersensitivity reaction and fluid overload. • Hyperventilation and headache may occur.
Serum albumin	Blood product or colloid: Contains albumin from plasma (main proteins found in blood); available in 5% and 25% solutions	• Infuse slowly. Start infusion with 25 g and repeat after 15 to 30 minutes as needed (without exceeding 250 g in 48 hours). • Watch for fluid overload, hypersensitivity reaction, and bleeding.
Lactated Ringer's solution	Crystalloid: Contains sodium, potassium, and calcium chlorides, sodium lactate, and water, closely approximating normal electrolyte contents	• Tailor dosage to patient's specific needs, depending on volume loss. • Can infuse rapidly (and while patient's blood is being typed and crossmatched). • Carries no risk of hypersensitivity reaction. • Watch for fluid overload.
0.9% sodium chloride solution	Crystalloid: Contains 0.9% sodium chloride and water	• Tailor dosage to patient's specific needs, depending on volume loss. • Can infuse rapidly (and while patient's blood is being typed and crossmatched). • Carries no risk of hypersensitivity reaction. • Watch for fluid overload. • Watch for electrolyte disturbances and potassium loss.

this nursing diagnosis, you'll establish these patient outcomes. The patient will:
• regain and maintain tissue perfusion and cellular oxygenation
• show no signs or symptoms of serious tissue hypoxia and residual deficits in vital organ function.

Decreased cardiac output related to hypovolemia resulting from GI hemorrhage. Based on this nursing diagnosis, you'll establish these patient outcomes. The patient will:
• attain hemodynamic stability, as evidenced by normal vital signs and relief of signs and symptoms of hypovolemia

• exhibit no serious adverse effects of decreased cardiac output, such as arrhythmias, chest pain, and altered mental status
• recover and maintain normal cardiac output.

Fluid volume deficit related to fluid loss and bleeding in the GI tract. Based on this nursing diagnosis, you'll establish these patient outcomes. The patient will:
• have his fluid volume deficit identified quickly and treated promptly
• recover and maintain a normal fluid and blood volume, as evidenced by stable vital signs.

NURSING INTERVENTIONS
• Notify the doctor immediately if GI hemorrhage is suspected.
• To improve tissue perfusion and oxygenation, insert a large-bore peripheral venous catheter to replace lost fluids and infuse blood products as ordered. Also administer supplemental oxygen therapy.
• Administer vasopressin and other medications as ordered.
• To determine the source of bleeding, prepare the patient for GI endoscopy or gastroscopy or a GI X-ray.
• Perform gastric lavage to arrest active bleeding as ordered.
• Insert a rectal tube to relieve bleeding, if necessary, from the lower GI tract.
• Once the patient is stabilized and the bleeding site identified, prepare him for surgery, if indicated.
• If surgery is planned, administer antibiotics beforehand, as ordered, to suppress the growth of intestinal bacteria and reduce the risk of peritonitis.
• If your patient doesn't require surgery, focus your care on permitting the bowel to rest and heal (if he had lower GI bleeding). Withhold all oral intake and keep the patient on complete bed rest to reduce intestinal motility.
• Provide measures to promote comfort and relieve pain.
• Help reduce the patient's anxiety by providing emotional support, supplying clear explanations of his condition, and informing him in advance about the procedures and treatments he'll receive.

Monitoring
• Frequently check the patient's vital signs for signs of hypovolemic shock (tachycardia, tachypnea, and hypotension).
• Evaluate arterial blood gases regularly as ordered.
• Monitor the patient's electrocardiogram for evidence of arrhythmias that may occur as a result of hemorrhage, including bradycardia, heart block, ventricular tachycardia, and ventricular fibrillation.
• Check fluid status and record central venous pressure (if available) and urine output hourly. Also measure vomitus and liquid stools as well as note color and consistency of stools and vomitus.
• Regularly assess the patient's pain level, noting quality, duration, and intensity. Evaluate effectiveness of pain relief measures.
• Monitor serial laboratory values.
• After surgery, observe the patient for bleeding, hypovolemia, and other postoperative complications.

Patient teaching
• Explain to the patient and his family how GI bleeding occurs and what treatments were ordered.
• Provide preoperative teaching for the patient scheduled for surgery.
• Teach the patient about signs and symptoms that suggest a recurrence of GI bleeding, and instruct him to report a suspected recurrence to his doctor immediately.
• Instruct the patient about any prescribed medication, including how to take the medication and possible adverse effects.
• Review causes of GI bleeding and stress the importance of eliminating these factors when possible. Also emphasize the importance of minimizing stress in everyday living.

INTESTINAL OBSTRUCTION

Commonly a medical emergency, intestinal obstruction is the partial or complete blockage of the small- or large-bowel lumen. Complete obstruction in any part of the bowel, if untreated, can cause death within hours from shock and vascular collapse. Intestinal obstruction is most likely after abdominal surgery or in persons with congenital bowel deformities.

CAUSES

Intestinal obstruction results from either mechanical or nonmechanical (neurogenic) blockage of the lumen. (See *Common causes of intestinal obstruction.*)

Although intestinal obstruction may occur in several forms, the underlying pathophysiology is similar. (See *What happens in intestinal obstruction,* page 206.)

COMPLICATIONS

Intestinal obstruction can lead to perforation, peritonitis, septicemia, secondary infection, metabolic alkalosis or acidosis, hypovolemic or septic shock and, if untreated, death.

ASSESSMENT

Investigation of the patient's history often reveals predisposing factors, such as surgery (especially abdominal surgery), radiation therapy, or gallstones. The history may also disclose certain illnesses, such as Crohn's disease, diverticular disease, or ulcerative colitis, that can lead to obstruction. Family history may reveal colorectal cancer among one or more relatives.

Hiccups are a common complaint in all types of bowel obstruction. Other specific assessment findings depend on the cause of obstruction—mechanical or nonmechanical—and its location in the bowel.

In *mechanical obstruction* of the small bowel, the patient may complain of colicky pain, nausea, vomiting, and constipation. If obstruction is complete, he may report vomiting of fecal matter. This results from vigorous peristaltic waves that propel bowel contents toward the mouth instead of the rectum.

Inspection of this patient may reveal a distended abdomen, the hallmark of all types of mechanical obstruction. Auscultation may detect bowel sounds, borborygmi, and rushes

(occasionally loud enough to be heard without a stethoscope). Palpation may disclose abdominal tenderness. Rebound tenderness may be noted in patients with obstruction that results from strangulation with ischemia.

In mechanical obstruction of the large bowel, a history of constipation is common, with a more gradual onset of signs and symptoms than in small-bowel obstruction. Several days after constipation begins, the patient may report the sudden onset of colicky abdominal pain, producing spasms that last less than 1 minute and recur every few minutes.

The patient history may reveal constant hypogastric pain, nausea and, in the later stages, vomiting. He may describe his vomitus as orange-brown and foul smelling, which is characteristic of large-bowel obstruction. On inspection, the abdomen may appear dramatically distended, with visible loops of large bowel. Auscultation may reveal loud, high-pitched borborygmi.

Partial obstruction usually causes similar signs and symptoms in a milder form. Leakage of liquid stools around the partial obstruction is common.

In *nonmechanical obstruction,* such as paralytic ileus, the patient usually describes diffuse abdominal discomfort instead of colicky pain. Typically, he also reports frequent vomiting, which may consist of gastric matter, bile and, rarely, fecal matter. He may also complain of constipation and hiccups.

If obstruction results from vascular insufficiency or infarction, the patient may complain of severe abdominal pain. On inspection, the abdomen is distended. Early in the disease, auscultation discloses decreased bowel sounds; this sign disappears as the disorder progresses.

DIAGNOSTIC TESTS

• *Abdominal X-rays* confirm intestinal obstruction and reveal the presence and location of intestinal gas or fluid. In small-bowel obstruction, a typical "stepladder" pattern emerges, with alternating fluid and gas levels apparent in 3 to 4 hours. In large-bowel obstruction, barium enema reveals a distended,

Common causes of intestinal obstruction

Causes of mechanical intestinal obstruction include adhesions and strangulated hernias (usually associated with small-bowel obstruction); tumors (associated with large-bowel obstruction); foreign bodies, such as fruit pits, gallstones, or worms; compression of the bowel wall from stenosis; intussusception; volvulus of the sigmoid or cecum; atresia; or diverticulitis.

Nonmechanical (neurogenic) obstruction usually results from paralytic ileus (the most common intestinal obstruction). Paralytic ileus is a physiologic form of intestinal obstruction that may develop in the small bowel after abdominal surgery. Other nonmechanical causes of obstruction include electrolyte imbalances; toxicity, such as that associated with uremia or generalized infection; neurogenic abnormalities, such as spinal cord lesions; and thrombosis or embolism of mesenteric vessels. Some common causes are illustrated below.

Adhesions

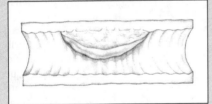

Hernia

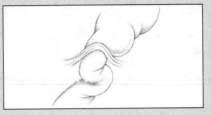

Occlusion of mesenteric vessels

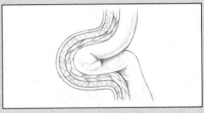

Neoplasm

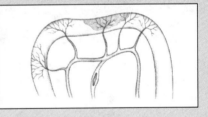

Intussusception

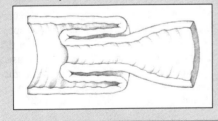

Diverticulitis

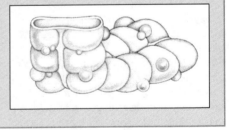

air-filled colon or a closed loop of sigmoid with extreme distention (in sigmoid volvulus).
• *Serum sodium, chloride,* and *potassium levels* may fall because of vomiting.

• *White blood cell counts* may be normal or slightly elevated if necrosis, peritonitis, or strangulation occurs.
• *Serum amylase level* may increase, possibly from irritation of the pancreas by a bowel loop.

What happens in intestinal obstruction

A partial or complete blockage of the small or large intestine results in obstruction.

Obstruction causes fluid, gas, and air to collect near the obstruction site. Peristalsis increases temporarily as the bowel tries to force its contents past the obstruction, injuring intestinal mucosa and causing further distention at and above the obstruction site.

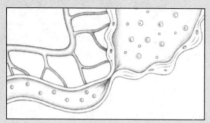

Distention impedes blood supply to the bowel wall and halts absorption. The bowel wall swells and—instead of absorbing—secretes water (H$_2$O), sodium (Na), and potassium (K) into pooled fluid in the bowel lumen, causing dehydration.

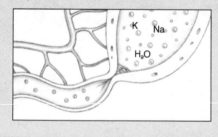

Gas-forming bacteria collect above the obstruction and further aggravate distention through fermentation.

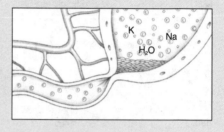

As more fluid pools, distention keeps extending proximal to the obstruction. If not treated early, this condition may lead to profound hypovolemia, shock, sepsis, and death.

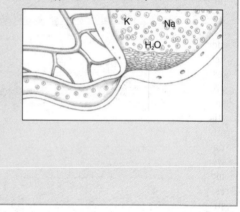

• *Hemoglobin concentration* and *hematocrit* may increase, indicating dehydration.
• *Sigmoidoscopy, colonoscopy,* or a *barium enema* may help determine the cause of obstruction; however, these tests are contraindicated if perforation is suspected.

TREATMENT

Surgery is usually the treatment of choice. One important exception is paralytic ileus, in which nonoperative therapy is usually attempted first. The type of surgery depends on the cause of blockage. For example, if a tumor is obstructing the intestine, a colon resection with anastomosis is performed; if adhesions are obstructing the lumen, these are lysed.

Surgical preparation is often lengthy, taking as long as 6 to 8 hours. It includes correction of fluid and electrolyte imbalances; decompression of the bowel to relieve vomiting and distention; treatment of shock and peritonitis; and administration of broad-spectrum antibiotics. Often, decompression is begun preoperatively with passage of a nasogastric (NG) tube attached to continuous suction. This tube relieves vomiting, reduces abdominal distention, and prevents aspiration. In strangulating obstruction, preoperative therapy also usually requires blood replacement and I.V. fluids.

Postoperative care involves careful patient monitoring and interventions geared to the type of surgery. Total parenteral nutrition may be ordered if the patient has a protein deficit from chronic obstruction, postoperative or paralytic ileus, or infection.

Nonsurgical treatment may be attempted in some patients with partial obstruction, particularly those who suffer recurrent partial obstruction or who develop it after surgery or a recent episode of diffuse peritonitis. Nonsurgical treatment usually includes decompression with an NG tube attached to low-pressure continuous suction, correction of fluid and electrolyte deficits, administration of broad-spectrum antibiotics and, occasionally, total parenteral nutrition. Rarely, a long nasointestinal tube is used for decompression.

Throughout nonsurgical treatment, the patient's condition must be closely monitored. If he fails to improve or his condition deteriorates, surgery is required.

Another indication for nonsurgical treatment is nonmechanical obstruction from paralytic ileus. Most of these cases occur postoperatively and disappear spontaneously in 2 to 3 days. However, if the disorder doesn't resolve in 48 hours, treatment consists of decompression with an NG tube attached to low-pressure continuous suction. Oral intake is restricted until bowel function resumes; then, the diet is gradually advanced.

In the patient with paralytic ileus, decompression occasionally responds to colonoscopy or rectal tube insertion. When paralytic ileus develops secondary to another illness, such as severe infection or electrolyte imbalance, the primary problem must also be treated. Again, if conservative treatment fails, surgery is required.

In both surgical and nonsurgical treatment, drug therapy includes antibiotics and analgesics or sedatives, such as meperidine or phenobarbital (but not opiates because they inhibit GI motility).

KEY NURSING DIAGNOSES AND PATIENT OUTCOMES

Decreased cardiac output related to shock and vascular collapse caused by complete intestinal obstruction. Based on this nursing diagnosis, you'll establish these patient outcomes. The patient will:
• attain hemodynamic stability, as evidenced by normal vital signs and relief of signs and symptoms of complete intestinal obstruction
• exhibit no serious complications of decreased cardiac output, such as arrhythmias, chest pain, and altered mental status
• recover and maintain normal cardiac output.

High risk for fluid volume deficit related to inability to ingest oral fluids. Based on this nursing diagnosis, you'll establish these patient outcomes. The patient will:
• maintain an adequate fluid volume balance, as evidenced by normal vital signs and an I.V. intake that equals his output
• demonstrate no signs or symptoms of hypovolemia
• ingest fluids orally after the obstruction is alleviated.

Pain related to the pressure and irritation resulting from an intestinal obstruction. Based on this nursing diagnosis, you'll establish these patient outcomes. The patient will:
• express relief of pain following analgesic administration
• become pain-free after the obstruction is alleviated.

NURSING INTERVENTIONS

• Because intestinal obstruction may be fatal and often causes overwhelming pain and distress, patients require skillful supportive care and keen observation.
• Allow the patient nothing by mouth, as ordered, but be sure to provide frequent mouth care to help keep mucous membranes moist. If surgery won't be performed, he may be allowed a small quantity of ice chips. Avoid using lemon-glycerin swabs, which can increase mouth dryness.

• Insert an NG tube to decompress the bowel, as ordered. Attach the tube to low-pressure, intermittent suction. Irrigate the tube with 0.9% sodium chloride solution if necessary to maintain patency.

• If ordered, assist with insertion of a weighted nasointestinal tube, such as a Miller-Abbott, Cantor, or Harris tube. Help the patient turn from side to side (or walk around, if he can) to facilitate passage of the tube.

• Begin and maintain I.V. therapy, as ordered. Provide I.V. fluids to keep levels within normal ranges. Provide blood replacement therapy as necessary.

• Administer analgesics, broad-spectrum antibiotics, and other medications, as ordered.

• Keep in mind that analgesics may be withheld until a diagnosis is confirmed. To ease discomfort, help the patient to change positions frequently.

• If you suspect bladder compression, catheterize the patient immediately after he has voided to remove residual urine.

• Keep the patient in semi-Fowler's or Fowler's position as much as possible. These positions help to promote pulmonary ventilation and ease respiratory distress from abdominal distention.

• If surgery is scheduled, prepare the patient as required.

Monitoring

• Look for signs of dehydration (thick, swollen tongue; dry, cracked lips; dry oral mucous membranes).

• Observe NG tube drainage for color, consistency, and amount.

• If a weighted tube has been inserted, check periodically to make sure it's advancing.

• Monitor intake and output. Maintain fluid and electrolyte balance by monitoring electrolyte, blood urea nitrogen, and creatinine levels.

• Assess vital signs frequently. A drop in blood pressure may indicate reduced circulating blood volume resulting from blood loss caused by a strangulated hernia. Remember, as much as 10 liters of fluid can collect in the small bowel, drastically reducing plasma volume.

Observe closely for signs of shock (pallor, rapid pulse, and hypotension).

• When administering medication, monitor the patient for the desired effects and for adverse reactions.

• Continually assess the patient's pain. Remember, colicky pain that suddenly becomes constant could signal perforation.

• Watch for signs of metabolic alkalosis (changes in sensorium, hypertonic muscles, tetany, and slow, shallow respirations) or acidosis (shortness of breath on exertion, disorientation and, later, weakness, malaise, and deep, rapid breathing). Watch for signs and symptoms of secondary infection, such as fever and chills.

• Monitor urine output carefully to assess renal function, circulating blood volume, and possible urine retention due to bladder compression by the distended intestine. Also measure abdominal girth frequently to detect progressive distention.

• Listen for bowel sounds, and watch for other signs of resuming peristalsis (passage of flatus and mucus through the rectum).

Patient teaching

• Teach the patient about his disorder, focusing on his type of intestinal obstruction, its cause, and signs and symptoms. Listen to his questions and take time to answer them.

• Explain necessary diagnostic tests and treatments. Make sure the patient understands that these procedures are necessary to relieve the obstruction and reduce pain. Instruct him in pretest guidelines; for example, advise him to lie on his left side for about a half hour before X-rays are taken.

• Prepare the patient and his family for the possibility of surgery. Provide preoperative teaching, and reinforce the doctor's explanation of the surgery. Demonstrate techniques for coughing and deep breathing, and teach the patient how to use incentive spirometry.

• Tell the patient what to expect postoperatively.

• Review the proper use of prescribed medications, focusing on their correct administration, desired effects, and possible adverse effects.

• Emphasize the importance of following a structured bowel elimination regimen, particularly if the patient had a mechanical obstruction from fecal impaction. Encourage him to eat a high-fiber diet and to exercise daily.
• Reassure the patient who had an obstruction from paralytic ileus that recurrence is unlikely. However, remind him to report any recurrence of abdominal pain, abdominal distention, nausea, or vomiting.

INTUSSUSCEPTION

Considered a pediatric emergency (although it can occur in adults), intussusception occurs when a portion of the bowel telescopes or invaginates into an adjacent bowel portion. Because this disorder leads to bowel obstruction and other serious complications, it can be fatal, especially if treatment is delayed for more than 24 hours.

Intussusception is most common in infants and occurs three times more often in males than in females; about 87% of children with intussusception are younger than age 2; about 70% of these children are between 4 and 11 months old.

CAUSES

In infants, intussusception usually arises from unknown causes. In older children, polyps, hemangioma, lymphosarcoma, lymphoid hyperplasia, Meckel's diverticulum, or alterations in intestinal motility may trigger the process. In adults, intussusception most commonly results from benign or malignant tumors (65% of patients); other possible causes include polyps, Meckel's diverticulum, gastroenterostomy with herniation, or an appendiceal stump.

In addition, studies suggest that intussusception may be linked to viral infections because seasonal peaks are noted—in the spring and summer, coinciding with peak incidence of enteritis, and in midwinter, coinciding with peak incidence of respiratory tract infections.

COMPLICATIONS

Without prompt treatment, strangulation of the intestine may occur, with gangrene, shock, perforation, and peritonitis. These complications can be fatal.

ASSESSMENT

If the patient is an infant or child, the history may reveal intermittent attacks of colicky pain. Typically, this pain causes the child to scream, draw his legs up to his abdomen, turn pale and diaphoretic, and possibly grunt. Parents may report that the child vomits—initially, stomach contents, and later, bile-stained or fecal material. Parents may describe the child's "currant jelly" stools, which contain a mixture of blood and mucus.

Inspection and palpation may reveal a distended, tender abdomen, with some guarding over the intussusception site. A sausage-shaped abdominal mass may be palpable in the right upper quadrant or in the midepigastrium if the transverse colon is involved. Rectal examination may show bloody mucus.

In the adult patient, the history may reveal nonspecific, chronic, and intermittent symptoms, such as colicky abdominal pain and tenderness, vomiting, diarrhea (occasionally constipation), bloody stools, and weight loss. He may describe abdominal pain that's localized in the right lower quadrant, radiates to the back, and increases with eating. The abdomen may be distended. Palpation may help pinpoint the tender area in the right lower quadrant.

In the adult patient, excruciating pain, abdominal distention, and tachycardia are signs that severe intussusception has led to strangulation.

DIAGNOSTIC TESTS

• *Barium enema* confirms colonic intussusception when it shows the characteristic coiled-spring sign; it also delineates the extent of intussusception.
• *Upright abdominal X-rays* may show a soft-tissue mass and signs of complete or partial obstruction, with dilated loops of bowel.

• *White blood cell count* up to 15,000/mm³ indicates obstruction; more than 15,000/mm³, strangulation; more than 20,000/mm³, bowel infarction.

TREATMENT

In children, therapy may include hydrostatic reduction or surgery. Surgery is indicated for children with recurrent intussusception, for those who show signs of shock or peritonitis, and for those in whom symptoms have been present longer than 24 hours. In adults, surgery is always the treatment of choice.

During hydrostatic reduction, the radiologist drips a barium solution into the rectum through a catheter from a height of not more than 3′ (0.9 m); fluoroscopy traces the progress of the barium. If the procedure is successful, the barium backwashes into the ileum and the mass disappears. If not, the procedure is stopped and the patient is prepared for surgery.

During surgery, manual reduction is attempted first. After compressing the bowel above the intussusception, the doctor attempts to milk the intussusception back through the bowel. However, if manual reduction fails or if the bowel is gangrenous or strangulated, the doctor will perform a resection of the affected bowel segment.

KEY NURSING DIAGNOSES AND PATIENT OUTCOMES

Altered GI tissue perfusion related to decreased blood flow. Based on this nursing diagnosis, you'll establish these patient outcomes. The patient will:
• seek early treatment for signs and symptoms of intussusception to minimize tissue damage
• regain normal GI tissue perfusion after the intussusception is alleviated.

High risk for fluid volume deficit related to adverse GI effects of intussusception. Based on this nursing diagnosis, you'll establish these patient outcomes. The patient will:
• maintain a normal fluid volume, as evidenced by stable vital signs and an I.V. intake that equals his output

• exhibit no signs or symptoms of dehydration
• stop vomiting or having diarrhea.

Pain related to intestinal pressure and ischemia. Based on this nursing diagnosis, you'll establish these patient outcomes. The patient will:
• express relief from pain following administration of an analgesic
• become pain-free.

NURSING INTERVENTIONS

• Offer reassurance and emotional support to the patient and, if the patient is a child, to his parents. Because this condition is considered a pediatric emergency, parents are often unprepared for their child's hospitalization and possible surgery. Similarly, the child is unprepared for an abrupt separation from his parents and familiar environment.
• Administer I.V. fluids, as ordered. If the patient is in shock, give blood or plasma, as ordered.
• A nasogastric (NG) tube is inserted to decompress the bowel. Replace volume lost as ordered.
• Prepare the patient for hydrostatic reduction, and answer questions to allay fears.
• Prepare the patient for surgery, if necessary, and provide postoperative care in the same manner as for the patient with a bowel resection and anastomosis.

Monitoring

• Frequently assess and record vital signs. A change in temperature may indicate sepsis; infants may become hypothermic at the onset of infection. Rising pulse rate and falling blood pressure may signal peritonitis.
• Check intake and output, and watch for signs of dehydration and bleeding.
• Monitor the amount and type of drainage from the NG tube.
• Watch the patient who has undergone hydrostatic reduction for passage of stools and barium, a sign that the reduction has been successful. Keep in mind that a few patients have a recurrence of intussusception; this usually occurs within the first 36 to 48 hours after the hydrostatic reduction.

Patient teaching

• Depending on the patient's age, explain to him or his parents what happens in intussuception. Review required diagnostic tests and treatments. If hydrostatic reduction by barium enema will be attempted, make sure the patient or his parents understand the procedure. Let them know that surgery will be necessary if the procedure isn't successful.

• If surgery is required, provide preoperative teaching. Reinforce the doctor's explanation of the surgery and its possible complications.

• To minimize the stress of hospitalization, encourage parents to participate in their child's care as much as possible. Be flexible about visiting hours.

VOLVULUS

Marked by sudden onset of severe abdominal pain, volvulus is a twisting of the intestine at least 180 degrees on itself. Potentially fatal, volvulus results in blood vessel compression and causes obstruction both proximal and distal to the twisted loop. (See *Recognizing volvulus*.)

Volvulus occurs in a bowel segment long enough to twist. The most common area, particularly in adults, is the sigmoid colon. Other common sites include the stomach and cecum.

CAUSES

In volvulus, twisting may result from an anomaly of bowel rotation in utero, an ingested foreign body, or an adhesion. Volvulus secondary to meconium ileus may occur in patients with cystic fibrosis. In some patients, however, the cause is unknown.

COMPLICATIONS

Without immediate treatment, volvulus can lead to strangulation of the twisted bowel loop, ischemia, infarction, perforation, and fatal peritonitis.

Recognizing volvulus

Although volvulus may occur anywhere in a bowel segment long enough to twist, the most common site, as the bottom illustration depicts, is the sigmoid colon. Here, a counterclockwise twist has occluded the colon, causing edema within the closed loop and obstruction at both its proximal and distal ends.

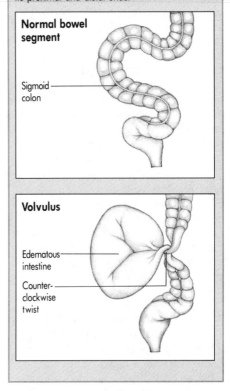

Normal bowel segment

Sigmoid colon

Volvulus

Edematous intestine

Counterclockwise twist

ASSESSMENT

The patient with volvulus complains of severe abdominal pain and may report bilious vomiting. The history may also reveal the passage of bloody stools.

On inspection, the patient appears to be in pain. Abdominal inspection and palpation may reveal distention and a palpable mass.

DIAGNOSTIC TESTS

• *Abdominal X-rays* may show multiple distended bowel loops and a large bowel without gas; in midgut volvulus, abdominal X-rays may be normal.

• *Barium enema* can help locate volvulus. In cecal volvulus, barium fills the colon distal to the section of cecum; in sigmoid volvulus, barium may twist to a point; and, in adults, it takes on an "ace of spades" configuration.

• *White blood cell (WBC) count* is elevated. In strangulation, the count is greater than $15,000/mm^3$; in bowel infarction, greater than $20,000/mm^3$.

TREATMENT

The severity and location of the volvulus determine therapy. For sigmoid volvulus, nonsurgical treatment includes proctoscopy to check for infarction and reduction by careful insertion of a flexible sigmoidoscope to deflate the bowel. Success of nonsurgical reduction is indicated by expulsion of gas and immediate relief of abdominal pain.

If the bowel is distended but viable, surgery consists of detorsion (untwisting); if the bowel is necrotic, surgery includes resection and anastomosis. Prolonged total parenteral nutrition and I.V. administration of antibiotics are usually necessary. Sedatives may be needed.

KEY NURSING DIAGNOSES AND PATIENT OUTCOMES

Altered GI tissue perfusion related to blood vessel compression. Based on this nursing diagnosis, you'll establish these patient outcomes. The patient will:

• seek emergency care at the onset of symptoms to minimize the risk of ischemia causing permanent damage to GI tissue

• not develop bowel necrosis

• regain adequate GI tissue perfusion with treatment.

High risk for infection related to potential for peritonitis to develop. Based on this nursing diagnosis, you'll establish these patient outcomes. The patient will:

• maintain a normal temperature and WBC count

• show no signs or symptoms of peritonitis.

Pain related to twisted bowel and obstruction. Based on this nursing diagnosis, you'll establish these patient outcomes. The patient will:

• express feelings of comfort following analgesic administration

• become pain-free when volvulus is resolved.

NURSING INTERVENTIONS

• Provide psychological support. Listen to the patient's concerns and offer reassurance; take time to answer his questions.

• Administer analgesics and broad-spectrum antibiotics, as ordered.

• Administer I.V. fluids, as ordered.

• Insert a nasogastric tube and connect to low-pressure intermittent suction, if ordered, to relieve abdominal distention.

• Prepare the patient for proctoscopy, as indicated.

• If the patient is scheduled for detorsion surgery, provide appropriate preoperative and postoperative care, as for any patient undergoing abdominal surgery.

Monitoring

• Observe the patient's response to administered analgesics and antibiotics, checking for desired effects and potential adverse reactions.

• Routinely monitor vital signs, intake and output, and fluid and electrolyte balance.

Patient teaching

• Explain what happens in volvulus, using teaching aids, if available. Review its signs and symptoms and possible complications. Discuss necessary diagnostic procedures and treatments.

• Reinforce the doctor's explanation of scheduled surgery and its possible complications. Provide preoperative teaching.

• If surgery was extensive, or if the patient's condition requires it, refer him and his family to the social service department and a local home health care agency.

•

PERITONITIS

An acute or chronic disorder, peritonitis is an inflammation of the peritoneum, the membrane that lines the abdominal cavity and covers the visceral organs. Such inflammation may extend throughout the peritoneum or be localized as an abscess. Peritonitis commonly decreases intestinal motility and causes intestinal distention with gas. Mortality is about 10%, with bowel obstruction the usual cause of death.

CAUSES

Although the GI tract normally contains bacteria, the peritoneum is sterile. In peritonitis, however, bacteria invade the peritoneum. Generally, such infection results from inflammation and perforation of the GI tract, allowing bacterial invasion. Usually, this is a result of appendicitis, diverticulitis, peptic ulcer, ulcerative colitis, volvulus, strangulated obstruction, abdominal neoplasm, or a stab wound. Peritonitis can also result from chemical inflammation after rupture of a fallopian tube, an ovarian cyst, or the bladder; after perforation of a gastric ulcer; or because of released pancreatic enzymes.

In both bacterial and chemical inflammation, fluid containing protein and electrolytes accumulates in the peritoneal cavity and makes the transparent peritoneum opaque, red, inflamed, and edematous. Because the peritoneal cavity is so resistant to contamination, such infection is often localized as an abscess instead of disseminated as a generalized infection.

COMPLICATIONS

Peritonitis can lead to abscess formation, septicemia, respiratory compromise, bowel obstruction, and shock.

ASSESSMENT

The patient's symptoms depend on whether the disorder is assessed early or late in its course. In the early phase, he may report vague, generalized abdominal pain. If peritonitis is localized, he may describe pain over a specific area (usually over the site of inflammation); if peritonitis is generalized, he may complain of diffuse pain over the abdomen.

As the disorder progresses, the patient typically reports increasingly severe and unremitting abdominal pain. Pain often increases with movement and respirations. Occasionally, pain may be referred to the shoulder or the thoracic area. Other signs and symptoms include abdominal distention, anorexia, nausea, vomiting, and an inability to pass feces and flatus.

Assessment of vital signs may reveal fever, tachycardia (a response to the fever), and hypotension. On inspection, the patient usually appears acutely distressed. He may lie very still in bed, often with his knees flexed to try to alleviate abdominal pain. He tends to breathe shallowly and move as little as possible to minimize pain. If he loses excessive fluid, electrolytes, and proteins into the abdominal cavity, you may observe excessive sweating, cold skin, pallor, abdominal distention, and such signs of dehydration as dry mucous membranes.

Early in peritonitis, auscultation usually discloses bowel sounds; as the inflammation progresses, these sounds tend to disappear. Abdominal rigidity is usually felt on palpation. If peritonitis spreads throughout the abdomen, palpation may disclose general tenderness; if peritonitis stays in a specific area, you may detect local tenderness. Rebound tenderness may also be present.

DIAGNOSTIC TESTS

• *White blood cell count* shows leukocytosis (commonly more than 20,000/mm^3).
• *Abdominal X-rays* demonstrate edematous and gaseous distention of the small and large bowel. With perforation of a visceral organ, the X-rays show air in the abdominal cavity.
• *Chest X-rays* may reveal elevation of the diaphragm.
• *Paracentesis* discloses the nature of the exudate and permits bacterial culture so that appropriate antibiotic therapy can be instituted.

TREATMENT

To prevent peritonitis, early treatment of GI inflammatory conditions and preoperative and postoperative antibiotic therapy are important. After peritonitis develops, emergency treatment must combat infection, restore intestinal motility, and replace fluids and electrolytes.

Antibiotic therapy depends on the infecting organism but usually includes administration of cefoxitin with an aminoglycoside, or penicillin G and clindamycin with an aminoglycoside. To decrease peristalsis and prevent perforation, the patient should receive nothing by mouth; instead, he requires supportive fluids and electrolytes parenterally.

Supplementary treatment includes administration of an analgesic, such as meperidine; nasogastric (NG) intubation to decompress the bowel; and possible use of a rectal tube to facilitate the passage of flatus.

The treatment of choice, surgery aims to eliminate the source of infection by evacuating the spilled contents and inserting drains. It should be performed as soon as the patient is stable enough to tolerate it.

The surgical procedure varies with the cause of peritonitis. For example, if appendicitis is the cause, an appendectomy is performed; if the colon is perforated, a colon resection may be performed. Occasionally, abdominocentesis may be necessary to remove accumulated fluid. Irrigation of the abdominal cavity with antibiotic solutions during surgery may be appropriate.

KEY NURSING DIAGNOSES AND PATIENT OUTCOMES

Altered GI tissue perfusion related to inflammatory process. Based on this nursing diagnosis, you'll establish these patient outcomes. The patient will:
• exhibit improved GI tissue perfusion as inflammation subsides with treatment
• regain and maintain normal GI function with treatment.

High risk for fluid volume deficit related to excessive fluid loss into abdomen. Based on this nursing diagnosis, you'll establish these patient outcomes. The patient will:
• maintain hemodynamic stability, as exhibited by normal vital signs
• have no signs or symptoms of ascites, dehydration, or hypovolemic shock
• maintain normal vascular fluid volume balance.

Pain related to inflammatory process. Based on this nursing diagnosis, you'll establish these patient outcomes. The patient will:
• express feelings of comfort after analgesic administration
• comply with antibiotic therapy to alleviate inflammation and pain.

NURSING INTERVENTIONS

• Provide psychological support, and offer encouragement when appropriate.
• Administer prescribed medications, such as analgesics and antibiotics, as ordered.
• Maintain parenteral fluid and electrolyte administration, as ordered.
• Maintain bed rest, and place the patient in semi-Fowler's position to help him breathe deeply with less pain and thus prevent pulmonary complications.
• Counteract mouth and nose dryness due to fever, dehydration, and NG intubation with regular hygiene and lubrication.
• Prepare the patient for surgery, as indicated.
• If necessary, refer the patient to the hospital's social service department or a home health care agency that can help him obtain needed services during convalescence.

Monitoring

• Observe the patient for the desired effects of medications and possible adverse reactions to them.
• Monitor the patient's WBC count.
• Assess fluid volume by checking skin turgor, mucous membranes, urine output, weight, vital signs, amount of NG tube drainage, and amount of I.V. infusion. Record intake and output, including NG tube drainage.
• Monitor the patient for surgical complications, if appropriate.

Patient teaching

• Teach the patient about peritonitis, what caused his problem, and necessary treatments.
• Provide preoperative teaching. Review postoperative care procedures.
• Discuss the proper use of prescribed medications, reviewing their correct administration, desired effects, and possible adverse effects.

PANCREATITIS

Inflammation of the pancreas, pancreatitis occurs in acute and chronic forms and may stem from edema, necrosis, or hemorrhage. In men, the disorder is commonly associated with alcoholism, trauma, or peptic ulcer; in women, with biliary tract disease. The prognosis is good when pancreatitis follows biliary tract disease but poor when it stems from alcoholism. Mortality reaches 60% when pancreatitis is associated with necrosis or hemorrhage.

CAUSES

The most common causes of pancreatitis are biliary tract disease and alcoholism, but the disorder can also result from abnormal organ structure, metabolic or endocrine disorders (such as hyperlipidemia or hyperparathyroidism), pancreatic cysts or tumors, penetrating peptic ulcers, or trauma (blunt or iatrogenic). This disorder also can develop after the use of certain drugs, such as glucocorticoids, sulfonamides, thiazides, and oral contraceptives.

Pancreatitis may be a complication of renal failure, kidney transplantation, open-heart surgery, and endoscopic retrograde cholangiopancreatography (ERCP). Heredity may be a predisposing factor and, in some patients, emotional or neurogenic factors are involved.

Regardless of the cause, pancreatitis involves autodigestion: The enzymes normally excreted by the pancreas digest pancreatic tissue.

COMPLICATIONS

If pancreatitis damages the islets of Langerhans, diabetes mellitus may occur. Fulminant pancreatitis causes massive hemorrhage and total destruction of the pancreas, resulting in diabetic acidosis, shock, or coma. Respiratory complications include adult respiratory distress syndrome, atelectasis, pleural effusion, and pneumonia. Proximity of the inflamed pancreas to the bowel may cause paralytic ileus. Other complications include GI bleeding, pancreatic abscess, pseudocysts and, rarely, cancer.

ASSESSMENT

Commonly, the patient describes intense epigastric pain centered close to the umbilicus and radiating to the back, between the 10th thoracic and 6th lumbar vertebrae. He typically reports that this pain is aggravated by eating fatty foods, consuming alcohol, or lying in a recumbent position. He may also complain of weight loss with nausea and vomiting.

Investigation may uncover predisposing factors, such as alcoholism, biliary tract disease, or pancreatic disease. Other medical problems, such as peptic ulcer disease or hyperlipidemia, may be discovered.

Assessment of vital signs may reveal decreased blood pressure, tachycardia, and fever. These signs, if present, indicate respiratory complications. Other signs of respiratory complications are dyspnea or orthopnea. Observe the patient for changes in behavior and sensorium; these signs may be related to alcohol withdrawal or may indicate hypoxia or impending shock.

Abdominal inspection may disclose generalized jaundice, Cullen's sign (bluish periumbilical discoloration), and Turner's sign (bluish flank discoloration). Inspection of stools may reveal steatorrhea, a sign of chronic pancreatitis.

During abdominal palpation, you may note tenderness, rigidity, and guarding. If you hear a dull sound while percussing, suspect pancreatic ascites. If bowel sounds are absent or decreased on abdominal auscultation, suspect paralytic ileus.

Critical test values in pancreatitis

The following findings confirm acute pancreatitis:
• Serum amylase levels above 180 Somogyi units/dl (130 U/L). This is the diagnostic hallmark that confirms acute pancreatitis. Characteristically, serum amylase reaches peak levels within 24 hours after onset of pancreatitis, then returns to normal within 48 to 72 hours despite continued symptoms.
• Urine amylase level above 80 amylase units/hr (17 U/h). Because urine amylase is reported in various units of measurement, values differ among laboratories. Check your hospital's normal range for urine amylase. Urine amylase levels remain elevated longer than serum amylase levels.
• Serum lipase level above 80 units/liter. Serum lipase levels remain elevated longer than serum amylase levels.

DIAGNOSTIC TESTS

For key abnormal laboratory test values, see *Critical test values in pancreatitis.*
• *Supportive laboratory studies* include elevated white blood cell count and serum bilirubin level. In many patients, hypocalcemia occurs and appears to be associated with the severity of the disease. Blood and urine glucose tests may reveal transient glucosuria and hyperglycemia. In chronic pancreatitis, significant laboratory findings include elevations in serum alkaline phosphatase, amylase, and bilirubin levels. Serum glucose levels may be transiently elevated. Stools contain elevated lipid and trypsin levels.
• *Abdominal and chest X-rays* differentiate pancreatitis from other diseases that cause similar symptoms and detect pleural effusions.
• *Computed tomography scan* and *ultrasonography* reveal an increased pancreatic diameter; these tests also identify pancreatic cysts and pseudocysts.

• *ERCP* shows the anatomy of the pancreas; identifies ductal system abnormalities, such as calcification or strictures; and differentiates pancreatitis from other disorders, such as pancreatic cancer.

TREATMENT

The goals are to maintain circulation and fluid volume, relieve pain, and decrease pancreatic secretions. Emergency treatment for shock (the most common cause of death in early-stage pancreatitis) consists of vigorous I.V. replacement of electrolytes and proteins. (For information on monitoring electrolyte levels, see *Vascular intermittent access system.*)

Metabolic acidosis secondary to hypovolemia and impaired cellular perfusion requires vigorous fluid volume replacement. Blood transfusions may be needed if shock occurs. Food and fluids are withheld to allow the pancreas to rest and to reduce pancreatic enzyme secretion.

In acute pancreatitis, nasogastric (NG) tube suctioning is usually required to decrease gastric distention and suppress pancreatic secretions. Prescribed medications may include:
• meperidine to relieve abdominal pain (this drug causes less spasm at the ampulla of Vater than opiates, such as morphine)
• antacids to neutralize gastric secretions
• histamine antagonists, such as cimetidine or ranitidine, to decrease hydrochloric acid production
• antibiotics, such as clindamycin or gentamicin, to treat bacterial infections
• anticholinergics to reduce vagal stimulation, decrease GI motility, and inhibit pancreatic enzyme secretion
• insulin to correct hyperglycemia, if present.

Once the crisis begins to resolve, oral low-fat, low-protein feedings are gradually implemented. Alcohol and caffeine are eliminated from the diet. If the crisis occurred during treatment with glucocorticoids, oral contraceptives, or thiazide diuretics, these drugs are discontinued.

Surgery usually isn't indicated in acute pancreatitis. However, if complications such as

Vascular intermittent access system

In patients who have an indwelling arterial or venous line, the vascular intermittent access system is used to measure electrolyte, hematocrit, glucose, and arterial blood gas levels automatically in 1 minute. Then it reinfuses the blood sample into the patient.

The vascular intermittent access system includes a sensor array, an I.V. administration set, I.V. solution with additives for sensor calibration, and a monitor that processes signals from the sensors. A pumping mechanism infuses the solution and withdraws blood samples.

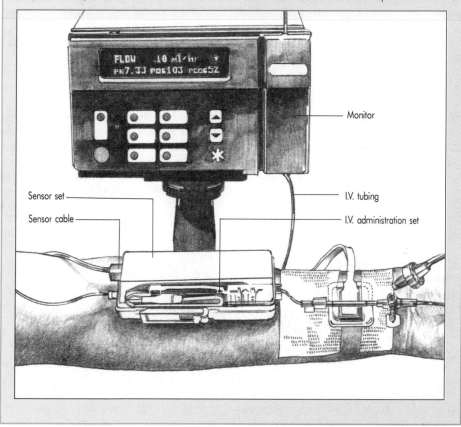

pancreatic abscess or pseudocyst occur, surgical drainage may be necessary. If biliary tract obstruction causes acute pancreatitis, a laparotomy may be required.

For chronic pancreatitis, treatment depends on the cause. Nonsurgical measures are appropriate if the patient isn't a suitable candidate for surgery or if he refuses this treatment. Measures to prevent and relieve abdominal pain are similar to those used in acute pancreatitis. Meperidine usually is the drug of choice; however, pentazocine also effectively relieves pain. Treatments for diabetes mellitus may include dietary modification, insulin replacement, or antidiabetic agents. Malabsorption and steatorrhea are treated with pancreatic enzyme replacement.

Surgical intervention relieves abdominal pain, restores pancreatic drainage, and reduces the frequency of acute pancreatitis attacks. Surgical drainage is required for an abscess or a pseudocyst. If biliary tract disease is the underlying cause, cholecystectomy or choledochotomy is performed. A sphincterotomy is indicated to enlarge a pancreatic sphincter that has become fibrotic. To relieve obstruction and allow drainage of pancreatic secretions, pancreaticojejunostomy (anastomosis of the jejunum with the opened pancreatic duct) may be required.

KEY NURSING DIAGNOSES AND PATIENT OUTCOMES

Fluid volume deficit related to massive hemorrhage caused by fulminant pancreatitis. Based on this nursing diagnosis, you'll establish these patient outcomes. The patient will:
• have his fluid volume deficit identified quickly and treated promptly
• recover and maintain a normal fluid and blood volume, as evidenced by stable vital signs.

Impaired gas exchange related to respiratory complications associated with acute pancreatitis. Based on this nursing diagnosis, you'll establish these patient outcomes. The patient will:
• demonstrate adequate gas exchange after therapy, as evidenced by normal arterial blood gas values and normal respiratory function
• recover from respiratory complications with no residual deficits.

Pain related to inflammatory process. Based on this nursing diagnosis, you'll establish these patient outcomes. The patient will:
• express feelings of comfort following analgesic administration
• avoid eating foods or engaging in activities that precipitate or increase pain
• experience no chronic pain.

NURSING INTERVENTIONS

• Administer meperidine or other analgesics, as ordered, and document the drugs' effectiveness.
• Maintain the NG tube for drainage or suctioning.
• In case of hypocalcemia, keep airway and suction apparatus handy and pad the side rails of the bed.
• Restrict the patient to bed rest, and provide a quiet and restful environment.
• Place the patient in a comfortable position, such as Fowler's position, that also allows maximal chest expansion.
• Keep water and other beverages at the bedside, and encourage the patient to drink plenty of fluids.
• Provide I.V. fluids and parenteral nutrition, as ordered. As soon as the patient can tolerate it, provide a diet high in carbohydrates, low in proteins, and low in fat.
• Prepare the patient for surgery, as indicated.
• If the patient has chronic pancreatitis, allow him to express feelings of anger, depression, and sadness related to his condition and help him to cope with these feelings. Encourage him to use appropriate physical outlets to express his emotions, such as pounding a punching bag or throwing pillows.
• Counsel the patient to contact a self-help group, such as Alcoholics Anonymous, if needed.

Monitoring

• Assess the patient's level of pain. Evaluate his response to administered analgesics, and monitor for adverse reactions.
• Assess pulmonary status at least every 4 hours to detect early signs of respiratory complications.
• Monitor fluid and electrolyte balance, and report any abnormalities. Maintain an accurate record of intake and output. Weigh the patient daily and record his weight.
• Evaluate the patient's present nutritional status and metabolic requirements.
• Monitor serum glucose levels, and administer insulin as ordered.

• Don't confuse thirst from hyperglycemia (indicated by serum glucose levels up to 350 mg/dl and glucose and acetone in the urine) with dry mouth due to NG intubation and anticholinergics.
• Watch for signs of calcium deficiency: tetany, cramps, carpopedal spasm, and seizures.

Patient teaching
• Emphasize the importance of avoiding factors that precipitate acute pancreatitis, especially alcohol.
• Refer the patient and his family to the dietitian. Stress the need for a diet high in carbohydrates and low in protein and fats. Caution the patient to avoid caffeinated beverages and irritating foods.
• Point out the need to comply with pancreatic enzyme replacement therapy. Instruct the patient to take the enzymes with meals or snacks to help digest food and to promote fat and protein absorption. Advise him to watch for and report any of the following signs and symptoms: fatty, frothy, foul-smelling stools; abdominal distention; cramping; and skin excoriation.
• If the patient has chronic pain, teach a family member how to give I.M. injections of analgesics as ordered.

LIVER ABSCESS

A relatively uncommon but often fatal disorder, liver abscess occurs when bacteria or protozoa destroy hepatic tissue. The damage produces a cavity, which fills with infectious organisms, liquefied hepatic cells, and leukocytes. Necrotic tissue then walls off the cavity from the rest of the liver.

Liver abscess carries a mortality of 30% to 50%. This mortality soars to more than 80% with multiple abscesses and to more than 90% with complications. Liver abscess affects both sexes and all age-groups, although it's slightly more prevalent in women (most commonly those between ages 40 and 60).

CAUSES
An amoebic abscess (the most common cause) results from infection with the protozoan *Entamoeba histolytica*, the organism that causes amebic dysentery. Amoebic liver abscesses usually occur singly in the right lobe.

In pyogenic liver abscesses, the common infecting organisms are *Escherichia coli*, *Klebsiella*, *Salmonella*, *Staphylococcus*, and enterococci. Such organisms may invade the liver directly after a liver wound, or they may spread from the lungs, skin, or other organs by the hepatic artery, portal vein, or biliary tract. Though multiple pyogenic abscesses are usual, a single abscess may occur.

Certain illnesses or conditions also may lead to abscess development, including cholecystitis, colon cancer, diverticulitis, peritonitis, regional enteritis, infective endocarditis, pelvic inflammatory disease, pneumonia, trauma, and septicemia.

COMPLICATIONS
Without treatment, liver abscess usually leads to death. Complications include abscess rupture into the peritoneum, pleura, or pericardium.

ASSESSMENT
The clinical manifestations of a liver abscess depend on the degree of involvement. Some patients are acutely ill; in others, the abscess is recognized only at autopsy, after death from another illness. Onset of symptoms of a pyogenic abscess is usually sudden; in an amoebic abscess, onset is more insidious. (See *Nursing care in liver abscess*, pages 220 and 221.)

The patient may report right abdominal and shoulder pain, chills, fever, diaphoresis, nausea, vomiting, and weight loss. If the abscess extends through the diaphragm, she may complain of dyspnea and chest pain (symptoms of pleural effusion); if she has developed anemia, she may report fatigue.

Inspection may detect jaundice, a sign of liver damage. On palpation, the liver may feel enlarged, indicating hepatic disease.

PRIORITY FLOWCHART

Nursing care in liver abscess

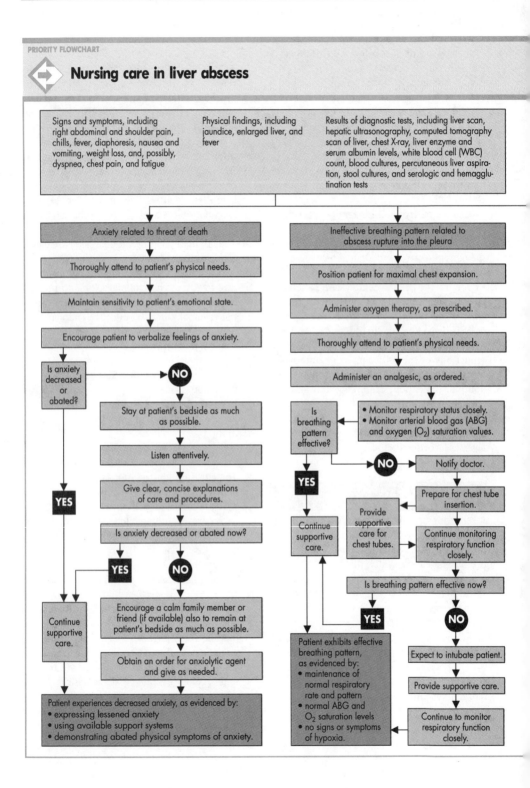

Signs and symptoms, including right abdominal and shoulder pain, chills, fever, diaphoresis, nausea and vomiting, weight loss, and, possibly, dyspnea, chest pain, and fatigue

Physical findings, including jaundice, enlarged liver, and fever

Results of diagnostic tests, including liver scan, hepatic ultrasonography, computed tomography scan of liver, chest X-ray, liver enzyme and serum albumin levels, white blood cell (WBC) count, blood cultures, percutaneous liver aspiration, stool cultures, and serologic and hemagglutination tests

Anxiety related to threat of death

Thoroughly attend to patient's physical needs.

Maintain sensitivity to patient's emotional state.

Encourage patient to verbalize feelings of anxiety.

Is anxiety decreased or abated?

NO

Stay at patient's bedside as much as possible.

Listen attentively.

Give clear, concise explanations of care and procedures.

Is anxiety decreased or abated now?

YES

YES   **NO**

Continue supportive care.

Encourage a calm family member or friend (if available) also to remain at patient's bedside as much as possible.

Obtain an order for anxiolytic agent and give as needed.

Patient experiences decreased anxiety, as evidenced by:
• expressing lessened anxiety
• using available support systems
• demonstrating abated physical symptoms of anxiety.

Ineffective breathing pattern related to abscess rupture into the pleura

Position patient for maximal chest expansion.

Administer oxygen therapy, as prescribed.

Thoroughly attend to patient's physical needs.

Administer an analgesic, as ordered.

Is breathing pattern effective?

• Monitor respiratory status closely.
• Monitor arterial blood gas (ABG) and oxygen (O₂) saturation values.

NO   Notify doctor.

YES

Continue supportive care.

Provide supportive care for chest tubes.

Prepare for chest tube insertion.

Continue monitoring respiratory function closely.

Is breathing pattern effective now?

YES   **NO**

Patient exhibits effective breathing pattern, as evidenced by:
• maintenance of normal respiratory rate and pattern
• normal ABG and O₂ saturation levels
• no signs or symptoms of hypoxia.

Expect to intubate patient.

Provide supportive care.

Continue to monitor respiratory function closely.

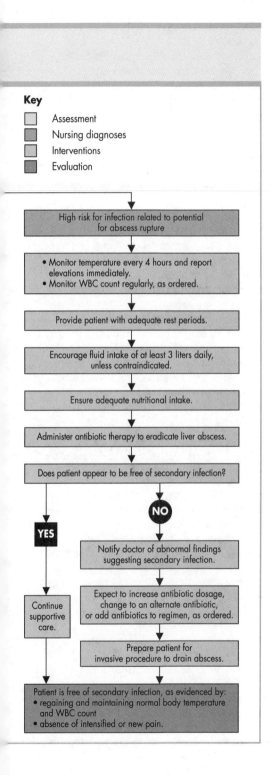

Key

☐ Assessment
▨ Nursing diagnoses
☐ Interventions
▨ Evaluation

High risk for infection related to potential for abscess rupture

• Monitor temperature every 4 hours and report elevations immediately.
• Monitor WBC count regularly, as ordered.

Provide patient with adequate rest periods.

Encourage fluid intake of at least 3 liters daily, unless contraindicated.

Ensure adequate nutritional intake.

Administer antibiotic therapy to eradicate liver abscess.

Does patient appear to be free of secondary infection?

NO

YES

Notify doctor of abnormal findings suggesting secondary infection.

Continue supportive care.

Expect to increase antibiotic dosage, change to an alternate antibiotic, or add antibiotics to regimen, as ordered.

Prepare patient for invasive procedure to drain abscess.

Patient is free of secondary infection, as evidenced by:
• regaining and maintaining normal body temperature and WBC count
• absence of intensified or new pain.

DIAGNOSTIC TESTS

• *Liver scan* showing filling defects at the abscess area larger than ¾" (2 cm), together with characteristic clinical features, confirms the diagnosis.
• *Hepatic ultrasonography* may indicate defects caused by the abscess but is less definitive than a liver scan.
• *Computed tomography scan* verifies the diagnosis after a liver scan or hepatic ultrasonography.
• *Chest X-ray* shows the diaphragm on the right side as raised and fixed.
• *Blood tests* demonstrate elevated levels of serum aspartate aminotransferase (formerly SGOT), serum alanine aminotransferase (formerly SGPT), alkaline phosphatase, and bilirubin. Serum albumin level is decreased. White blood cell count is elevated (usually more in pyogenic than in amoebic abscess).
• *Blood cultures* and *percutaneous liver aspiration* may help to identify the causative bacteria in pyogenic abscess.
• *Stool cultures* and *serologic* and *hemagglutination tests* can isolate *E. histolytica* in amoebic abscess.

TREATMENT

If the organism causing the liver abscess is unknown, long-term antibiotic therapy begins immediately with aminoglycosides, cephalosporins, clindamycin, or chloramphenicol. If cultures demonstrate that the infectious organism is *E. coli,* treatment includes ampicillin; if *E. histolytica,* emetine, chloroquine hydrochloride, chloroquine phosphate, or metronidazole. The therapy continues for 2 to 4 months. Surgery is usually avoided, but it may be required for a single pyogenic abscess or for an amoebic abscess that fails to respond to antibiotics.

KEY NURSING DIAGNOSES AND PATIENT OUTCOMES

Anxiety related to potential threat of death from liver abscess. Based on this nursing diagnosis, you'll establish these patient outcomes. The patient will:
• express fears and concerns about dying

• use available support systems to cope with overwhelming anxiety
• exhibit abated physical signs and symptoms of anxiety.

Ineffective breathing pattern related to abscess rupture into the pleura. Based on this nursing diagnosis, you'll establish these patient outcomes. The patient will:
• have her changed condition detected quickly and treated promptly
• achieve maximum lung expansion with adequate ventilation during treatment
• exhibit a respiratory rate and pattern and arterial blood gas values that return to baseline and remain within this normal range.

High risk for infection related to potential for abscess rupture. Based on this nursing diagnosis, you'll establish these patient outcomes. The patient will:
• exhibit no signs or symptoms of sepsis
• maintain normal body function
• have abscess eradicated with antibiotic therapy or surgery before rupture can occur.

NURSING INTERVENTIONS

• Provide supportive care and maintain fluid and nutritional intake.
• Administer analgesics, as ordered. Apply heat or cold, as ordered, to minimize or relieve pain. Help the patient into a comfortable position, using pillows to splint or support painful areas.
• Administer antibiotics, as ordered.
• Wash your hands before and after providing patient care. Wear gloves to maintain asepsis when providing direct care, such as dressing changes.
• Prepare the patient for surgery, if indicated.
• Provide the patient and family opportunities to express their feelings and concerns. Provide support and, whenever possible, allay their anxiety and fears.

Monitoring

• Closely monitor vital signs, especially respirations.
• Assess the patient's pain level regularly. Evaluate and document the effectiveness of administered analgesics and note any adverse reactions.
• Check the patient's hydration status regularly by measuring intake and output and assessing skin turgor.
• Obtain and record the patient's weight at the same time every day to ensure the most accurate readings.
• Inspect the patient's skin every shift; document skin condition and report any changes.
• Watch carefully for complications of abdominal surgery, such as hemorrhage and infection.

Patient teaching

• Explain all diagnostic and surgical procedures to the patient.
• Stress the importance of compliance with antibiotic drug therapy. Review the medication's purpose, correct use, potential adverse effects, and any special considerations.
• Teach the patient how to perform skin care. Advise her to use nonirritating soap; pat rather than rub her skin dry; inspect skin on a regular basis; and avoid prolonged exposure to environmental elements, such as the sun and wind.

PSEUDOMEMBRANOUS ENTEROCOLITIS

An acute inflammation and necrosis of the small and large intestines, pseudomembranous enterocolitis usually affects the mucosa but may extend into the submucosa and, rarely, other layers. This rare condition, marked by severe diarrhea, can be fatal in 1 to 7 days because of severe dehydration and toxicity, peritonitis, or perforation.

CAUSES

What triggers the acute inflammation and necrosis characteristic of this disorder is unknown; however, *Clostridium difficile* may produce a toxin that plays a role in its development. The disease typically occurs in patients who are undergoing treatment with broad-spectrum antibiotics or who have received such therapy within the past 4 weeks.

Nearly all broad-spectrum antibiotics, especially clindamycin, ampicillin, and the cephalosporins, have been linked with its onset. Possible exceptions are vancomycin and aminoglycosides.

Pseudomembranous enterocolitis may also occur postoperatively in debilitated patients who have undergone abdominal surgery. Whatever the cause, the necrotic mucosa is replaced by a pseudomembrane filled with staphylococci, leukocytes, mucus, fibrin, and inflammatory cells.

COMPLICATIONS

Severe dehydration, electrolyte imbalance, hypotension, shock, colonic perforation, and peritonitis are among the potentially fatal complications associated with this disorder.

ASSESSMENT

The patient's history usually reveals current or recent antibiotic treatment. Typically, the patient reports the sudden onset of copious, watery or, rarely, bloody diarrhea; abdominal pain; and fever. Palpation may reveal abdominal tenderness.

Careful consideration of the patient history is essential because the abrupt onset of enterocolitis and the emergency situation it creates may make diagnosis difficult.

DIAGNOSTIC TESTS

Rectal biopsy through sigmoidoscopy confirms pseudomembranous enterocolitis. Stool cultures can identify *C. difficile.*

TREATMENT

If the patient is receiving broad-spectrum antibiotic treatment, the first priority is immediate discontinuation of the offending drug. Usually, the patient is then treated with oral metronidazole or oral vancomycin. Metronidazole generally is used first; if it's ineffective, vancomycin is given. Anion exchange resins such as cholestyramine, which bind the toxin produced by *C. difficile,* may be ordered for patients with mild pseudomembranous enterocolitis. However, patient response to this treatment has proved inferior to that with oral vancomycin or metronidazole.

Supportive treatments maintain fluid and electrolyte balance and combat hypotension and shock with vasopressors, such as dopamine and norepinephrine.

KEY NURSING DIAGNOSES AND PATIENT OUTCOMES

Diarrhea related to inflammation of the intestines. Based on this nursing diagnosis, you'll establish these patient outcomes. The patient will:
• control diarrhea with treatment
• develop no complications of diarrhea, such as skin breakdown or fluid and electrolyte imbalance
• regain and maintain a normal elimination pattern.

Fluid volume deficit related to loss of fluids from diarrhea. Based on this nursing diagnosis, you'll establish these patient outcomes. The patient will:
• restore and maintain fluid and electrolyte balance
• have no signs or symptoms of hypovolemic shock.

Pain related to inflammation of the intestines. Based on this nursing diagnosis, you'll establish these patient outcomes. The patient will:
• express increased feelings of comfort with therapy
• use nonpharmacologic measures to alleviate or minimize abdominal pain
• become pain-free when pseudomembranous enterocolitis is cured.

NURSING INTERVENTIONS

• If ordered, administer I.V. fluids to restore and maintain fluid and electrolyte balance.
• Administer medications as ordered.
• Keep the patient as comfortable as possible. Administer analgesics to decrease abdominal pain and antipyretics to control high fever. Teach the patient how to perform relaxation techniques, such as distraction or guided imagery, to help him cope with abdominal pain.
• Keep a bedpan within the patient's reach to help prevent embarrassing accidents.

Monitoring

• Frequently assess and record vital signs and skin color. Monitor level of consciousness. Immediately report signs of shock.
• Record fluid intake and output, including fluid lost in stools. Watch for indications of dehydration (poor skin turgor, sunken eyes, and decreased urine output).
• Check serum electrolyte levels daily, and watch for clinical signs of hypokalemia (especially malaise) and a weak, rapid, irregular pulse.
• Monitor the patient for the desired effects of administered medications and for adverse reactions.

Patient teaching

• Teach the patient about the disorder and its possible causes; discuss signs and symptoms, ordered diagnostic tests, and treatments.
• Review prescribed medications, explaining their desired effects, potential adverse effects, and proper administration.
• Point out that because pseudomembranous enterocolitis recurs in about 20% of cases, the patient must immediately report symptoms of recurrence. Reassure him that a second course of therapy resolves the disorder.
• If the disorder was antibiotic-related, instruct the patient to caution doctors who might prescribe similar medications in the future.

BLUNT AND PENETRATING ABDOMINAL INJURIES

Because these injuries may damage major blood vessels and internal organs, they can be immediately life-threatening. The prognosis depends on the extent of injury and the organs damaged but is improved by prompt diagnosis and surgical repair.

CAUSES

Blunt (nonpenetrating) abdominal injuries usually result from motor vehicle accidents, fights, falls from heights, and sports accidents; penetrating abdominal injuries, from stabbings and gunshots.

COMPLICATIONS

Immediate life-threatening complications include hemorrhage and hypovolemic shock. Later complications include infection and dysfunction of major organs, such as the liver, spleen, pancreas, and kidneys.

ASSESSMENT

The patient's history reveals an accidental or forcibly inflicted abdominal injury. Symptoms vary with the degree of injury and the organs damaged. The patient with a blunt or penetrating abdominal injury typically is in obvious discomfort or pain.

A patient with a blunt abdominal injury may report severe pain that radiates beyond the abdomen to the shoulders, nausea, and vomiting. A penetrating abdominal wound may be obvious, especially if the patient is bleeding in the abdominal area. (If you observe the wound in the upper abdominal area, consider it a thoracoabdominal injury until proved otherwise.)

Inspection pinpoints the type of abdominal injury and helps determine its severity. Depending on the severity of the injury, the patient may be pale or cyanotic, short of breath or dyspneic. Inspection also reveals bruises, abrasions, contusions, and distention.

For a patient with a penetrating abdominal injury, inspection reveals the type of wound and associated blood loss.

Palpation may reveal the extent of pain and tenderness and, in blunt abdominal injuries, abdominal splinting or rigidity. Rib fractures often accompany blunt abdominal injuries. Auscultation of the chest may disclose tachycardia and decreased breath sounds. The patient also may have hypotension.

DIAGNOSTIC TESTS

Specific tests vary with the patient's condition but usually include abdominal X-rays and examination of the stools and stomach contents for blood.
• *Chest X-rays*, preferably done with the patient upright, show free air.

• *Blood studies* include hematocrit and hemoglobin levels, coagulation studies, white blood cell (WBC) count, arterial blood gas (ABG) analysis, and serum amylase, aspartate aminotransferase (formerly SGOT), and alanine aminotransferase (formerly SGPT) levels. Typing and crossmatching precede blood transfusion.

Decreased hematocrit and hemoglobin levels point to blood loss. Coagulation studies evaluate clotting ability. WBC count normally is elevated but doesn't necessarily point to infection. ABG analysis evaluates respiratory status.

A patient with pancreatic injury typically has elevated serum amylase levels. Also, levels of aspartate aminotransferase and alanine aminotransferase increase with tissue injury and cell death.

• *Excretory urography* and *cystourethrography* show renal and urinary tract damage.

• *Radioisotope scanning* and *ultrasound examination* detect liver, kidney, and spleen injuries.

• *Angiography* detects specific injuries, especially to the kidneys.

• *Peritoneal lavage* is performed to check for blood, urine, ascitic fluid, bile, and chyle (a milky fluid absorbed by the intestinal lymph vessels during digestion).

• *Computed tomography scanning* helps detect the extent of the injury and other injuries that may have occurred.

• *Exploratory laparotomy* detects specific injuries when other clinical evidence is incomplete.

TREATMENT

The patient needs an immediate infusion of I.V. fluids and blood components to control hemorrhage and prevent hypovolemic shock. He also may require intubation and mechanical ventilation or supplemental oxygen, as well as a nasogastric (NG) tube and an indwelling urinary catheter.

When administering emergency care to a patient with a penetrating abdominal injury, don't remove the penetrating object. Not only could that cause further damage, but it could also make determining the cause of the injury more difficult. Instead, secure the penetrating object and leave it in place until the surgical team is ready to remove it.

After stabilization, most abdominal injuries require surgical repair. Analgesics, withheld until after a definitive diagnosis, increase patient comfort, and antibiotics prevent infection.

The patient will probably require hospitalization; if he's asymptomatic, he may require observation for only 6 to 24 hours.

KEY NURSING DIAGNOSES AND PATIENT OUTCOMES

Altered cardiopulmonary, cerebral, or renal tissue perfusion related to reduced cardiac output caused by blood loss. Based on this nursing diagnosis, you'll establish these patient outcomes. The patient will:

• develop no chest pain, cardiac arrhythmias, or shortness of breath

• stay alert and oriented to time, person, and place

• maintain urine output of at least 30 ml/hour

• regain or maintain normal GI function

• regain normal peripheral pulses, color, and temperature.

Decreased cardiac output related to development of hypovolemic shock caused by fluid and blood loss. Based on this nursing diagnosis, you'll establish these patient outcomes. The patient will:

• regain normal cardiac output, as evidenced by normal blood, central venous, right atrial, pulmonary artery, and pulmonary artery wedge pressure readings

• exhibit no residual deficits as a result of decreased cardiac output.

Fluid volume deficit related to blood loss from abdominal injury. Based on this nursing diagnosis, you'll establish these patient outcomes. The patient will:

• respond quickly to measures used to control and stop bleeding

• recover and maintain normal fluid volume, as evidenced by stable vital signs and adequate urine output

• recover normal hemoglobin and hematocrit levels, red blood cell and platelet counts, electrolyte levels, and urine specific gravity.

NURSING INTERVENTIONS

• Provide emergency care as needed to support the patient's vital functions.
• To maintain airway and breathing, intubate the patient and provide mechanical ventilation, as needed; otherwise, provide oxygen.
• When possible, explain each procedure to the patient before performing it.
• Using a large-bore needle, start one or more I.V. lines for rapid fluid infusion, using lactated Ringer's solution. Then draw a blood sample for laboratory studies. Also, insert an NG tube and, if necessary, an indwelling urinary catheter.
• Apply a sterile dressing to any open wounds. Splint a suspected pelvic injury by tying the patient's legs together with a pillow between them. Move the patient as little as possible.
• If evisceration has occurred, minimize movement of the patient. Apply a wet saline dressing to exposed abdominal contents.
• Give analgesics, as ordered. Narcotics usually aren't recommended. If the pain is severe, give narcotics in small, titrated I.V. doses, as ordered.
• Give tetanus prophylaxis and prophylactic I.V. antibiotics, as ordered.
• Prepare the patient for surgery. Obtain a consent form signed by the patient or a responsible relative.
• If the injury was caused by a motor vehicle accident, make sure the police are notified. If the patient suffered a gunshot or stab wound, also notify the police, place all his clothes in a bag, and retain them for the police. Document the number and sites of the wounds.

Monitoring

• Obtain vital signs for baseline data. Continue checking them every 15 minutes until the patient's condition stabilizes. Continuously monitor cardiac rhythm.
• Monitor the patient's vital organ function for signs of abnormalities.
• Assess the patient's central venous pressure, right atrial pressure, pulmonary artery pressure, pulmonary artery wedge pressure, and cardiac output hourly or as ordered.

• Monitor the patient's hydration status. Measure intake and output and check skin turgor.
• Check the patient's ABG and electrolyte levels frequently as ordered.
• During treatment, assess skin color and temperature, and note any changes. Cold, clammy skin may signal continuing peripheral vascular constriction, indicating progressive shock.
• Assess the patient frequently for signs of complications. Check stomach aspirate and urine for blood.
• Evaluate the patient's pain level and response to administered analgesics.
• Assess the patient regularly for signs and symptoms of infection at the injury site and early signs of sepsis.

Patient teaching

• Tell the patient with a blunt abdominal injury that he may be assessed and discharged from the emergency department. But some injuries, such as delayed rupture of the spleen, may not become apparent for several hours or days.
• Instruct the patient to notify the doctor if he experiences increased localized or generalized abdominal pain; shoulder pain that's not the result of shoulder trauma (Kehr's sign); malaise, lethargy, or dizziness (signs of slow blood loss); unexplained fever; nausea or vomiting, particularly if it's persistent; hematemesis or melena; or light-headedness, restlessness, diaphoresis, or hemoptysis.
• Tell the patient to take analgesics as ordered.
• Advise the patient to avoid contact sports until the doctor permits him to resume such activities.

9
Renal disorders

By producing and eliminating urine, the kidneys play a vital role in maintaining homeostasis. These essential organs regulate the volume, electrolyte concentration, and acid-base balance of body fluids; detoxify the blood and eliminate wastes; regulate blood pressure; and aid in erythropoiesis. Disorders that alter renal function can become life-threatening because they can lead to renal shutdown. This shutdown results in electrolyte imbalance, metabolic acidosis, and other severe effects as the patient becomes increasingly uremic and renal dysfunction disrupts other body systems. If left untreated, the patient will die. Even with treatment, life-threatening complications can occur.

This section includes three potentially life-threatening renal disorders: acute renal failure, acute pyelonephritis, and acute poststreptococcal glomerulonephritis.

Because renal shutdown can occur quickly, you'll need to monitor the patient closely for signs and symptoms suggesting renal dysfunction. You may also need to prepare the patient for emergency diagnostic tests, such as kidney ultrasonography or excretory urography, or assist with lifesaving treatment, such as peritoneal dialysis or hemodialysis. In addition, supportive measures, such as emotional support and early recognition and treatment of complications, will be an essential part of your nursing care for the patient with renal compromise.

Initial renal care

Check for:
- [ ] history of chronic renal disorders
- [ ] medication history and history of medical conditions that affect the renal system
- [ ] history of urinary tract obstruction or infection
- [ ] recent history of trauma, abdominal surgery, infection, or a life-threatening event that resulted in hypovolemia or impaired systemic circulation
- [ ] recent history of chills and fever, fluid retention, flank pain, hematuria or other change in urine appearance, urinary urgency and frequency, unusual urine odor, burning during urination, dysuria, or nocturia
- [ ] fluid intake unequal to output
- [ ] neurologic dysfunction, especially impaired mental status
- [ ] abnormal vital signs and heart sounds, reflecting infection or congestive heart failure
- [ ] peripheral edema and possibly lung crackles
- [ ] abdominal or flank pain
- [ ] abnormal results of renal function studies, urinalysis, and renal radiography.

Intervene by:
- [ ] notifying the doctor of abnormal findings
- [ ] initiating fluid and sodium restriction
- [ ] inserting a peripheral I.V. line
- [ ] monitoring vital signs and condition continuously
- [ ] measuring intake and output hourly
- [ ] placing the patient on strict bed rest
- [ ] obtaining urine and blood samples for culture.

Prepare for:
- [ ] medication administration
- [ ] measures to correct electrolyte and acid-base imbalances
- [ ] emergency peritoneal dialysis or hemodialysis.

ACUTE RENAL FAILURE

About 5% of all hospitalized patients develop acute renal failure—the sudden interruption of renal function resulting from obstruction, reduced circulation, or renal parenchymal disease. This condition is classified as prerenal, intrarenal, or postrenal and normally consists of three distinct phases: oliguric, diuretic, and recovery. It's usually reversible with medical treatment. If not treated, it may progress to end-stage renal disease, uremia, and death.

CAUSES

Each type of acute renal failure has different causes. Prerenal failure results from conditions that diminish blood flow to the kidneys. Between 40% and 80% of all cases of acute renal failure are caused by prerenal azotemia. Intrarenal failure (also called intrinsic or parenchymal renal failure) results from damage to the kidneys themselves, usually from acute tubular necrosis. Postrenal failure results from bilateral obstruction of urine flow. (See *Causes of acute renal failure.*)

COMPLICATIONS

Ischemic acute tubular necrosis can lead to renal shutdown. Electrolyte imbalance, metabolic acidosis, and other severe effects follow as the patient becomes increasingly uremic and renal dysfunction disrupts other body systems. If left untreated, the patient will die. Even with treatment, the older patient is particularly susceptible to volume overload, precipitating acute pulmonary edema, hypertensive crisis, hyperkalemia, and infection.

ASSESSMENT

The patient's history may include a disorder that can cause renal failure, and he may have a recent history of fever; chills; GI problems, such as anorexia, nausea, vomiting, diarrhea, and constipation; and central nervous system (CNS) problems such as headache.

The patient may appear irritable, drowsy, and confused or demonstrate other alterations in his level of consciousness. In ad-

vanced stages, seizures and coma may occur. Depending on the stage of renal failure, he may be oliguric (urine output of less than 400 ml/ 24 hours) or anuric (urine output of less than 100 ml/24 hours).

Inspection may uncover evidence of bleeding abnormalities, such as petechiae and ecchymoses. Hematemesis may occur. The skin may be dry and pruritic and, rarely, you may note uremic frost. Mucous membranes may be dry, and the patient's breath may have a uremic odor. If the patient has hyperkalemia, muscle weakness may occur.

Auscultation may detect tachycardia and, possibly, an irregular rhythm. Bibasilar crackles may be heard if the patient has congestive heart failure (CHF).

Palpation and percussion may reveal abdominal pain, if pancreatitis or peritonitis occurs, and peripheral edema, if the patient has CHF.

DIAGNOSTIC TESTS

• *Blood test results* indicating acute intrarenal failure include elevated blood urea nitrogen, serum creatinine, and potassium levels, and low blood pH, bicarbonate, hematocrit, and hemoglobin levels.
• *Urine specimens* show casts, cellular debris, decreased specific gravity and, in glomerular diseases, proteinuria and urine osmolality close to serum osmolality. The urine sodium level is under 20 mEq/liter if oliguria results from decreased perfusion and above 40 mEq/ liter if it results from an intrarenal problem. A creatinine clearance test measures the glomerular filtration rate and allows for an estimate of the number of remaining functioning nephrons.
• *Electrocardiography (ECG)* reveals tall, peaked T waves, a widening QRS complex, and disappearing P waves if hyperkalemia is present.

Other studies that help determine the cause of renal failure include *kidney ultrasonography, plain X-rays of the abdomen, kidney-ureter-bladder radiography, excretory urography, renal scan, retrograde pyelography, computed tomography scans,* and *nephrotomography.*

Causes of acute renal failure

Acute renal failure can be classified as prerenal, intrarenal, or postrenal. All conditions that lead to prerenal failure impair renal perfusion, resulting in decreased glomerular filtration rate and increased proximal tubular reabsorption of sodium and water. Intrarenal failure results from damage to the kidneys themselves; postrenal failure, from obstruction of urine flow.

PRERENAL FAILURE	INTRARENAL FAILURE	POSTRENAL FAILURE
Cardiovascular disorders	*Acute tubular necrosis*	*Bladder obstruction*
• Arrhythmias	• Ischemic damage to renal paren-	• Anticholinergic drugs
• Cardiac tamponade	chyma from unrecognized or poorly	• Autonomic nerve dysfunction
• Cardiogenic shock	treated prerenal failure	• Infection
• Congestive heart failure	• Nephrotoxins – analgesics (such as	• Tumor
• Myocardial infarction	aspirin given in high doses and long-	
	term); anesthetics (such as methoxy-	*Ureteral obstruction*
Hypovolemia	flurane); antibiotics (such as gentami-	• Blood clots
• Burns	cin); heavy metals (such as lead);	• Calculi
• Dehydration	radiographic contrast media; organic	• Edema or inflammation
• Diuretic abuse	solvents	• Necrotic renal papillae
• Hemorrhage	• Obstetric complications – eclampsia,	• Retroperitoneal fibrosis or hemor-
• Hypovolemic shock	postpartum renal failure, septic abor-	rhage
• Trauma	tion, uterine hemorrhage	• Surgery (accidental ligation)
	• Crush injury, myopathy, sepsis, trans-	• Tumor
Peripheral vasodilation	fusion reaction	• Uric acid crystals
• Antihypertensive drugs		
• Sepsis	*Other parenchymal disorders*	*Urethral obstruction*
	• Acute glomerulonephritis	• Benign prostatic hyperplasia or
Renovascular obstruction	• Acute interstitial nephritis	tumor
• Arterial embolism	• Acute pyelonephritis	• Strictures
• Arterial or venous thrombosis	• Bilateral renal vein thrombosis	
• Tumor	• Malignant nephrosclerosis	
	• Papillary necrosis	
Severe vasoconstriction	• Periarteritis nodosa	
• Disseminated intravascular co-	• Renal myeloma	
agulation	• Sickle cell disease	
• Eclampsia	• Systemic lupus erythematosus	
• Malignant hypertension	• Vasculitis	
• Vasculitis		

TREATMENT

Supportive measures include a diet high in calories and low in protein, sodium, and potassium, with supplemental vitamins and restricted fluids. Meticulous electrolyte monitoring is essential to detect hyperkalemia. If hyperkalemia occurs, acute therapy may include hypertonic glucose-and-insulin infusions and sodium bicarbonate – all administered I.V. – and sodium polystyrene sulfonate by mouth or enema to remove potassium from the body. Early initiation of diuretic therapy during the oliguric phase may benefit the patient.

If these measures fail to control uremic symptoms, the patient may require hemodialysis or peritoneal dialysis.

KEY NURSING DIAGNOSES
AND PATIENT OUTCOMES

Fluid volume excess related to decreased ability of the kidneys to excrete water and sodium. Based on this nursing diagnosis, you'll establish these patient outcomes. The patient will:
• adhere to fluid restrictions
• exhibit no signs or symptoms of CHF
• regain and maintain normal fluid volume with alleviation of acute renal failure.

High risk for infection related to renal dysfunction. Based on this nursing diagnosis, you'll establish these patient outcomes. The patient will:
• maintain a normal temperature and white blood cell count
• demonstrate appropriate infection-control measures
• show no signs or symptoms of sepsis.

High risk for injury related to potential for hyperkalemia. Based on this nursing diagnosis, you'll establish these patient outcomes. The patient will:
• adhere to a potassium-restricted diet
• maintain a normal serum potassium level
• show no signs or symptoms of hyperkalemia.

NURSING INTERVENTIONS

• Use infection-control measures during care because the patient with acute renal failure is highly susceptible to infection. Don't allow staff members or visitors with upper respiratory tract infections to have contact with the patient. Also use universal precautions when handling all blood and body fluids.
• Replace blood components as ordered.

◆ NURSING ALERT. Don't use whole blood for a patient with acute renal failure if he's prone to CHF and can't tolerate extra fluid volume. Packed red blood cells deliver the necessary blood components without added volume.
• Maintain proper electrolyte balance. Avoid administering medications that contain potassium.
• Maintain nutritional status. Provide a diet high in calories and low in protein, sodium,

and potassium. Provide vitamin supplements. Give the anorexic patient small, frequent meals.
• Prevent complications of immobility by encouraging frequent coughing and deep breathing and by performing passive range-of-motion exercises. Help the patient walk as soon as possible. Add lubricating lotion to his bathwater to combat skin dryness.
• Provide mouth care frequently to lubricate dry mucous membranes. If stomatitis occurs, use an antibiotic solution, if ordered, and have the patient swish it around in his mouth before swallowing.
• Administer medications carefully, especially antacids and stool softeners.
• Provide meticulous perineal care to reduce the risk of ascending urinary tract infection in women and to prevent impaired skin integrity caused by loose, irritating stools, particularly when sodium polystyrene sulfonate is used.
• Use appropriate safety measures, such as side rails and restraints, because the patient with CNS involvement may become dizzy or confused.
• Prepare the patient for hemodialysis or peritoneal dialysis, as indicated.
• Administer any prescribed medications after hemodialysis is completed. Many medications are removed from the blood during treatment.
• Provide emotional support to the patient and his family.

Monitoring

• Measure and record intake and output of all fluids, including wound drainage, nasogastric tube output, and diarrhea.
• Weigh the patient daily. You also may need to measure abdominal girth every day. Mark the skin with indelible ink so that measurements can be taken in the same place.
• Monitor renal function studies, electrolyte levels (especially potassium), and hematocrit and hemoglobin levels regularly, as ordered.
• Monitor vital signs. Watch for and report signs of pericarditis (pleuritic chest pain, tachycardia, and pericardial friction rub), inadequate renal perfusion (hypotension), and acidosis.

• Watch for signs of hyperkalemia (malaise, anorexia, paresthesia, muscle weakness, and ECG changes), and report them immediately.
• Assess the patient frequently, especially during emergency treatment to lower potassium levels. If he receives hypertonic glucose-and-insulin infusions, monitor potassium and glucose levels. If you give sodium polystyrene sulfonate rectally, make sure the patient doesn't retain it and become constipated. This can lead to bowel perforation.
• Monitor for GI bleeding by testing all stools for occult blood, using the guaiac test.
• Evaluate the patient's nutritional status.
• Assess the patient's ability to resume normal activities of daily living, and plan for the gradual resumption of activity.

Patient teaching

• Reassure the patient and his family by clearly explaining all diagnostic tests, treatments, and procedures.
• Tell the patient about his prescribed medications, and stress the importance of complying with the regimen.
• Stress the importance of following the prescribed diet and fluid allowance.
• Instruct the patient to weigh himself daily and to report changes of 3 lb (1.4 kg) or more immediately.
• Advise the patient against overexertion. If he becomes dyspneic or short of breath during normal activity, tell him to notify his doctor.
• Teach the patient how to recognize edema, and tell him to report this finding to the doctor.

ACUTE PYELONEPHRITIS

Also called acute infective tubulointerstitial nephritis, acute pyelonephritis is one of the most common renal diseases. In this disorder, sudden inflammation is caused by bacterial invasion, mainly in the interstitial tissue and the renal pelvis and occasionally in the renal tubules. It may affect one or both kidneys and is potentially life-threatening if septic shock develops. However, with treatment

and continued follow-up care, the prognosis is good and extensive permanent damage is rare.

Pyelonephritis occurs more often in women than in men, probably because the shorter urethra and the proximity of the urinary meatus to the vagina and rectum allow bacteria to reach the bladder more easily. Women also lack the antibacterial prostatic secretions that men produce.

Typically, the infection spreads from the bladder to the ureters and then to the kidneys, commonly through vesicoureteral reflux. Vesicoureteral reflux may result from congenital weakness at the junction of the ureter and the bladder. Bacteria refluxed to intrarenal tissues may create colonies of infection within 24 to 48 hours.

CAUSES

Acute pyelonephritis results from bacterial infection of the kidneys. Infecting bacteria usually are normal intestinal and fecal flora that grow readily in urine. The most common causative organism is *Escherichia coli,* but *Proteus, Pseudomonas, Staphylococcus aureus,* and *Streptococcus faecalis* (enterococcus) also may cause such infections. Infection may result from procedures that involve the use of instruments (such as catheterization, cystoscopy, and urologic surgery) or from a hematogenic infection (such as septicemia and endocarditis).

Pyelonephritis may result from an inability to empty the bladder (for example, in patients with neurogenic bladder), urinary stasis, and urinary obstruction caused by tumors, strictures, or benign prostatic hyperplasia. Incidence increases with age and is higher in the following groups:
• sexually active women. Intercourse increases the risk of bacterial contamination.
• pregnant women. About 5% of pregnant women develop asymptomatic bacteriuria; if untreated, about 40% of these women develop pyelonephritis.
• people with obstructive diseases. Resulting hydronephrosis increases the risk of urinary tract infection (UTI), which can lead to pyelonephritis.

• people with neurogenic bladder. Seen in diabetes mellitus, spinal cord injury, multiple sclerosis, and tabes dorsalis, neurogenic bladder causes incomplete emptying and urinary stasis. Frequent catheterization increases the risk of introducing bacteria. Glycosuria may support bacterial growth in urine.
• people with other renal diseases. Compromised renal function increases susceptibility to acute pyelonephritis.

COMPLICATIONS
Associated complications include secondary arteriosclerosis, calculus formation, further renal damage, renal abscesses with possible metastasis to other organs, septic shock, and chronic pyelonephritis.

ASSESSMENT
A patient with acute pyelonephritis commonly looks quite ill. She usually complains of pain over one or both kidneys, urinary urgency and frequency, burning during urination, dysuria, nocturia, and hematuria (usually microscopic but possibly gross).

Palpating the flank area may increase pain. Urine may appear cloudy and have an ammonia-like or fishy odor. Other common signs include a temperature of 102° F (38.9° C) or higher, shaking chills, anorexia, and general fatigue.

The patient usually reports that symptoms developed rapidly over a few hours or a few days. Although these symptoms may disappear within days, even without treatment, residual bacterial infection is likely and may cause recurrence of symptoms.

DIAGNOSTIC TESTS
Diagnosis requires a urinalysis and culture and sensitivity testing. Typical findings include the following:
• pyuria (leukocytes singly, in clumps, and in casts and possibly a few red blood cells)
• significant bacteriuria (more than 100,000 organisms/mm³ of urine revealed in urine culture)
• low specific gravity and osmolality resulting from a temporarily decreased ability to concentrate urine

• slightly alkaline urine pH
• proteinuria, glycosuria, and ketonuria (less common).

Blood tests and X-rays also help in the evaluation of acute pyelonephritis. A complete blood count shows an elevated white blood cell count (up to 40,000/mm³) and an elevated neutrophil count. The erythrocyte sedimentation rate also is elevated.

Kidney-ureter-bladder radiography may reveal calculi, tumors, or cysts in the kidneys and the urinary tract. Excretory urography may show asymmetrical kidneys.

TREATMENT
Appropriate treatment centers on antibiotic therapy appropriate to the specific infecting organism after identification by urine culture and sensitivity studies. For example, *S. faecalis* requires treatment with ampicillin, penicillin G, or vancomycin. *S. aureus* requires penicillin G or, if the bacterium is resistant, a semisynthetic penicillin, such as nafcillin, or a cephalosporin. *E. coli* may be treated with sulfisoxazole, nalidixic acid, or nitrofurantoin; *Proteus*, with ampicillin, sulfisoxazole, nalidixic acid, or a cephalosporin; and *Pseudomonas*, with gentamicin, tobramycin, or carbenicillin.

When the infecting organism can't be identified, therapy usually consists of a broad-spectrum antibiotic, such as ampicillin or cephalexin. Antibiotics must be prescribed cautiously for older patients because of the combined effects of aging and pyelonephritis on renal function. Antibiotics also are used with caution in pregnant patients. In these patients, urinary analgesics, such as phenazopyridine, can help relieve pain.

Symptoms may disappear after several days of antibiotic therapy. Although urine usually becomes sterile within 48 to 72 hours, the course of such therapy ranges from 10 to 14 days. Follow-up treatment includes reculturing urine 1 week after drug therapy stops and then periodically for the next year to detect residual or recurring infection. A patient with an uncomplicated infection usually responds well to therapy and doesn't suffer reinfection.

If infection results from obstruction or vesicoureteral reflux, antibiotics may be less effective and surgery may be necessary to relieve the obstruction or correct the anomaly.

A patient at high risk for recurring urinary tract and kidney infections—for example, a patient with a long-term indwelling urinary catheter or one on maintenance antibiotic therapy—requires long-term follow-up medical care.

KEY NURSING DIAGNOSES AND PATIENT OUTCOMES

Decreased cardiac output related to septic shock. Based on this nursing diagnosis, you'll establish these patient outcomes. The patient will:
• have septic shock detected early and emergency interventions administered to alleviate it
• maintain hemodynamic stability
• regain and maintain adequate cardiac output.

Hyperthermia related to inflammatory process. Based on this nursing diagnosis, you'll establish these patient outcomes. The patient will:
• regain normal body temperature with antipyretic and antibiotic therapy
• show no signs or symptoms of complications associated with hyperthermia, such as seizures and dehydration.

Pain related to dysuria. Based on this nursing diagnosis, you'll establish these patient outcomes. The patient will:
• state and carry out appropriate interventions for pain relief
• express feelings of comfort and relief from pain with eradication of pyelonephritis.

NURSING INTERVENTIONS

• Administer antipyretics for fever.
• Force fluids to achieve a urine output of more than 2,000 ml/day. This helps empty the bladder of contaminated urine and is the best way to prevent calculus formation. Don't encourage intake of more than 2 to 3 qt (or liters) because this may decrease the effectiveness of the antibiotics.
• Provide an acid-ash diet to prevent calculus formation.

• Observe strict sterile technique during catheter insertion and care.
• Refrigerate or culture a urine specimen within 30 minutes of collection to prevent overgrowth of bacteria.

Monitoring

• Assess the patient's temperature regularly to determine his response to administered antipyretics.
• Check the patient's voiding pattern and urine characteristics for evidence of improvement or complications. Measure his intake and output.

Patient teaching

• Instruct a female patient to avoid bacterial contamination by wiping from front to back after bowel movements.
• Teach proper technique for collecting a clean-catch urine specimen.
• Stress the need to complete the prescribed antibiotic regimen even after symptoms subside. Encourage long-term follow-up care for a high-risk patient.
• Advise routine checkups for a patient with a history of UTIs. Teach her to recognize signs and symptoms of infection, such as cloudy urine, burning on urination, and urinary urgency and frequency, especially when accompanied by a low-grade fever and back pain. Emphasize the importance of seeking prompt medical attention if such signs and symptoms occur.

ACUTE POSTSTREPTOCOCCAL GLOMERULONEPHRITIS

Also called acute glomerulonephritis, acute poststreptococcal glomerulonephritis is relatively common. This disorder, a bilateral inflammation of the glomeruli, follows a streptococcal infection of the respiratory tract or, less often, a skin infection such as impetigo. Up to 70% of adults recover fully; the rest, especially older patients, may progress to life-threatening chronic renal failure within months.

CAUSES

Acute poststreptococcal glomerulonephritis results from the entrapment and collection of antigen-antibody complexes (produced as an immunologic mechanism in response to a group A beta-hemolytic streptococcus) in the glomerular capillary membranes, inducing inflammatory damage and impeding glomerular function.

Sometimes the immune complement further damages the glomerular membrane. The damaged and inflamed glomeruli lose the ability to be selectively permeable, allowing red blood cells (RBCs) and proteins to filter through as the glomerular filtration rate (GFR) falls. Uremic poisoning may result from this further immunologic damage.

COMPLICATIONS

Renal function progressively deteriorates in 33% to 50% of adults who contract sporadic acute poststreptococcal glomerulonephritis, often in the form of glomerulosclerosis accompanied by hypertension. The more severe the disorder, the more likely that complications will follow.

ASSESSMENT

In most cases, acute poststreptococcal glomerulonephritis begins within 1 to 3 weeks after an untreated streptococcal infection of the respiratory tract. The patient—or the patient's parents—may report decreased urination, smoky or coffee-colored urine, and fatigue.

The patient also may experience shortness of breath, dyspnea, and orthopnea. These symptoms of pulmonary edema point to congestive heart failure (CHF) resulting from hypervolemia.

Assessment findings may show oliguria (urine output of less than 400 ml/24 hours) and mild to moderate periorbital edema. Findings also may reveal mild to severe hypertension resulting from either sodium or water retention (caused by decreased GFR) or inappropriate renin release.

An older patient may complain of vague, nonspecific symptoms, such as nausea, malaise, and arthralgia. Auscultation of the lungs may reveal bibasilar crackles if CHF is present.

DIAGNOSTIC TESTS

• *Blood studies* may reveal elevated electrolyte, blood urea nitrogen (BUN), and creatinine levels and decreased serum protein levels. Elevated antistreptolysin-O titers (in 80% of patients with this disorder), elevated streptozyme and anti-DNase B titers, and low serum complement levels verify recent streptococcal infection.
• *Urinalysis* may show RBCs, white blood cells, mixed cell casts, and protein, which could indicate renal failure. (Proteinuria in an older patient usually isn't as pronounced.) Urine frequently contains high levels of fibrin-degradation products and C3 protein.
• *Throat culture* may show group A beta-hemolytic streptococci.
• *Kidney-ureter-bladder radiography* shows bilateral kidney enlargement.
• *Renal biopsy* may be necessary to confirm the diagnosis of acute poststreptococcal glomerulonephritis or to assess renal tissue status.

TREATMENT

Therapy aims to relieve symptoms and prevent complications from acute poststreptococcal glomerulonephritis. Vigorous supportive care bed rest, fluid and dietary sodium restrictions, and correction of electrolyte imbalances (possibly with dialysis, although this procedure seldom is necessary).

Treatment may include loop diuretics, such as metolazone or furosemide, to reduce extracellular fluid overload, and vasodilators, such as hydralazine or nifedipine. If the patient with this disorder has a documented staphylococcal infection, antibiotics are recommended for 7 to 10 days; otherwise, their use is controversial.

KEY NURSING DIAGNOSES AND PATIENT OUTCOMES

Altered urinary elimination related to changes in renal function. Based on this nursing diagnosis, you'll establish these patient outcomes. The patient will:

• identify any abnormal changes in his urine elimination pattern and seek prompt medical attention

• communicate his clear understanding of the treatment prescribed to restore renal function

• regain and maintain his normal urine elimination pattern.

Fluid volume excess related to inability of kidneys to excrete fluid adequately. Based on this nursing diagnosis, you'll establish these patient outcomes. The patient will:

• show no signs or symptoms of severe fluid retention, such as CHF

• adhere to fluid and sodium restrictions to minimize fluid retention

• regain and maintain normal renal function and normal fluid balance.

High risk for injury related to potential for permanent kidney damage. Based on this nursing diagnosis, you'll establish these patient outcomes. The patient will:

• express an understanding of the prescribed treatment and the need for compliance with treatment to minimize or prevent kidney damage

• regain and maintain his normal renal function.

NURSING INTERVENTIONS

• Acute poststreptococcal glomerulonephritis usually resolves within 2 weeks, so nursing care primarily is supportive.

• Provide bed rest during the acute phase. Perform passive range-of-motion exercises for the patient on bed rest. Allow the patient to resume normal activities *gradually* as symptoms subside.

• Consult the dietitian about a diet high in calories and low in protein, sodium, potassium, and fluids.

• Protect the debilitated patient against secondary infection by providing good nutrition and good hygienic technique. You should also prevent the patient from having any contact with infected people.

• Provide emotional support for the patient with acute poststreptococcal glomerulonephritis and his family. Encourage the patient to verbalize his concerns about his inability to perform in his expected role. Assure him that activity restrictions are temporary.

Monitoring

• Check the patient's vital signs and electrolyte values. Assess renal function daily through serum creatinine and BUN levels and urine creatinine clearance tests. Immediately report signs of acute renal failure to the doctor. Such signs may include oliguria, azotemia, and acidosis.

• Monitor intake and output and daily weight. Report peripheral edema or the formation of ascites.

Patient teaching

• Stress to the patient or his family that follow-up examinations are necessary to detect chronic renal failure.

• Emphasize the need for regular blood pressure, urine protein, and renal function assessments during the convalescent months to detect recurrence of acute poststreptococcal glomerulonephritis.

• Explain to the patient that after acute poststreptococcal glomerulonephritis, gross hematuria may recur during nonspecific viral infections and abnormal urinary findings may persist for years.

• If the patient is scheduled for dialysis, explain the procedure fully. Tell him that dialysis removes toxic wastes and other impurities from the blood.

• Explain that in hemodialysis blood is removed from the body through a surgically created access site, pumped through a filtration unit to remove toxins, and then returned to the body.

• Teach the patient that peritoneal dialysis uses the patient's peritoneal membrane as a semipermeable dialyzing membrane. In this procedure, a hypertonic dialyzing solution is instilled through a catheter that is inserted into the patient's peritoneal cavity. Substances diffuse through the peritoneal membrane. Waste products remain in the solution and are removed.

• Advise a patient with a history of chronic upper respiratory tract infections to report signs and symptoms of infection, such as fever and sore throat, immediately.

• Encourage a pregnant patient with a history of acute poststreptococcal glomerulonephritis to have frequent medical evaluations because pregnancy further stresses the kidneys and increases the risk of chronic renal failure.

• Explain to the patient taking diuretics that he may experience orthostatic hypotension and dizziness when he changes positions too quickly.

10

Metabolic and endocrine disorders

Complex chemical and hormonal regulation is critical in maintaining homeostasis. When disturbances in acid-base balance cause a decreased pH (acidosis) or an increased pH (alkalosis) or when endocrine dysfunction results in a hormonal imbalance, lethal consequences are possible. To prevent these life-threatening events, early detection and appropriate intervention are vital.

This section describes a variety of life-threatening metabolic conditions, including diabetic ketoacidosis, metabolic acidosis, and metabolic alkalosis. Life-threatening endocrine conditions covered here include hyperosmolar nonketotic syndrome, acute hypoglycemia, thyroid storm, myxedema crisis, adrenal crisis, and diabetes insipidus.

The signs and symptoms of a metabolic or endocrine disorder are frequently nonspecific or misleading. For example, in a patient with hyperosmolar nonketotic syndrome, severe dehydration and neurologic deficits may suggest a cerebrovascular accident. Until the patient's blood glucose level is found to be dangerously high, the disorder can't be clearly identified.

The information in this section will help you identify the signs and symptoms of acute metabolic and endocrine disorders and the diagnostic studies that confirm the diagnosis. You'll also learn what type of emergency care can help the patient regain homeostasis.

PRIORITY CHECKLIST

Initial metabolic and endocrine care

Check for:
- □ history of chronic metabolic or endocrine disorders and risk factors
- □ medication history, especially current use of hormonal agents, aspirin, alcohol, or antacids
- □ history of noncompliance with treatment
- □ recent stress, trauma, infection, or surgery
- □ recent extracellular fluid volume depletion
- □ abnormal neurologic findings
- □ restlessness, anxiety, and agitation
- □ neuromuscular weakness
- □ polydipsia, polyphagia, polyuria, or weight loss
- □ dehydration and output greater than intake
- □ abnormal vital signs
- □ Kussmaul's respirations and fruity breath odor
- □ abnormal arterial blood gas values, electrolyte studies, and blood glucose or hormonal levels
- □ ketonuria
- □ abnormal electrocardiogram findings.

Intervene by:
- □ notifying the doctor of abnormal findings
- □ maintaining patent airway and initiating cardio-pulmonary resuscitation if needed
- □ inserting large-bore needle for peripheral I.V. line
- □ performing fingerstick for analysis of blood glucose level and testing urine for ketone bodies
- □ drawing blood for laboratory analysis.

Prepare for:
- □ medication administration
- □ aggressive fluid replacement or restriction therapy
- □ electrolyte replacement therapy
- □ possible intubation and mechanical ventilation.

DIABETIC KETOACIDOSIS

Also called diabetic coma, diabetic ketoacidosis (DKA) is an acute complication of diabetes mellitus marked by pronounced hyperglycemia and ketonemia. Reflecting an insulin deficiency, it usually occurs in patients with Type I (insulin-dependent) diabetes mellitus. For instance, it may arise if the patient has an illness that increases his insulin needs or if he omits or reduces his regular insulin dose. In some patients, DKA is the first manifestation of Type I diabetes.

DKA carries a mortality of 5% to 10%. Any delay in recognizing the condition and treating the patient may jeopardize his life.

CAUSES

DKA results from a severe insulin deficiency and secretion of excess contra-insulin hormones (epinephrine, cortisol, glucagon, and growth hormones). Causes of severe insulin deficiency include undiagnosed Type I diabetes and, in a patient with Type I diabetes, failure to receive extra insulin during times of acute physiologic stress or failure to take insulin because of noncompliance or misinformation. For example, a Type I diabetic may think he shouldn't take his insulin when he's unable to eat because of a GI illness.

Common causes of excess contra-insulin hormones include surgery, stress resulting from infection (especially pneumonia and flu-like illnesses), trauma, and intercurrent illnesses such as myocardial infarction or stroke.

Although uncommon, DKA can affect patients with Type II diabetes who experience severe stress and secrete large amounts of contra-insulin hormones, which antagonize the effects of insulin.

DKA begins when a lack of insulin prevents glucose from entering body cells, resulting in a rise in the blood glucose level. When the blood glucose level exceeds the renal threshold, osmotic diuresis occurs. This leads to loss of water and electrolytes, promoting dehydration and intravascular volume depletion.

Insulin normally controls the release of free fatty acids (FFAs) from fat cells. Without adequate insulin, fat catabolism begins to compensate for deficient carbohydrate fuels. However, fat catabolism is incomplete; FFAs are released and carried to the liver. The liver then begins to break down stored glycogen to glucose (glycogenolysis) and to synthesize new glucose from amino and lactic acids and fats (gluconeogenesis). Both processes worsen hyperglycemia.

In response to hyperglycemia and excessive contra-insulin hormones, the liver releases additional fuels and also uses FFAs as fuel. This release results in excessive ketone bodies in the blood—a condition called ketonemia. Although some tissues can use ketone bodies for fuel, most of these ketone bodies cannot be metabolized. Metabolic acidosis rapidly sets in, and ketone bodies are excreted into the urine (ketonuria) as the kidneys try to compensate for acidosis.

Lack of insulin also affects protein metabolism. Transport of amino acids into body cells decreases, and protein catabolism occurs. Muscle tissues then release amino acids for use as fuel, and the liver metabolizes them. Muscle tissue loses nitrogen in this reaction, characteristically causing loss of lean body mass and elevations in blood urea nitrogen (BUN) and serum creatinine levels. (See *How insulin deficiency affects protein, carbohydrate, and fat metabolism.*)

COMPLICATIONS

DKA leads to severe dehydration (volume depletion), hyperosmolality, metabolic acidosis, and electrolyte disturbances (such as potassium deficiency). Life-threatening arrhythmias may develop from potassium depletion. Lactic acidosis may occur if the patient has severe metabolic acidosis without severe ketonemia or renal failure. Volume depletion may cause vascular thrombosis.

Other complications may arise from treatment of DKA. For example, reducing the patient's blood glucose level too rapidly or too much may cause hypoglycemia. A rapid blood glucose drop brought on by insulin and fluid

How insulin deficiency affects protein, carbohydrate, and fat metabolism

Insulin is required to maintain normal metabolism of proteins, carbohydrates, and fats. Without effective insulin, catabolism occurs, eventually leading to hypovolemia and electrolyte disturbances. A lack of effective insulin can trigger the reactions in the chart below.

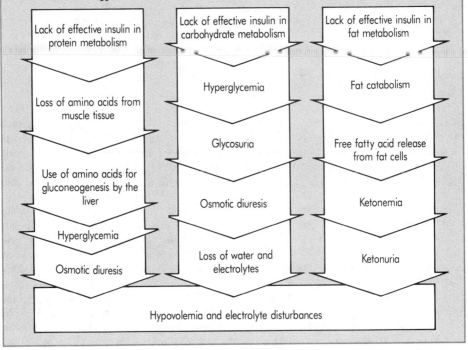

administration may cause fluid shifts within the brain, triggering cerebral edema.

ASSESSMENT

Expect a history of increased fatigue, lethargy, dry mouth, and increased thirst and urination over the last few hours or days. The patient may or may not know he has diabetes. If Type I diabetes is reported, the patient may relate having decreased or discontinued his insulin therapy recently. He also may report having a recent illness or infection and complain of flulike symptoms, such as abdominal discomfort, nausea or vomiting, and generalized myalgia.

The patient with DKA will appear acutely ill and severely dehydrated. Inspection may reveal muscle weakness, fatigue, and an altered level of consciousness (LOC), ranging from confusion to coma. Signs of dehydration, including dry mucous membranes, poor skin turgor, and warm, dry, flushed skin will be present. Measurement of the patient's blood pressure may reveal intravascular volume depletion if his systolic pressure drops 20 mm Hg or more when he moves from a supine to a sitting or standing position. Also neck vein filling probably will be reduced from dehydration. Inspection also will reveal the classic signs of DKA—acetone (fruity) breath odor and Kussmaul's respirations (rapid but deep respirations).

Auscultation of the patient's abdomen may reveal diminished or absent bowel sounds.

DOSAGE FINDER

Identifying insulin dosage in diabetic ketoacidosis

To treat severe ketoacidosis and diabetic coma, give an adult 2.4 to 7.2 units of insulin by direct injection initially; then give 2.4 to 7.2 units/hour by continuous infusion. Base the dosage on the patient's response and his serum glucose level.

As an alternative, give 50 to 100 units of insulin by direct injection, usually along with the same subcutaneous dose. Base further doses on the patient's response and serum glucose level.

Abdominal tenderness, guarding, or rebound tenderness on palpation may also occur. These signs and symptoms probably stem from ketosis and usually resolve as the patient's biochemical status improves.

DIAGNOSTIC TESTS

A urine dipstick test shows +4 glycosuria and moderate to extensive ketonuria. Blood study results may reveal:
• elevated serum glucose levels (300 mg/dl or more) reflecting marked hyperglycemia
• arterial blood gas (ABG) measurements that show below-normal pH (usually less than 7.3) and a serum carbon dioxide level of less than 18 mm Hg, indicating metabolic acidosis
• abnormal serum ketone levels (measured by mixing serum with tap water in various dilutions)—a significant number of ketone bodies in a 1:2 dilution indicates ketonemia
• normal or below-normal serum sodium levels
• high, low, or normal serum potassium values, even though total body potassium levels may decrease
• serum phosphate levels that may be normal on admission but may later drop as phosphate moves from cells into the extracellular space. Total body phosphate decreases as a result of osmotic diuresis.
• BUN levels that rise secondary to volume depletion
• falsely elevated serum creatinine levels because of production of acetone (a ketone body).

TREATMENT

Primarily, treatment consists of replacing fluid and electrolytes while giving supportive care. Rapid I.V. fluid replacement, usually in the form of 0.9% sodium chloride solution or 0.45% sodium chloride solution, is given at 1 liter/hour until the patient's blood pressure stabilizes and his urine output measures 60 ml/hour. Typically, this takes 1 to 2 hours. Then I.V. fluid therapy is continued at a slower rate with 0.45% sodium chloride solution. When the blood glucose level falls to approximately 250 mg/dl, dextrose is added to the solution to prevent hypoglycemia.

Regular insulin therapy is usually initiated with an I.V. bolus dose followed by a continuous I.V. insulin infusion. The infusion is administered at a rate that will lower the serum glucose level by 80 to 100 mg/dl/hour. Adjustments in the infusion rate will be made periodically according to the patient's blood glucose levels. (See *Identifying insulin dosage in diabetic ketoacidosis.*)

Potassium replacement therapy is usually required. Initially, potassium is administered I.V. in the form of potassium chloride after fluid and insulin therapy begins. Potassium phosphate may be used subsequently to prevent transient hyperchloremic acidosis if potassium needs continue to be high.

Hydration and insulin therapy alone usually correct acidosis. However, if acidosis is severe (pH less than 7.1), sodium bicarbonate may be required.

If the patient is suspected of having an infection, appropriate antibiotic therapy will be prescribed.

KEY NURSING DIAGNOSES AND PATIENT OUTCOMES

Fluid volume deficit related to osmotic diuresis. Based on this nursing diagnosis, you'll establish these patient outcomes. The patient will:
• regain and maintain normal fluid volume
• experience no signs or symptoms of hypovolemic shock.

High risk for injury related to electrolyte imbalance. Based on this nursing diagnosis,

you'll establish these patient outcomes. The patient will:
• have electrolyte imbalances detected early and receive appropriate treatment
• regain and maintain normal electrolyte balance with resolution of DKA
• experience no residual adverse effects from electrolyte imbalance.

Ineffective breathing pattern related to Kussmaul's respirations. Based on this nursing diagnosis, you'll establish these patient outcomes. The patient will:
• regain and maintain a normal respiratory rate and pattern
• have ABG levels return to baseline
• report breathing comfort.

NURSING INTERVENTIONS
• Initiate fluid replacement therapy with insertion of a large-bore catheter for a peripheral I.V. line, and begin administering the prescribed I.V. fluid. Expect to administer potassium chloride in I.V. solution, as needed.
• Prepare and administer regular insulin, as prescribed. Maintain a continuous insulin infusion via infusion pump at all times. Adjust the flow rate according to the patient's serum glucose level, as ordered.
• Expect to administer sodium bicarbonate *only* if the patient has severe acidosis.
• Provide supportive care as indicated by the patient's condition. For example, administer oxygen therapy and treat infection and other underlying disorders with antibiotics.
• Begin to reestablish the patient's preillness subcutaneous insulin regimen once he can tolerate oral food. As ordered, discontinue the insulin infusion 30 minutes after administering the first dose of subcutaneous insulin.
• Gradually progress from clear liquids to the patient's prehospitalization diet unless his diet exacerbated or provoked his condition.
• Attempt to determine the underlying cause of DKA, and take corrective measures to prevent its recurrence.
• Teach the patient and his family about DKA, including how to avoid future episodes. Make sure that they know how to manage diabetes during illness. (See *Diabetes sick-day guidelines.*)

Diabetes sick-day guidelines

If your patient has diabetes mellitus, stress the importance of adhering to sick-day guidelines to prevent diabetic ketoacidosis and other crises. Instruct the patient to follow these directions.
• *Never* omit your insulin. Call your health care professional during illness because he may need to adjust the dosage. For instance, he may instruct you to take extra insulin to counter the stress of illness and the effects of the counter-regulatory hormones that increase your blood glucose level.
• Test your blood glucose level at least four times a day because it may rise rapidly during illness.
• Drink plenty of fluids to prevent severe dehydration. You may want to take frequent, small sips.
• Do a urine dipstick test for ketone bodies, and notify your health care professional if the results are moderate or high.
• Contact your health care professional if your illness interferes with your food intake or if you have a fever above 101° F (38.3° C). Also seek medical advice if you experience persistent vomiting or diarrhea (longer than 24 hours) or if your illness lasts more than 24 hours.
• Have a family member or another person check on you frequently when you're ill because coma may develop rapidly.

Monitoring
• Assess the patient's serum glucose level hourly. Also monitor serum electrolyte and ABG levels frequently, as ordered.
• Monitor the patient's response to therapy. Be especially alert for signs and symptoms of complications such as hypoglycemia and cerebral edema.
• Frequently monitor fluid status. Measure intake and output and assess skin turgor. Obtain vital signs often, and stay alert for tachycardia and hypotension, which suggest hypovolemic shock.

• Monitor the patient's electrocardiogram for signs of life-threatening arrhythmias from potassium depletion.
• Continually assess neurologic status. If the patient's LOC remains decreased 8 to 10 hours after treatment begins, suspect increased intracranial pressure from fluid shifts within the brain, and notify the doctor immediately.

Patient teaching
• Assess the patient's ability to perform self-care activities, and give him instructions in diabetes self-care skills, such as administering insulin, monitoring blood glucose levels, planning meals, testing for urine ketone bodies, and recognizing, treating, and preventing hypoglycemia and hyperglycemia.
• Arrange for follow-up teaching and care at an outpatient diabetes clinic or with a home health care nurse.

HYPEROSMOLAR NONKETOTIC SYNDROME

Hyperosmolar nonketotic syndrome (HNKS) is a severe hyperglycemic state characterized by profound intravascular volume depletion, marked dehydration (serum osmolality above 350 mOsm), and central nervous system (CNS) depression. This syndrome may involve coma, prerenal azotemia, and electrolyte depletion. The patient's blood glucose level typically rises above 800 mg/dl. HNKS is potentially fatal.

HNKS commonly strikes patients over age 60 who have Type II diabetes and become debilitated, develop mild renal insufficiency, or lack normal thirst mechanisms or access to water.

CAUSES
HNKS may occur when insulin tolerance is stressed—for example, in infection, congestive heart failure, myocardial infarction (MI), cerebrovascular accident (CVA), burns, pancreatitis, pancreatic cancer, thyrotoxicosis, subdural hematoma, Cushing's syndrome, or uremia.

Other causes include the use of certain medications (including thiazide diuretics,

diazoxide, diphenylhydantoin, furosemide, propranolol, and glucocorticoids), medical procedures (such as peritoneal dialysis, total parenteral nutrition, and parenteral and enteral feedings), and insufficient insulin or oral antidiabetic administration.

Hyperglycemia and hyperosmolality are the cardinal events in HNKS. Hyperglycemia normally causes osmotic diuresis, leading to water and electrolyte loss. In response to hyperglycemia and such stressors as infection and dehydration, hepatic glucose production increases. Physiologic stressors also promote production of counterregulatory hormones, which contribute to the increased blood glucose level and heightened hepatic glucose production.

When the blood glucose level exceeds the renal threshold, glycosuria results, causing osmotic diuresis, dehydration, and loss of water and electrolytes. These conditions trigger additional hepatic glucose production, resulting in severe hyperglycemia.

HNKS doesn't involve ketoacidosis—probably because enough insulin is present to prevent lipolysis, thus averting ketone body formation and subsequent metabolic acidosis.

COMPLICATIONS
HNKS can result in death, typically from a thromboembolic disorder, such as MI or CVA, rather than from an acute metabolic disturbance. Cerebral edema is a rare complication, but it can also lead to death.

ASSESSMENT
Typically, an altered level of consciousness (LOC), reported by a friend or family member, is the patient's chief sign. A history of Type II diabetes may or may not be reported. Frequently, the precipitating factor in HNKS, such as recent infection or a new medication, is revealed during history taking.

Inspection reveals diffuse and focal CNS deficits, such as hallucinations, aphasia, nystagmus, hemianopia, hemiplegia, hemisensory deficits, and focal or generalized tonic-clonic seizures. An altered LOC or even coma may be present. You'll also see signs of dehydration, such as dry oral mucous membranes,

Comparing signs and symptoms of DKA, HNKS, and hypoglycemia

Patients with diabetic ketoacidosis (DKA), hyperosmolar nonketotic syndrome (HNKS), or hypoglycemia typically have a history of diabetes. However, the symptoms of these three disorders may be so similar that telling them apart is difficult. This chart can help you identify the distinctive features of each disorder.

FINDINGS	D.K.A.	H.N.K.S.	HYPOGLYCEMIA
Onset	• Over several hours to days	• Over several days	• Over several minutes
Skin	• Warm, dry, flushed skin	• Warm, dry, flushed skin	• Cool, clammy skin • Sweating
Urologic and renal	• Polyuria	• Polyuria	—
Metabolic	• Polydipsia • Acetone (fruity) breath odor	• Polydipsia • No acetone breath odor	• Hunger
Musculoskeletal	• Myalgia	• Myalgia	—
GI	• Flulike symptoms • Abdominal pain • Nausea, vomiting	• Flulike symptoms • Lower incidence of abdominal discomfort, nausea, and vomiting than in DKA	—
Respiratory	• Kussmaul's respirations	—	—
Cardiac	• Orthostatic hypotension	—	• Tachycardia • Palpitations
Neurologic	• Lethargy • Hyporeflexia • Hypotonia • Stupor • Coma	• Lethargy • Hyporeflexia • Hypotonia • Stupor • Coma • Wider variety of mental status changes than in DKA (hallucinations, seizures, aphasia)	• Nervousness, agitation • Headache • Confusion • Visual disturbances (such as blurred vision) • Paresthesia • Mental dullness • Seizures • Coma

branes, sunken eyes, poor skin turgor, and low blood pressure. (See *Comparing signs and symptoms of DKA, HNKS, and hypoglycemia.*)

DIAGNOSTIC TESTS

Laboratory values that suggest HNKS include a markedly elevated blood glucose level (above 800 mg/dl, perhaps reaching 2,000 mg/dl), an elevated blood urea nitrogen level, and an above-normal serum sodium level, and a normal to slightly elevated serum potassium level (despite total body potassium loss). The serum potassium level will be elevated as the potassium moves out of the cells and into the extracellular space, thereby depleting intracellular or total body potassium. Expect increased serum osmolality—usually above 350 mOsm. Urine ketone bodies are absent, and arterial pH and carbon dioxide levels may be normal.

Serum calcium, magnesium, and phosphate levels usually are below normal in HNKS. Creatine kinase levels may be elevated from rhabdomyolysis (muscle disintegration brought on by hyperosmolality).

A complete blood count typically shows above-normal values for white blood cells, hemoglobin, and hematocrit, reflecting dehydration.

TREATMENT

Emergency treatment of HNKS is similar to that of DKA and includes aggressive fluid replacement therapy with 0.9% or 0.45% sodium chloride solution, regular insulin therapy first as a bolus dose followed by a continuous infusion to slowly bring the serum glucose level back to normal, and electrolyte replacement as indicated.

▲ NURSING ALERT. Administer only regular insulin. Don't give any other type.

When the patient's blood glucose level drops to about 250 mg/dl, dextrose is added to the sodium chloride solution. Then the doctor discontinues the insulin infusion initiated during emergency treatment. These measures prevent hypoglycemia from developing.

The patient also needs ongoing treatment for any diagnosed infection as well as stabilizing measures, such as heparin or another anticoagulant therapy, to treat any vascular events.

Finally, the doctor reestablishes the patient's prehospital routine, including his usual diabetic diet and oral antidiabetic therapy, if appropriate. If HNKS was the presenting event in diabetes, a diabetic diet may serve as the sole therapy, monitored by close follow-up care.

KEY NURSING DIAGNOSES AND PATIENT OUTCOMES

Decreased cardiac output related to fluid volume deficit. Based on this nursing diagnosis, you'll establish these patient outcomes. The patient will:
• maintain hemodynamic stability
• have no serious complications of decreased cardiac output, such as arrhythmias, chest pain, or syncope
• regain and maintain normal cardiac output.

Fluid volume deficit related to osmotic diuresis. Based on this nursing diagnosis, you'll establish these patient outcomes. The patient will:
• regain and maintain a normal fluid volume
• have no signs or symptoms of hypovolemic shock.

High risk for injury related to electrolyte imbalance. Based on this nursing diagnosis, you'll establish these patient outcomes. The patient will:
• have electrolyte imbalance detected early and receive appropriate treatment
• regain and maintain normal electrolyte balance with resolution of HNKS
• experience no residual adverse effects from electrolyte imbalance.

NURSING INTERVENTIONS

• Initiate fluid replacement therapy by inserting a large-bore needle for a peripheral I.V. line and administering the prescribed I.V. fluid. Expect to administer potassium chloride in I.V. solution, as needed.
• Prepare and administer regular insulin, as prescribed. Maintain a continuous insulin infusion via infusion pump at all times. Adjust the flow rate according to the patient's serum glucose level, as ordered.
• Provide supportive care as indicated by the patient's condition. For example, take appropriate measures to treat any diagnosed infection or other underlying condition.
• Attempt to determine the underlying cause of HNKS, and take corrective measures to prevent its recurrence.

Monitoring

• Assess the patient's serum glucose level hourly. Monitor serum electrolytes frequently, as ordered.
• Monitor the patient's response to therapy, watching for complications.
• Frequently monitor fluid status. Measure intake and output and assess skin turgor. Obtain vital signs often, watching for tachycardia, tachypnea, and hypotension, which suggest hypovolemic shock.

• Monitor the patient's electrocardiogram for signs of life-threatening arrhythmias from potassium depletion.
• Continually assess the patient's neurologic status for evidence of deterioration or for new findings.

Patient teaching

• Begin discharge planning as soon as the patient receives initial rehydration and his blood glucose and electrolyte levels have stabilized. With the patient and his family, review the events that led to hospitalization. Teach them how to recognize signs and symptoms of hyperglycemia. Review diabetes sick-day guidelines. Teach the patient how to monitor his blood glucose levels at home, and make sure he understands his prescribed dietary and medication regimens.
• If the patient has newly diagnosed diabetes, teach him beginning management skills. These include meal planning, recognition of signs and symptoms of hyperglycemia, follow-up laboratory measurement of blood glucose values, and prevention or delay of long-term complications of diabetes (for example, eye, kidney, and vascular problems) by controlling his blood glucose level. Provide emotional support, and allow time for him to ask questions.

ACUTE HYPOGLYCEMIA

An abnormally low blood glucose level, acute hypoglycemia occurs when glucose burns up too rapidly, when the glucose release rate falls behind tissue demands, or when excessive insulin enters the bloodstream. When the brain is deprived of glucose, as with oxygen deprivation, its functioning becomes deranged. Prolonged glucose deprivation can lead to tissue damage or even death.

Hypoglycemia may be classified as reactive, pharmacologic, or fasting. *Reactive hypoglycemia* results from the reaction to the disposition of meals. Blood glucose levels typically fall 2 to 4 hours after a meal.

Pharmacologic hypoglycemia results from the response to a drug that does one of the following: increases the amount of insulin circulating in the blood, enhances insulin action, or impairs the liver's glucose-producing capacity. Blood glucose levels may fall slowly or rapidly.

Fasting hypoglycemia causes discomfort during periods of abstinence from food. Blood glucose levels fall gradually. Signs and symptoms don't occur until 5 hours or more after a meal. This rare type of hypoglycemia occurs most often during the night.

Manifestations of hypoglycemia tend to be vague and depend on how quickly the patient's glucose levels drop. Gradual onset of hypoglycemia produces predominantly central nervous system (CNS) signs and symptoms (headache, dizziness, restlessness, and decreased mental capability); a more rapid decline in plasma glucose levels results predominantly in adrenergic signs and symptoms (hunger, weakness, diaphoresis, tachycardia, pallor, anxiety, tremor, and possibly rebound hyperglycemia). If hypoglycemia isn't treated promptly, coma, seizures, permanent brain damage, or even death may follow.

CAUSES

Reactive hypoglycemia has several possible causes. Most commonly, it results from alimentary hyperinsulinism caused by dumping syndrome. Fructose or galactose ingestion may cause hypoglycemia in patients with fructose intolerance or galactosemia. Reactive hypoglycemia may also occur secondary to the imminent onset of Type II diabetes mellitus or impaired glucose tolerance. In some patients, reactive hypoglycemia may have no known cause (idiopathic reactive).

Pharmacologic hypoglycemia most commonly results from the use of insulin or oral sulfonylureas. Other causes include the use of beta blockers and excessive alcohol ingestion.

Fasting hypoglycemia most commonly results from hepatic disease or a tumor. Insulinomas, small islet cell tumors in the pancreas, secrete excessive amounts of insulin, which inhibits hepatic glucose production. These tumors are usually benign (in 90% of patients). Extrapancreatic tumors, though uncommon, can also cause hypoglycemia by

DOSAGE FINDER

Identifying glucagon dosage in acute hypoglycemia

To treat severe hypoglycemia in diabetic patients, give an adult 0.5 to 1 unit (0.5 to 1 mg) of glucagon I.M., S.C, or I.V. Larger doses may be necessary. If the patient doesn't awaken within 20 minutes, repeat the dose. If necessary, repeat the dose again.

increasing glucose utilization and inhibiting glucose output. Such tumors occur primarily in the mesenchyma, liver, adrenal cortex, GI system, and lymphatic system. They may be benign or malignant.

Other nonendocrine causes of fasting hypoglycemia are severe hepatic diseases, including hepatitis, cancer, cirrhosis, and liver congestion associated with heart failure. All of these conditions reduce the uptake and release of glycogen from the liver.

Some endocrine causes include destruction of pancreatic islet cells; adrenocortical insufficiency, which contributes to hypoglycemia by reducing the production of cortisol and cortisone needed for gluconeogenesis; and pituitary insufficiency, which reduces corticotropin and growth hormone levels.

COMPLICATIONS

Prolonged or severe hypoglycemia (blood glucose levels of 20 mg/dl or less) can cause permanent brain damage and may be fatal.

ASSESSMENT

When taking the history of a patient with suspected hypoglycemia, note the pattern of food intake for the preceding 24 hours, as well as any drug and alcohol use. The medical or surgical history may reveal causative factors, such as gastrectomy or hepatic disease.

A patient with reactive hypoglycemia may report adrenergic symptoms, such as diaphoresis, anxiety, hunger, nervousness, and weakness, indicating a rapid decline in his blood glucose levels. A patient with fasting hypoglycemia may report signs and symptoms of

CNS disturbance, such as dizziness, headache, clouding of vision, restlessness, and mental status changes, indicating a slow decline in blood glucose levels. The history of a patient with prolonged glucose deprivation may reveal seizures, decreasing level of consciousness (LOC), and coma. A patient with pharmacologic hypoglycemia may experience a rapid or slow decline in blood glucose levels, with characteristic signs and symptoms.

Inspection may reveal adrenergic signs, such as diaphoresis, pallor, and tremor; or CNS signs, such as restlessness, loss of fine-motor skills, and altered LOC. Palpation may detect tachycardia.

DIAGNOSTIC TESTS

• *Bedside glucose readings* provide quick screening of blood glucose levels. Laboratory testing confirms the diagnosis by showing decreased blood glucose values of less than 40 mg/dl before a meal or less than 50 mg/dl after a meal.
• A *5-hour glucose tolerance test* may provoke reactive hypoglycemia. Following a 12-hour fast, laboratory testing to detect *plasma insulin and plasma glucose levels* may identify fasting hypoglycemia.
• A *C-peptide assay* helps diagnose fasting hypoglycemia. It also differentiates fasting hypoglycemia caused by an insulinoma from fasting hypoglycemia caused by insulin injections.

TREATMENT

For *severe hypoglycemia* (producing confusion or coma), initial treatment is usually I.V. administration of a bolus dose of 25 or 50 g of glucose as a 50% solution. This is followed by a continuous infusion of glucose until the patient can eat a meal. Glucagon may be administered to treat severe hypoglycemia in diabetic patients. (See *Identifying glucagon dosage in acute hypoglycemia.*)

A patient who experiences adrenergic reactions without CNS symptoms may receive oral carbohydrates (parenteral therapy isn't required).

Reactive hypoglycemia requires dietary modification to help delay glucose absorption and gastric emptying. Usually, this includes small, frequent meals, avoidance of simple carbohydrates, and ingestion of high-protein meals with added fiber. The patient may also receive anticholinergic drugs to slow gastric emptying and intestinal motility and to inhibit vagal stimulation of insulin release.

For *fasting hypoglycemia,* surgery and drug therapy may be required. In patients with insulinoma, removal of the tumor is the treatment of choice. Drug therapy may include diazoxide or octreotide for inoperable insulinomas. Hormone replacement therapy may be needed for pituitary or adrenal gland insufficiency. In many cases of recurrent hypoglycemia, the only treatment needed is avoidance of fasting.

KEY NURSING DIAGNOSES AND PATIENT OUTCOMES

Anxiety related to potential threat of death caused by frequent or severe hypoglycemic episodes. Based on this nursing diagnosis, you'll establish these patient outcomes. The patient will:
• identify and express feelings of anxiety
• request information about hypoglycemia
• exhibit fewer physical signs of anxiety.

High risk for injury related to neurologic damage. Based on this nursing diagnosis, you'll establish these patient outcomes. The patient will:
• comply with treatments to prevent hypoglycemia-induced injury
• exhibit normal neurologic function after hypoglycemic episodes
• avoid neurologic damage.

Knowledge deficit related to acute hypoglycemia's potential to be life-threatening. Based on this nursing diagnosis, you'll establish these patient outcomes. The patient will:
• express a need for information about complications of hypoglycemia
• participate in patient-teaching sessions that address hypoglycemia's potentially life-threatening effects
• articulate an understanding of the seriousness of hypoglycemia.

NURSING INTERVENTIONS
• Treat hypoglycemic episodes quickly. Implement measures to protect the unconscious patient, such as maintaining a patent airway.
• For the patient experiencing an acute hypoglycemic episode who is awake and able to swallow, administer 10 to 15 g of a simple carbohydrate (three to five pieces of hard candy, two to three packets of sugar, or 4 oz of orange juice). Repeat this amount every 15 minutes until the patient's symptoms disappear. If the next meal is more than an hour away, have the patient eat a snack to prevent recurrence of the symptoms. If the patient can't swallow, prepare to administer glucagon S.C. or I.M.
• For severe hypoglycemia (suggested by confusion or coma), expect to administer 25 or 50 g of 50% glucose solution by I.V. bolus, followed by a continuous glucose infusion until the patient can eat.
• Administer other medications, as prescribed.
• Avoid delays in meal times and provide an appropriate diet. Arrange to have a dietitian visit the patient to teach him about proper diet.
• Prepare the insulinoma patient for surgery, if indicated. Provide the same preoperative and postoperative care as for a patient undergoing abdominal surgery.

Monitoring
• Watch for and report signs of hypoglycemia in high-risk patients. If possible, measure blood glucose levels before correcting hypoglycemia to verify its presence and severity.
• Monitor any infusion of hypertonic glucose to avoid hyperglycemia, circulatory overload, and cellular dehydration.
• Measure blood glucose levels, as ordered.
• Assess the effects of drug therapy, and watch for adverse reactions.

Patient teaching
• Explain the purpose, preparation, and procedure for any diagnostic tests.
• Emphasize the importance of preventing or promptly treating hypoglycemic episodes to avoid severe complications. Be sure the pa-

tient understands the key danger with hypoglycemia: Once it occurs, he may quickly lose his ability to think clearly. If this should happen while he's driving a car or operating machinery, a serious accident could result.

• Tell the patient to note the early symptoms he typically experiences with hypoglycemia. Family, friends, and co-workers should also be able to recognize the warning signs so that immediate treatment can be initiated.

• Review with the patient and his family treatment measures for a hypoglycemic episode. If the patient is conscious, he should consume a readily available source of glucose, such as three to five pieces of hard candy; 4 oz of apple juice, orange juice, cola, or another soft drink; or 1 tbs of honey or grape jelly. If he's unconscious, he should be given a subcutaneous injection of glucagon. Teach the family how to administer glucagon. Advise the patient and his family to notify the doctor if hypoglycemic episodes don't respond to treatment or if they occur frequently.

• Emphasize the importance of carefully following the prescribed diet to prevent a rapid drop in blood glucose levels. Advise the patient to eat small meals throughout the day, and mention that bedtime snacks also may be necessary to keep blood glucose at an even level. Instruct him to avoid alcohol and caffeine because they may trigger severe hypoglycemic episodes.

• If the patient is obese and has impaired glucose tolerance, suggest ways to restrict his caloric intake and lose weight. If necessary, help him find a weight-loss support group.

• Warn the patient with fasting hypoglycemia not to postpone or skip meals and snacks. Instruct him to call his doctor for instructions if he doesn't feel well enough to eat.

• Discuss the patient's lifestyle and personal habits to help him identify precipitating factors, such as poor diet, stress, or noncompliance with diabetes mellitus treatment. Explain ways that he can change or avoid each precipitating factor. If necessary, teach him stress-reduction techniques, and encourage him to join a support group.

• Teach the patient about precautions to take when exercising; for example, tell him to consume extra calories and not to exercise alone or when his blood glucose level is likely to drop.

• Inform the patient that he should carry a source of fast-acting carbohydrate, such as hard candy, with him at all times. Advise him to wear a medical identification bracelet or to carry a medical identification card that describes his condition and its emergency treatment measures.

• For the patient with pharmacologic hypoglycemia from insulin or oral antidiabetic agents, review the essentials of managing diabetes mellitus, if indicated.

• If warranted, teach the patient about prescribed drug therapy or surgery.

• Because hypoglycemia is a chronic disorder, encourage the patient to see his doctor regularly.

• Encourage the patient and his family to discuss their concerns about the patient's condition and treatment.

THYROID STORM

An acute form of severe hyperthyroidism, thyroid storm (thyrotoxic crisis) is marked by sudden and excessive release of thyroid hormones into the bloodstream. It's the most serious complication of thyroid hyperfunction. (See *Understanding thyroid storm.*)

Without immediate intervention, the patient may suffer delirium, coma, or death. Mortality from thyroid storm is roughly 20%. Make sure that you know what steps to take to avert grave consequences. (See *Nursing care in thyroid storm*, pages 250 and 251.)

CAUSES

Thyroid storm typically is triggered by stressful conditions, such as trauma, surgery, infection, or emotional distress. Other precipitating factors include myocardial infarction, pulmonary embolism, abrupt withdrawal of antithyroid agents, initiation of therapy with radioiodine (^{131}I) or iodine-containing agents, preeclampsia, thyroid tumor, and subtotal thyroidectomy with excessive intake of synthetic thyroid hormone.

Normally, the hypothalamus triggers the thyroid gland to release thyrotropin-releasing hormone, which in turn causes the anterior pituitary gland to secrete thyroid-stimulating hormone (TSH). This pituitary activity enhances the release of the thyroid hormones triiodothyronine (T_3) and thyroxine (T_4) into the bloodstream.

In hyperthyroid disorders, however, excessive thyroid hormones are released, causing systemic adrenergic activity. Epinephrine overproduction leads to severe hypermetabolic decompensation, which usually affects the cardiovascular, GI, and sympathetic nervous systems but may involve all body systems.

COMPLICATIONS

Thyroid storm may lead to heart failure, shock, hyperthermia, fatal arrhythmias, and coma.

ASSESSMENT

The patient's history may reveal abrupt onset of symptoms after a typical precipitating event, such as physical stress, infection, or an acute emotional shock. A family history of hyperthyroidism (Graves' disease) is a common finding in patients with thyroid storm. The patient or an accompanying family member may report such classic symptoms as nervousness, heat intolerance, weight loss despite increased appetite, excessive sweating, diarrhea, tremor, and palpitations. Angina pain may be reported.

Inspection may reveal hypermetabolic sympathetic activity such as fine tremors, agitation, and restlessness progressing to manic or psychotic behavior. Tachypnea may be present as well as obvious respiratory distress. Body temperature initially may measure 100° F (37.8° C), then rise to 106° F (41.1° C). In addition, the patient may appear to be dehydrated.

Auscultation of the patient's heart rate may reveal tachyarrhythmias, starting at 130 beats/minute and increasing to 300 beats/minute. Atrial arrhythmias such as atrial fibrillation may result in an irregular heartbeat.

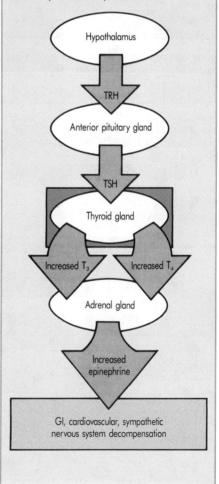

Understanding thyroid storm

Normally, the hypothalamus stimulates the release of thyrotropin-releasing hormone (TRH), which causes the anterior pituitary gland to release thyroid-stimulating hormone (TSH). The thyroid gland then secretes triiodothyronine (T_3) and thyroxine (T_4).

In thyroid storm, however, the thyroid overproduces I_3 and I_4, and systemic adrenergic activity increases. This causes epinephrine overproduction and severe hypermetabolism, leading rapidly to GI, cardiovascular, and sympathetic nervous system decompensation.

Hypothalamus

TRH

Anterior pituitary gland

TSH

Thyroid gland

Increased T_3 Increased T_4

Adrenal gland

Increased epinephrine

GI, cardiovascular, sympathetic nervous system decompensation

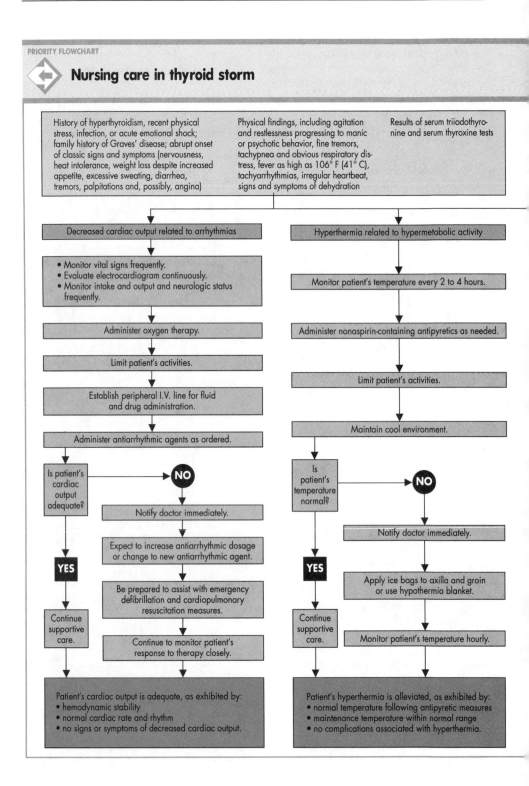

PRIORITY FLOWCHART

Nursing care in thyroid storm

History of hyperthyroidism, recent physical stress, infection, or acute emotional shock; family history of Graves' disease; abrupt onset of classic signs and symptoms (nervousness, heat intolerance, weight loss despite increased appetite, excessive sweating, diarrhea, tremors, palpitations and, possibly, angina)	Physical findings, including agitation and restlessness progressing to manic or psychotic behavior, fine tremors, tachypnea and obvious respiratory distress, fever as high as 106° F (41° C), tachyarrhythmias, irregular heartbeat, signs and symptoms of dehydration	Results of serum triiodothyronine and serum thyroxine tests

Decreased cardiac output related to arrhythmias

- Monitor vital signs frequently.
- Evaluate electrocardiogram continuously.
- Monitor intake and output and neurologic status frequently.

Administer oxygen therapy.

Limit patient's activities.

Establish peripheral I.V. line for fluid and drug administration.

Administer antiarrhythmic agents as ordered.

Is patient's cardiac output adequate? → **NO**

NO → Notify doctor immediately.

Expect to increase antiarrhythmic dosage or change to new antiarrhythmic agent.

Be prepared to assist with emergency defibrillation and cardiopulmonary resuscitation measures.

Continue to monitor patient's response to therapy closely.

YES

Continue supportive care.

Patient's cardiac output is adequate, as exhibited by:
- hemodynamic stability
- normal cardiac rate and rhythm
- no signs or symptoms of decreased cardiac output.

Hyperthermia related to hypermetabolic activity

Monitor patient's temperature every 2 to 4 hours.

Administer nonaspirin-containing antipyretics as needed.

Limit patient's activities.

Maintain cool environment.

Is patient's temperature normal? → **NO**

NO → Notify doctor immediately.

Apply ice bags to axilla and groin or use hypothermia blanket.

Monitor patient's temperature hourly.

YES

Continue supportive care.

Patient's hyperthermia is alleviated, as exhibited by:
- normal temperature following antipyretic measures
- maintenance temperature within normal range
- no complications associated with hyperthermia.

Key

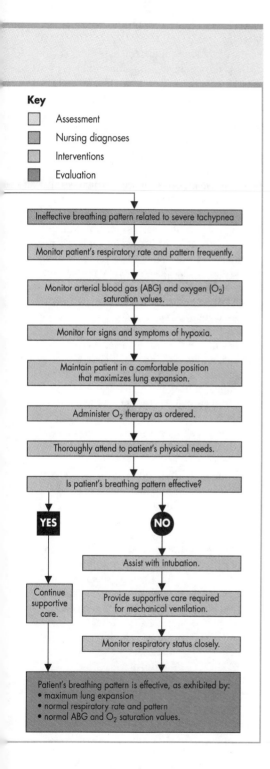

☐ Assessment
☐ Nursing diagnoses
☐ Interventions
■ Evaluation

Ineffective breathing pattern related to severe tachypnea

Monitor patient's respiratory rate and pattern frequently.

Monitor arterial blood gas (ABG) and oxygen (O_2) saturation values.

Monitor for signs and symptoms of hypoxia.

Maintain patient in a comfortable position that maximizes lung expansion.

Administer O_2 therapy as ordered.

Thoroughly attend to patient's physical needs.

Is patient's breathing pattern effective?

YES   **NO**

Continue supportive care.

Assist with intubation.

Provide supportive care required for mechanical ventilation.

Monitor respiratory status closely.

Patient's breathing pattern is effective, as exhibited by:
• maximum lung expansion
• normal respiratory rate and pattern
• normal ABG and O_2 saturation values.

DIAGNOSTIC TESTS

Emergency diagnosis relies on clinical findings and the results of serum T_3 and T_4 tests. After the acute crisis, the doctor may order a TSH test to identify an underlying thyroid, pituitary, or hypothalamic disorder. He also may order a ^{131}I uptake test and a thyroid scan to gauge thyroid size and help establish how much ^{131}I to prescribe later.

TREATMENT

Immediate interventions aim to maintain the airway and tissue oxygenation, reverse hypovolemia, prevent further hypermetabolic decompensation, and decrease thyroid hyperfunction.

Oxygen therapy helps the patient meet his high metabolic demands. I.V. fluids containing dextrose reverse hypovolemia and prevent further glycogen depletion. Antipyretic measures, such as ice packs, hypothermia blankets, and antipyretics, are used to reduce the patient's high temperature.

Drug therapy used to halt cardiovascular and other hypermetabolic activity may include a beta-adrenergic blocker such as propranolol to reduce sympathetic nervous system activity and relieve arrhythmias; digoxin and diuretics to prevent or treat cardiac failure; and, possibly, hydrocortisone therapy if the patient is in shock or has adrenal insufficiency. Antithyroid agents are prescribed to halt conversion of thyroid hormone to T_3 and T_4. The doctor may prescribe propylthiouracil or methimazole orally or by nasogastric tube followed by an iodine preparation to prevent release of stored thyroid hormones.

Additional supportive treatment may be required depending on the patient's underlying condition. For example, if the patient is suspected of having an infection, antibiotic therapy will be prescribed.

KEY NURSING DIAGNOSES AND PATIENT OUTCOMES

Decreased cardiac output related to arrhythmias. Based on this nursing diagnosis, you'll establish these patient outcomes. The patient will:

• maintain hemodynamic stability
• regain and maintain a normal cardiac rate and rhythm
• exhibit no serious signs of decreased cardiac output, such as hypotension and altered tissue perfusion.

Hyperthermia related to hypermetabolic activity. Based on this nursing diagnosis, you'll establish these patient outcomes. The patient will:
• exhibit a reduced temperature after antipyretic measures
• avoid complications associated with hyperthermia such as seizures
• regain and maintain a temperature within the normal range.

Ineffective breathing pattern related to severe tachypnea. Based on this nursing diagnosis, you'll establish these patient outcomes. The patient will:
• achieve maximum lung expansion with adequate ventilation after effective treatment
• regain and maintain a normal respiratory rate and pattern and normal arterial blood gas (ABG) values.

NURSING INTERVENTIONS
• Notify the doctor immediately if you suspect thyroid storm.
• Administer oxygen via nasal cannula or mask. Be prepared to assist with intubation and mechanical ventilation if the patient's respiratory function deteriorates.
• Help the patient into a position that facilitates respiration and turn him occasionally from side to side.
• Administer the prescribed antithyroid agent and iodine preparation. Give the iodine preparation 1 to 3 hours after the antithyroid agent to minimize hormone formation from the iodine. Mix it with milk or fruit juice to make it more palatable, and provide a straw to prevent tooth staining.
• Use caution when administering antithyroid agents to a pregnant or breast-feeding patient. These drugs may cause goiter and cretinism in a fetus and may impair thyroid hormone production in a breast-feeding infant. Also administer these agents cautiously to a patient receiving anticoagulants because they may

cause hypoprothrombinemia and subsequent bleeding problems.
• Be prepared to administer medications such as I.V. propranolol, digoxin, diuretics, and hydrocortisone to halt cardiovascular and other hypermetabolic activity.
• Institute measures to reduce the patient's temperature such as ice packs, fans, a hypothermia blanket, and antipyretic therapy.

◆ NURSING ALERT. Give only nonaspirin-containing antipyretics, such as acetaminophen, because aspirin further displaces thyroid hormones, which worsens the hypermetabolic state.

• Administer I.V. fluids as prescribed. Ensure a fluid intake of 3 to 4 liters daily (unless contraindicated by the patient's age or a preexisting cardiovascular disease) to compensate for excessive diaphoresis and to help correct hypovolemic states caused by polyuria, diarrhea, and vomiting.
• When the patient can tolerate oral intake, supply a diet high in calories, carbohydrates, proteins, vitamins, and minerals. If necessary, provide up to six full meals a day. Minimize intake of fiber and highly seasoned foods because they increase peristalsis and cause diarrhea.
• Assume a calm, reassuring manner when providing care. Provide periods of uninterrupted rest.
• Help the patient's family cope with the patient's altered behavior and appearance.
• Provide a safe environment for the patient by reducing environmental hazards. Keep noises to a minimum; keep the room temperature cool and the lights dim; and limit procedures to counter the effects of hypermetabolism. If possible, arrange for a private room to minimize external noise and prevent the patient from disturbing others. Provide safety measures, such as side rails and soft restraints, and perform frequent bed checks.

Monitoring
• Assess the patient's respiratory rate and pattern every 1 to 2 hours. Note tachypnea, dyspnea, pallor, or cyanosis. Auscultate breath sounds regularly for crackles. Evaluate ABG

and oxygen saturation values regularly, as ordered.

• Monitor the patient's heart rate and rhythm and electrocardiogram for evidence of tachyarrhythmias. Be alert for signs of decreased cardiac output, such as hypotension and mental status changes.

• Measure the patient's temperature hourly, and watch for chills, which can further increase the body's metabolic rate.

• Closely monitor fluid status. Measure intake and output and assess for signs of dehydration.

• Monitor for drug toxicity when administering antithyroid agents. During high-dose therapy, the patient is at risk for agranulocytosis, pancytopenia, and thrombocytopenia. Assess him periodically for fever, rash, sore throat, epistaxis, and unexplained bruising or bleeding.

• Review laboratory test results, checking particularly for increased levels of T_3, T_4, and blood glucose, and a decreased level of plasma cortisol.

• Assess the patient for a possible precipitating factor, such as an infection. Obtain blood cultures, as ordered.

• Be alert for complications.

Patient teaching

• After the crisis resolves, teach the patient about thyroid storm and review hyperthyroidism.

• Emphasize the importance of reporting changes in temperature, pulse rate, and weight to the doctor. Stress that the patient must comply with the prescribed medication regimen to help prevent recurrence of thyroid storm. Describe potential adverse drug effects, such as fever, sore throat, and rash, and emphasize the need to report these at once. Provide him with a written treatment plan, and review it with him and family members.

• Teach the patient how to recognize the signs and symptoms of hypothyroidism.

• Urge the patient to make and keep appointments for frequent follow-up medical visits.

MYXEDEMA CRISIS

In myxedema crisis (myxedema coma), the rare clinical presentation of severe hypothyroidism, the patient passes into a hypothermic, stuporous state. Progression is usually gradual, but when stress aggravates hypothyroidism, coma may develop abruptly. This disorder occurs most commonly in older patients with preexisting, although often undiagnosed, hypothyroidism who experience a stressful event. The patient's prognosis depends on the coma's duration and the promptness of treatment. The outcome is fatal for 50% to 80% of patients.

CAUSES

Hypothyroidism may result in myxedema crisis if it's left untreated for a prolonged time, is severe, or is coupled with severe stress, such as infection, exposure to cold, and trauma. Other precipitating factors include thyroid medication withdrawal; use of sedatives, narcotics, or anesthetics; surgery; cardiac disease; and hemorrhage.

COMPLICATIONS

Potential complications associated with myxedema crisis include dilutional hyponatremia from fluid retention; acute respiratory failure from carbon dioxide narcosis; hypotension and shock from decreased cardiac output; and coma from cerebral hypoxia, hypothermia, and hypoglycemia. Ultimately, myxedema crisis can be lethal.

ASSESSMENT

The patient's history may reveal hypothyroidism or hyperthyroidism that was treated with surgery or ^{131}I resulting in hypothyroidism. Inspection reveals characteristic thickened, puffy, dry skin; yellow-orange complexion; coarsened facial features; facial (especially periorbital) and peripheral edema; droopy upper eyelids; diminished level of consciousness (ranging from slow mentation to stupor and coma); and decreased respiratory rate and effort. The patient's hair may be dry and sparse with patchy hair loss, and his nails may be thick and brittle. A neck scar from previous thyroid surgery may be present. You may also observe ataxia and intention tremor.

Palpation may detect rough, doughy skin that feels cool; a weak pulse and bradycardia; muscle weakness; nonpitting sacral or peripheral edema; and delayed reflex relaxation time (especially in the Achilles tendon). Palpation of the neck may reveal a thyroid goiter. Palpation of the abdomen may disclose tender areas that may be sites of infection. Palpation and percussion of the abdomen may detect abdominal distention related to ascites, ileus, or fecal impaction.

Auscultation may show absent or decreased bowel sounds, hypotension, a gallop or distant heart sounds, and adventitious breath sounds. Additional assessment may reveal an abnormally low body temperature, possibly below 93° F (33.9° C). Shivering may be absent.

DIAGNOSTIC TESTS

The diagnosis of myxedema crisis is usually based solely on the patient's history and physical assessment. This is because thyroid function study results take hours or days, and treatment must begin immediately for the patient to survive. The diagnosis is later confirmed when triiodothyronine and thyroxine test results are abnormally low. The thyroid-stimulating hormone level will be elevated in primary hypothyroidism and normal or low in secondary hypothyroidism.

Additional studies include a complete blood count, which may reveal anemia, and tests for cholesterol, triglycerides, serum creatine kinase, aspartate aminotransferase (formerly SGOT), and lactate dehydrogenase levels, all of which are elevated in myxedema crisis.

TREATMENT

In myxedema crisis, treatment aims to prevent respiratory failure, increase cardiac output, and restore normal metabolism. Immediate treatment involves maintaining airway patency and providing oxygen therapy with a ventilator, if necessary; infusing I.V. plasma expanders; and administering large doses of I.V. thyroid hormone, as ordered.

Additional treatment may include I.V. administration of corticosteroids, such as hydrocortisone, to meet the body's demands as metabolism increases and to prevent adrenal crisis in patients with coexisting adrenal insufficiency. Other treatments are transfusion of packed red blood cells (RBCs) if the patient is anemic, administration of antibiotics if the patient has an infection, and other measures to treat an underlying illness.

KEY NURSING DIAGNOSES AND PATIENT OUTCOMES

Decreased cardiac output related to abnormal sympathetic responses of the myocardium secondary to thyroid hormone deficiency. Based on this nursing diagnosis, you'll establish these patient outcomes. The patient will:
• regain and maintain adequate cardiac output exhibited by normal heart rate and blood pressure
• report no chest pain and demonstrate no ischemic changes on electrocardiogram (ECG).

Impaired gas exchange related to hypoventilation and respiratory acidosis. Based on this nursing diagnosis, you'll establish these patient outcomes. The patient will:
• have a respiratory rate within normal limits
• regain and maintain arterial blood gas (ABG) values within the normal range
• regain and maintain normal cerebral function exhibited by being alert and oriented to person, place, and time.

Fluid volume excess related to increased extracellular fluid and capillary permeability secondary to hypometabolism. Based on this nursing diagnosis, you'll establish these patient outcomes. The patient will:
• regain and maintain normal fluid and electrolyte values
• show a decrease in edema and weight
• maintain normal renal function as exhibited by a urine output of at least 30 ml/hour.

NURSING INTERVENTIONS

• Maintain airway patency, administer oxygen, and assist with intubation, if necessary. Provide supportive ventilatory care, as indicated. Take aspiration precautions.
• Establish a peripheral I.V. line and administer ordered I.V. fluids, such as plasma expanders, to maintain circulation and treat shock.
• Restrict fluids, as ordered, if edema is excessive and shock isn't present.
• Expect to replace thyroid hormone intravenously, as ordered.
• Administer corticosteroids, as ordered.
• Transfuse packed RBCs as needed.
• Passively warm the patient with blankets.

▲ NURSING ALERT. Don't use a hypothermia blanket because it might increase peripheral vasodilation, causing shock.

• Provide additional supportive measures, such as skin care and passive range-of-motion exercises to prevent contractures, as indicated.
• Institute seizure precautions.

Monitoring

• Monitor vital signs every 15 to 30 minutes, especially noting the patient's respiratory status.
• If the patient is intubated and on a ventilator, monitor ventilator settings, including tidal volume, flow rate, and percentage of oxygen.
• Monitor the patient's ABG values to detect hypoxia and metabolic acidosis; also monitor his ECG to assess cardiac status.
• Monitor body temperature.
• Compare laboratory values with baseline measurements to assess improvement.
• Measure the patient's intake and urine output to ensure accurate fluid balance.
• Frequently assess the patient's level of consciousness.
• Weigh the patient daily.
• Monitor closely for signs and symptoms of hypoglycemia.

Patient teaching

• If the patient isn't acutely ill, briefly teach him about his condition and why it's occurring. Describe treatment measures and explain each new procedure before beginning.
• If the patient is intubated and on a ventilator, explain how the ventilator will help him breathe and how he can communicate through notes.
• When the patient's condition stabilizes, instruct him about hypothyroidism and its treatment. Also teach him the signs and symptoms of recurring myxedema crisis, hypothyroidism, and hyperthyroidism and the importance of reporting them.
• Emphasize the importance of obtaining prompt medical care for respiratory problems and chest pain. Teach the patient precautions to prevent infections and to avoid exposure to cold.
• Stress the importance of medication compliance even when the patient feels well. Encourage him to have regular follow-up care for his underlying hypothyroidism for the rest of his life.
• Advise the patient to always wear a medical identification bracelet and to carry his medication with him.

ADRENAL CRISIS

Also called addisonian crisis or acute adrenal insufficiency, adrenal crisis is the rapid and severe onset of adrenal hypofunction or insufficiency. The patient experiences metabolic and endocrine imbalances (hyponatremia, hypoglycemia, and hyperkalemia); his blood pressure falls severely; and his fluid volume drops profoundly.

Adrenal crisis is the most serious complication of adrenocortical insufficiency. Left untreated, the condition is fatal.

CAUSES

Adrenal crisis typically occurs when a patient doesn't respond to hormone replacement therapy or undergoes pronounced stress (such as from infection, trauma, or surgery) without

Complications of adrenal crisis

As this flowchart shows, adrenal crisis may lead to a group of complications known as the five H's: hypoglycemia, hypotension, hyponatremia, hyperkalemia, and hypovolemia.

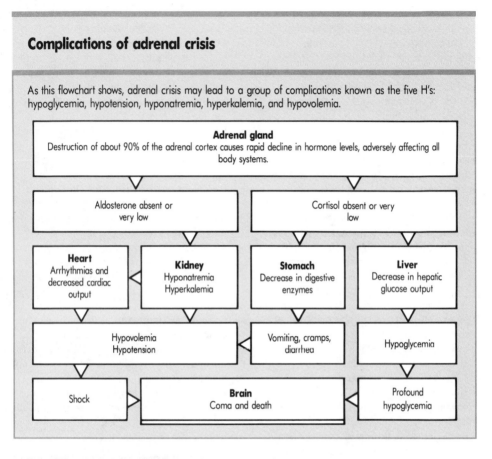

sufficient glucocorticoid replacement. In a patient who's been receiving high or long-term glucocorticoid doses, this emergency may occur after abrupt drug withdrawal.

Other precipitating factors include adrenal tumor, burns, hemorrhage associated with anticoagulant therapy, hypermetabolic states, bilateral adrenalectomy, sudden cessation of antineoplastic therapy, hypopituitarism, and hypothalamic suppression.

Normally, the hypothalamus secretes corticotropin-releasing factor, which triggers the anterior pituitary gland to secrete corticotropin. This, in turn, induces cortisol production by the adrenal cortex. Meanwhile, renin secreted by the kidneys is converted to angiotensin I, which is then converted to angiotensin II. This latter substance stimulates the adrenal cortex to release aldosterone, which helps the kidneys conserve sodium and water and promotes potassium excretion.

In adrenal crisis, these mechanisms are disrupted. Insufficient production of cortisol causes hypotension and hypoglycemia; insufficient release of aldosterone leads to hyponatremia, hypovolemia, and hyperkalemia.

COMPLICATIONS

Adrenal crisis may lead to hypoglycemia, hypotension, hyponatremia, hypovolemia, and hyperkalemia. (See *Complications of adrenal crisis*.)

ASSESSMENT

A history of adrenal insufficiency is a strong indicator of adrenal crisis when the patient exhibits signs and symptoms of this disorder. The history also may reveal use of steroids, previous adrenal surgery, a recent infection, or pronounced physical or emotional stress. The medication history may reveal noncompliance with a prescribed steroid regimen.

Other history findings may include nausea, vomiting, diarrhea, abdominal pain, anxiety, irritability, fatigue, anorexia, muscle cramps, excessive thirst, headache, fever, or progressive muscle weakness. These signs and symptoms reflect hyponatremia, hyperkalemia, and hypoglycemia from adrenal crisis. The patient may also report reduced urine output, which reflects hypovolemia.

Inspection may reveal signs of dehydration (such as dry skin and mucous membranes), flaccid extremities, lethargy, confusion, restlessness, or a progressively diminishing level of consciousness. You also may detect coordination problems. Measurements of the patient's vital signs may reveal an elevated temperature, low blood pressure, a weak and irregular pulse, and an increased respiratory rate.

If the patient has a long-standing history of chronic adrenal insufficiency, you may see a bronze coloration similar to a deep suntan on his elbows, knees, knuckles, and possibly on his lips, buccal mucosa, and on any scars. Vitiligo (depigmented skin patches) or abnormal hyperpigmentation may be evident. Hyperpigmentation results from excessive secretion of melanocyte-stimulating hormone and corticotropin (an effect of reduced cortisol secretion).

DIAGNOSTIC TESTS

The diagnosis of adrenal crisis is confirmed by laboratory studies—but treatment should begin before laboratory test results arrive. Laboratory indicators of adrenal crisis include:
• above-normal serum potassium and calcium levels
• increased blood urea nitrogen (BUN) levels
• elevated hematocrit and hemoglobin levels
• above-normal lymphocyte, eosinophil, and white blood cell counts
• below-normal serum sodium and glucose levels
• below-normal serum and urine cortisol levels.

DOSAGE FINDER

Identifying hydrocortisone dosage in adrenal crisis

To treat adrenal insufficiency, give an adult 15 to 240 mg of hydrocortisone sodium phosphate I.V. daily. Or give 100 to 500 mg of hydrocortisone sodium succinate I.V.; then repeat the dose every 2 to 10 hours, as needed.

The patient with adrenal insufficiency also has a decreased corticotropin level. Electrocardiogram abnormalities may include tall, peaked T waves; wide QRS complexes; and ST-segment depression. Caused by hyperkalemia, these changes predispose the patient to dangerous arrhythmias.

TREATMENT

Emergency treatment for the patient in adrenal crisis has three primary goals: reversing shock, replacing fluids, and replacing cortisol.

Rapid fluid therapy will be initiated with dextrose 5% in 0.9% sodium chloride solution. Up to 3 liters may be given over the first few hours. Hydrocortisone will be administered I.V. to replace cortisol. The doctor will order maintenance hydrocortisone (100 mg I.V. every 8 hours or as a continuous infusion) until acute symptoms subside. (See *Identifying hydrocortisone dosage in adrenal crisis.*) When the patient can tolerate oral intake, oral doses will begin on an 8-hour schedule. Ideally, glucocorticoid administration should mimic the body's natural cortisol secretion pattern. For this reason, the doctor may direct you to give two-thirds of the total daily dose in the early morning and the remainder in the afternoon.

To maintain normal electrolyte levels and blood pressure, the doctor may place the patient on fludrocortisone, an oral mineralocorticoid. The typical dosage is 0.1 to 0.2 mg/day.

Additional supportive treatment may include oxygen therapy, plasma administration, and short-term vasopressor therapy. If the patient has an infection, antibiotics will be prescribed.

If the patient fails to regain normal adrenal function, he'll need lifelong replacement therapy on cortisone or fluorohydrocortisone and additional salt intake during periods of GI upset. If he does regain normal adrenal function, the doctor will taper drug administration gradually to prevent steroid-induced adrenal crisis. The patient will continue to be at risk for adrenal crisis for 1 year or more after receiving corticosteroids because this condition causes a sudden, marked decrease in hormones. If surgery is anticipated during this time, he'll need I.V. corticosteroid therapy.

KEY NURSING DIAGNOSES
AND PATIENT OUTCOMES

Decreased cardiac output related to hypovolemia. Based on this nursing diagnosis, you'll establish these patient outcomes. The patient will:
• regain and maintain hemodynamic stability
• exhibit no serious effects of decreased cardiac output, such as chest pain or altered mental status
• regain adequate cardiac output.

Fluid volume deficit related to hypovolemia. Based on this nursing diagnosis, you'll establish these patient outcomes. The patient will:
• have fluid and blood volume return to normal
• produce adequate urine and regain normal vital signs after fluid replacement therapy is initiated
• exhibit no signs or symptoms of hypovolemic shock.

High risk for injury related to hypoglycemia. Based on this nursing diagnosis, you'll establish these patient outcomes. The patient will:
• have hypoglycemia detected quickly and receive prompt treatment
• regain and maintain a normal blood glucose level
• exhibit no residual neurologic deficits following resolution of hypoglycemia.

NURSING INTERVENTIONS

• Notify the doctor immediately if you suspect adrenal crisis.
• Insert a large-bore needle to establish a peripheral I.V. line, and expect to implement aggressive fluid replacement therapy.
• Administer hydrocortisone replacement therapy, as prescribed.
• Initiate oxygen therapy, as ordered.
• Explain all procedures and treatments in advance to decrease anxiety.
• Provide frequent rest periods to prevent fatigue.
• Take steps to prevent infection, and protect the patient against exposure to potential sources of infection.
• To help prevent pressure ulcers, turn and reposition the patient every 2 hours, avoiding pressure over bony prominences.
• Maintain a quiet, calm environment to prevent recurrence of adrenal crisis. Urge family members and others to minimize stress when visiting the patient.
• Encourage the patient to use relaxation techniques to reduce stress.
• During the first 24 hours, you'll need to perform all activities of daily living for the patient. Gradually add activities according to his tolerance.
• Encourage the patient to dress in layers to retain body heat because he'll have a decreased tolerance for cold. Urge him to adjust room temperature, if possible.

Monitoring

• Monitor fluid and electrolyte balance carefully. Weigh the patient daily and routinely assess his skin turgor, mucous membranes, and urine output.
• Watch for cushingoid signs caused by adverse effects of glucocorticoids.
• Measure blood pressure frequently. If systolic pressure drops 20 mm Hg or more, suspect fluid volume deficit. Also, assess laboratory test results to monitor fluid and electrolyte balances, such as sodium, potassium, calcium, BUN, and cortisol levels.
• Monitor the patient closely for complications.

Patient teaching

• Once adrenal crisis resolves, supply explicit oral and written instructions to promote compliance with therapy. Make sure that the patient understands why he may need lifelong steroid replacement therapy. Instruct him to check with the doctor during periods of stress because his dosage may need to be increased then. Caution him not to stop taking his medication suddenly.

• Warn the patient that infection, injury, or profuse sweating may trigger adrenal crisis.

• Instruct the patient to take steroids with antacids or meals to minimize gastric irritation.

• Advise the patient to carry a medical identification card describing his condition and his drug therapy and listing his doctor's name.

• Advise the patient and his family to keep an emergency kit available with a prepared syringe of hydrocortisone in case of an unexpected trauma or resurgence of adrenal crisis. Teach them how to give the injection.

• Explain that adrenal insufficiency causes mood swings and mental status changes, but reassure the patient and his family that these symptoms will subside with steroid replacement therapy.

DIABETES INSIPIDUS

A deficiency of vasopressin (also called antidiuretic hormone) causes this metabolic disorder characterized by excessive fluid intake and hypotonic polyuria. Diabetes insipidus may start in childhood or early adulthood (the median age of onset is 21) and occurs more commonly in men than in women.

In uncomplicated diabetes insipidus, with adequate water replacement, the prognosis is good, and patients usually lead normal lives. However, in patients with an underlying disorder, such as cancer, the prognosis varies and the disorder can become life-threatening.

CAUSES

The most common cause of diabetes insipidus is failure of vasopressin secretion in response to normal physiologic stimuli (pituitary or neurogenic diabetes insipidus). A less common cause is failure of the kidneys to respond to vasopressin (congenital nephrogenic diabetes insipidus).

Two types of pituitary diabetes insipidus exist: primary and secondary. The primary form affects about 50% of patients. The secondary form results from conditions or procedures that damage the neurohypophyseal structures, such as intracranial neoplastic or metastatic lesions, hypophysectomy or other types of neurosurgery, a skull fracture, or head trauma. This disorder can also result from infection, granulomatous disease, and vascular lesions.

A transient form of diabetes insipidus may also occur during pregnancy, usually after the fifth or sixth month of gestation. The condition usually reverses spontaneously after delivery.

COMPLICATIONS

Untreated diabetes insipidus can produce hypovolemia, hyperosmolality, circulatory collapse, unconsciousness, and central nervous system damage. These complications are most likely to occur if the patient has an impaired or absent thirst mechanism.

A prolonged increase in urine flow may produce chronic complications, such as bladder distention, enlarged calyces, hydroureter, and hydronephrosis. Complications may result from underlying conditions, such as metastatic brain lesions, head trauma, and infections.

ASSESSMENT

The patient's history shows an abrupt onset of extreme polyuria (usually 4 to 16 liters/day of dilute urine, but sometimes as much as 30 liters/day), extreme thirst, and consumption of extraordinary volumes of fluid. The patient may report weight loss, dizziness, weakness, constipation, slight to moderate nocturia and, in severe cases, fatigue from inadequate rest caused by frequent voiding and excessive thirst.

On inspection, you may notice signs of dehydration, such as dry skin and mucous membranes, fever, and dyspnea. Urine is pale and voluminous. Palpation may reveal poor skin turgor, tachycardia, and decreased muscle strength. Hypotension may be present on blood pressure auscultation.

DIAGNOSTIC TESTS

To distinguish diabetes insipidus from other types of polyuria, the doctor may order the following tests:
• *Urinalysis* reveals almost colorless urine of low osmolality (50 to 200 mOsm/kg of water, less than that of plasma) and of low specific gravity (less than 1.005).
• *Dehydration test* helps diagnose diabetes insipidus and differentiate vasopressin deficiency from other forms of polyuria. This simple, reliable test compares urine osmolality after dehydration with urine osmolality after vasopressin administration. In diabetes insipidus, the rise in urine osmolality after vasopressin administration exceeds 9%. Patients with pituitary diabetes insipidus respond to exogenous vasopressin with decreased urine output and increased urine specific gravity. Those with nephrogenic diabetes insipidus show no response to vasopressin.
• *Plasma and urinary vasopressin evaluations* are too expensive and time-consuming to use regularly but are occasionally necessary if osmolality measures are inconclusive.

In critically ill patients, diagnosis may be based on the following laboratory values only:
• urine osmolality – below 200 mOsm/kg of water
• urine specific gravity – below 1.005
• serum osmolality – above 300 mOsm/kg of water
• serum sodium – above 147 mEq/liter.

TREATMENT

Until the cause of diabetes insipidus is identified and eliminated, administration of vasopressin or a vasopressin stimulant can control fluid balance and prevent dehydration.

Aqueous vasopressin is a replacement agent administered by subcutaneous injection in doses of 5 to 10 units with a duration of action of 3 to 6 hours. It's used in the initial management of diabetes insipidus after head trauma or a neurosurgical procedure.

Vasopressin tannate, an I.M. preparation of vasopressin in peanut oil in a 5 unit/ml suspension, is administered in doses of 0.3 to 1 ml, as required.

Desmopressin acetate, a synthetic vasopressin analogue, exerts prolonged antidiuretic activity and has no pressor effects. It's given intranasally in doses of 0.1 to 0.4 ml or subcutaneously in doses of 2 to 4 mcg. Duration of action is 12 to 24 hours, making it the drug of choice.

Lypressin is a synthetic vasopressin replacement given as a short-acting nasal spray. It has significant disadvantages: variable absorption rate, nasal congestion and irritation, ulcerated nasal passages (with repeated use), substernal chest tightness, coughing, and dyspnea (after accidental inhalation of large doses).

Chlorpropamide, an oral antidiabetic agent used in patients who have residual release of vasopressin, stimulates or potentiates the action of submaximal amounts of vasopressin on the renal tubules and reduces polyuria. It may be given with clofibrate.

KEY NURSING DIAGNOSES AND PATIENT OUTCOMES

Altered urinary elimination related to polyuria. Based on this nursing diagnosis, you'll establish these patient outcomes. The patient will:
• express an understanding of how the prescribed medication can control polyuria
• regain and maintain normal urine output with drug therapy.

Fluid volume deficit related to massive fluid loss caused by secondary diabetes insipidus. Based on this nursing diagnosis, you'll establish these patient outcomes. The patient will:
• regain and maintain normal fluid volume as evidenced by equal intake and output
• develop no signs or symptoms of hypovolemic shock.

High risk for injury related to complications. Based on this nursing diagnosis, you'll establish these patient outcomes. The patient will:

• have complications detected early and appropriate treatment given
• show no signs or symptoms of permanent deficits
• comply with the prescribed medical treatment and follow-up visits.

NURSING INTERVENTIONS

• Institute safety precautions if the patient complains of dizziness or weakness.
• Make sure that the patient has easy access to the bathroom or bedpan, and answer his call signals promptly.
• Give vasopressin cautiously to a patient with coronary artery disease because the drug may cause vasoconstriction.
• If the patient is taking chlorpropamide, provide adequate calories, and keep orange juice or another carbohydrate handy to treat hypoglycemic episodes.
• Provide meticulous skin and mouth care. Use a soft toothbrush and mild mouthwash to avoid trauma to the oral mucosa, and apply petroleum jelly to cracked or sore lips. Use alcohol-free skin care products and apply emollient lotion after baths.
• Urge the patient to verbalize his feelings. Offer encouragement and a realistic assessment of his situation. Identify his strengths for use in developing coping strategies. Refer him to a mental health professional for counseling, if necessary.

Monitoring

• Keep accurate records of hourly fluid intake and urine output, vital signs, and daily weight.
• Monitor urine specific gravity and serum electrolyte and blood urea nitrogen levels.
• During dehydration testing, watch for signs of hypovolemic shock. Monitor blood pressure, pulse rate, body weight, and changes in mental or neurologic status.
• Monitor patients taking chlorpropamide for signs of hypoglycemia. Watch for decreasing urine output and increasing urine specific gravity between doses. Check laboratory values for hyponatremia and hypoglycemia.
• If the patient is receiving vasopressin for coronary artery disease, monitor for electrocardiogram changes and exacerbation of angina.

Patient teaching

• Encourage the patient to maintain adequate fluid intake during the day to prevent severe dehydration, but to limit fluids in the evening to prevent nocturia.
• Instruct the patient and his family to identify and report signs of severe dehydration and impending hypovolemia.
• Tell the patient to record his weight daily, and teach him and his family how to monitor intake and output and how to use a hydrometer to measure urine specific gravity.
• Inform the patient and his family about long-term hormone replacement therapy. Inform them that the medication must be taken as prescribed and must not be discontinued abruptly without the doctor's advice. Teach them how to give subcutaneous or I.M. injections and how to use nasal applicators. Discuss the drug's adverse effects and when to report them.
• Advise the patient to wear a medical identification bracelet and to carry his medication with him at all times.

METABOLIC ACIDOSIS

Produced by an underlying disorder, metabolic acidosis is a physiologic state of excess acid accumulation and deficient base bicarbonate. Symptoms result from the body's attempts to correct the acidotic condition through compensatory mechanisms in the lungs, kidneys, and cells. Severe or untreated metabolic acidosis can be fatal.

CAUSES

Metabolic acidosis usually results from excessive burning of fats in the absence of usable carbohydrates. This can be caused by diabetic ketoacidosis (DKA), chronic alcoholism, malnutrition, or a low-carbohydrate, high-fat diet – all of which produce more keto acids than the metabolic process can handle. Other causes include:

• *anaerobic carbohydrate metabolism.* A decrease in tissue oxygenation or perfusion (as occurs with pump failure after myocardial infarction or with pulmonary or hepatic disease, shock, or anemia) forces a shift from aerobic to anaerobic metabolism, causing a corresponding rise in lactic acid level.

• *renal insufficiency and failure (renal acidosis).* Underexcretion of metabolized acids or inability to conserve base bicarbonate results in excess acid accumulation or deficient base bicarbonate.

• *diarrhea and intestinal malabsorption.* Loss of sodium bicarbonate from the intestines causes the bicarbonate buffer system to shift to the acidic side.

• *massive rhabdomyolysis.* High quantities of organic acids added to the body with the breakdown of cells cause high anion gap acidosis.

• *poisoning and drug toxicity.* Common causative agents, such as salicylates, ethylene glycol, and methyl alcohol, may produce acid-base imbalance.

• *hypoaldosteronism or use of potassium-sparing diuretics.* These conditions inhibit distal tubular secretion of acid and potassium.

COMPLICATIONS

If untreated, metabolic acidosis may lead to coma, arrhythmias, and cardiac arrest.

ASSESSMENT

The history of a patient with metabolic acidosis may point to risk factors, including associated disorders or the use of medications that contain alcohol or aspirin. Information about the patient's urine output, fluid intake, and dietary habits (including any recent fasting) may help to establish the underlying cause and severity of metabolic acidosis.

The patient's history (obtained from a family member, if necessary) also may reveal central nervous system signs and symptoms, such as changes in level of consciousness (LOC)

that range from lethargy, drowsiness, and confusion to stupor and coma.

Inspection findings may include Kussmaul's respirations (as the lungs attempt to compensate by "blowing off" carbon dioxide). Underlying diabetes mellitus may cause a fruity breath odor from catabolism of fats and excretion of accumulated acetone through the lungs.

Palpation may reveal cold and clammy skin. As acidosis grows more severe, the skin feels warm and dry, indicating ensuing shock. Auscultation may detect hypotension and arrhythmias. Neuromuscular assessment may reveal diminished muscle tone and deep tendon reflexes.

DIAGNOSTIC TESTS

If your patient has metabolic acidosis, expect the following test values:

• pH below 7.35

• decreased partial pressure of arterial carbon dioxide, representing compensation for acidosis

• bicarbonate level below 24 mEq/liter in acute metabolic acidosis (see *Comparing ABG values in acid-base disorders*)

• anion gap value above 14 mEq/liter from increased acid production or renal insufficiency.

Several other characteristic laboratory findings include:

• urine pH of 4.5 in the absence of renal disease

• elevated serum potassium levels as hydrogen ions move into the cells and potassium moves out of the cells to maintain electroneutrality

• increased blood glucose levels in diabetes

• increased serum ketone body levels in diabetes mellitus

• elevated plasma lactic acid levels in lactic acidosis.

TREATMENT

In acute metabolic acidosis, treatment may include I.V. administration of sodium bicarbonate (when arterial pH is less than 7.2) to neutralize blood acidity. In chronic metabolic acidosis, oral sodium bicarbonate may be given.

Comparing ABG values in acid-base disorders

Metabolic acidosis is an acid-base disturbance marked by an abnormally low pH (increased hydrogen ion concentration) and a low plasma bicarbonate concentration. Arterial blood gas (ABG) values, the primary assessment tool used to identify metabolic acidosis and alkalosis, indicate the body's attempt to correct acidosis using the lungs as a compensatory mechanism. When analyzing your patient's pH, partial pressure of carbon dioxide in arterial blood ($PaCO_2$), and bicarbonate (HCO_3^-) values, keep in mind the following normal values:

• pH: 7.35 to 7.45
• $PaCO_2$: 35 to 45 mm Hg
• HCO_3^-: 21 to 25 mEq/liter.
  If the patient isn't compensating for the disorder, the $PaCO_2$ value will be normal.

METABOLIC DISORDER	pH	$PaCO_2$ IF COMPENSATED	HCO_3^-
Metabolic acidosis	Below 7.35	Below 35 mm Hg	Below 21 mEq/liter
Metabolic alkalosis	Above 7.45	Above 45 mm Hg	Above 25 mEq/liter

Other treatment measures include careful evaluation and correction of electrolyte imbalances and, ultimately, correction of the underlying cause. For example, DKA requires insulin administration and fluid replacement.

Mechanical ventilation may be required to ensure adequate respiratory compensation.

KEY NURSING DIAGNOSES AND PATIENT OUTCOMES

Altered thought processes related to neurologic dysfunction. Based on this nursing diagnosis, you'll establish these patient outcomes. The patient will:
• remain safe and free from injury
• be oriented to time, person, and place.

Decreased cardiac output related to arrhythmias. Based on this nursing diagnosis, you'll establish these patient outcomes. The patient will:
• remain hemodynamically stable
• avoid manifestations of profoundly decreased cardiac output, such as shock or ischemia
• regain a normal sinus rhythm and normal cardiac output.

Ineffective breathing pattern related to pulmonary dysfunction. Based on this nurs-

ing diagnosis, you'll establish these patient outcomes. The patient will:
• regain a normal respiratory rate and pattern
• exhibit no signs or symptoms of hypoxia
• maintain adequate ventilation.

NURSING INTERVENTIONS

• Provide care to eliminate the underlying cause of metabolic acidosis. For example, administer insulin and I.V. fluids, as ordered, to reverse DKA.
• Administer sodium bicarbonate, as prescribed, and keep sodium bicarbonate ampules handy for emergency administration.
• Position the patient to promote chest expansion. If he's stuporous, turn him frequently.
• Orient the patient, as needed. Reduce unnecessary environmental stimulation. Ensure a safe environment if he's confused. Keep the bed in the lowest position, with the side rails raised.
• Provide good oral hygiene. Use sodium bicarbonate washes to neutralize mouth acids, and lubricate the patient's lips with lemon and glycerin swabs.

Monitoring

• Frequently assess the patient's vital signs, laboratory test results, and LOC because changes can occur rapidly.
• Monitor the patient's respiratory function. Check his arterial blood gas values frequently.
• If the patient has DKA, watch for secondary changes caused by hypovolemia, such as falling blood pressure.
• Record the patient's intake and output accurately to monitor renal function. Watch for signs of excessive serum potassium, such as weakness, flaccid paralysis, and arrhythmias (which may lead to cardiac arrest). After treatment, check for overcorrection resulting in hypokalemia.

Patient teaching

• To prevent DKA, teach the patient with diabetes how to routinely test blood glucose levels or how to test urine for glucose and acetone. Encourage strict adherence to insulin or oral antidiabetic therapy, and reinforce the need to follow the prescribed dietary regimen.
• As needed, teach the patient and his family about prescribed medications, including their mechanism of action, dosage, and possible adverse effects. Provide verbal and written instructions.

METABOLIC ALKALOSIS

Always secondary to an underlying cause, metabolic alkalosis is a clinical state marked by decreased amounts of acid or increased amounts of base bicarbonate. It's usually associated with hypocalcemia and hypokalemia, which may account for signs and symptoms. With early diagnosis and prompt treatment, the prognosis is good. However, untreated metabolic alkalosis may be fatal.

CAUSES

Metabolic alkalosis results from the loss of acid or the increase of base. Causes of acid loss include vomiting, nasogastric (NG) tube drainage or lavage without adequate electrolyte replacement, fistulas, and the use of ste-

roids and certain diuretics (furosemide, thiazides, and ethacrynic acid). Hyperadrenocorticism is another cause of severe acid loss. Cushing's disease, primary hyperaldosteronism, and Bartter's syndrome, for example, all lead to retention of sodium and chloride and urinary loss of potassium and hydrogen.

Excessive retention of base can result from excessive intake of bicarbonate of soda or other antacids (usually for treatment of gastritis or peptic ulcer), excessive intake of absorbable alkali (as in milk-alkali syndrome, often seen in patients with peptic ulcers), administration of excessive amounts of I.V. fluids with high concentrations of bicarbonate or lactate, massive blood transfusions, or respiratory insufficiency.

COMPLICATIONS

Untreated metabolic alkalosis may result in coma, atrioventricular arrhythmias, and death.

ASSESSMENT

The patient's history (obtained from a family member, if necessary) may disclose such risk factors as excessive ingestion of alkaline antacids. The history may include extracellular fluid (ECF) volume depletion, which is frequently associated with conditions leading to metabolic alkalosis (for example, vomiting or NG tube suctioning). The patient or a family member may report irritability, belligerence, and paresthesia.

Inspection may reveal the presence of tetany if serum calcium levels are borderline or low. The rate and depth of the patient's respirations may be decreased as a compensatory mechanism; however, this mechanism is limited because of the development of hypoxemia, which stimulates ventilation.

Assessment of the patient's level of consciousness (LOC) may find apathy, confusion, seizures, stupor, or coma if alkalosis is severe. Neuromuscular assessment may discover hyperactive reflexes and muscle weakness if serum potassium is markedly low. Auscultation may detect cardiac arrhythmias occurring with hypokalemia.

DIAGNOSTIC TESTS

• *Arterial blood gas analysis* may reveal a blood pH over 7.45 and a bicarbonate level over 25 mEq/liter in metabolic alkalosis. A partial pressure of carbon dioxide in arterial blood over 45 mm Hg indicates attempts at respiratory compensation.

• *Serum electrolyte studies* usually show low potassium, calcium, and chloride levels.

• *Electrocardiogram (ECG)* findings disclose a low T wave merging with a P wave and atrial or sinus tachycardia.

TREATMENT

Correcting the underlying cause of metabolic alkalosis is the goal of treatment. Mild metabolic alkalosis generally requires no treatment. Rarely, therapy for severe alkalosis includes cautious I.V. administration of ammonium chloride to release hydrogen chloride and restore concentration of ECF and chloride levels. Potassium chloride and 0.9% sodium chloride solution (except with heart failure) are usually sufficient to replace losses from gastric drainage.

Electrolyte replacement with potassium chloride and discontinuation of diuretics correct metabolic alkalosis resulting from potent diuretic therapy.

Oral or I.V. acetazolamide, which enhances renal bicarbonate excretion, may be prescribed to correct metabolic alkalosis without rapid volume expansion. Because acetazolamide also enhances potassium excretion, potassium administration before giving this drug may be necessary.

KEY NURSING DIAGNOSES AND PATIENT OUTCOMES

Altered thought processes related to neurologic dysfunction. Based on this nursing diagnosis, you'll establish these patient outcomes. The patient will:

• remain safe and protected from injury

• become oriented to time, person, and place with effective treatment.

Decreased cardiac output related to atrioventricular arrhythmias. Based on this nursing diagnosis, you'll establish these patient outcomes. The patient will:

• maintain hemodynamic stability

• exhibit no signs of profoundly decreased cardiac output, such as shock and tissue ischemia

• exhibit correction of arrhythmias and improved cardiac output with treatment.

High risk for injury related to tetany. Based on this nursing diagnosis, you'll establish these patient outcomes. The patient will:

• maintain a normal calcium level

• show no signs or symptoms of tetany.

NURSING INTERVENTIONS

• When administering I.V. solutions containing potassium salts, dilute potassium with the prescribed I.V. solution and use an I.V. infusion pump. Infuse ammonium chloride 0.9% I.V. no faster than 1 liter over 4 hours; faster administration may cause hemolysis of red blood cells (RBCs). Avoid administering excessive amounts of these solutions because this could cause overcorrection leading to metabolic acidosis. Don't give ammonium chloride to a patient who has signs of hepatic or renal disease.

• Observe seizure precautions, and provide a safe environment for the patient with altered thought processes. Orient the patient as needed.

• Irrigate the patient's NG tube with 0.9% sodium chloride solution instead of plain water to prevent loss of gastric electrolytes.

Monitoring

• Monitor I.V. fluid concentrations of bicarbonate or lactate. Observe the infusion rate of I.V. solutions containing potassium salts to prevent damage to blood vessels. Monitor I.V. solutions containing ammonium chloride to prevent hemolysis of RBCs. Watch for signs of phlebitis.

• Assess the patient's laboratory values, including pH, serum bicarbonate, serum potassium, and serum calcium levels. Notify the doctor if you detect significant changes or if the patient responds poorly to treatment.

• Observe the ECG for arrhythmias.

• Watch closely for signs of muscle weakness, tetany, or decreased activity.
• Check the patient's vital signs frequently, and record intake and output to evaluate respiratory, fluid, and electrolyte status. Keep in mind that the respiratory rate usually slows in an effort to compensate for alkalosis. Tachycardia may indicate electrolyte imbalance, especially hypokalemia.
• Assess the patient's LOC frequently.

Patient teaching

• To prevent metabolic alkalosis, warn the patient not to overuse alkaline agents.
• If the patient has an ulcer, teach him how to recognize signs of milk-alkali syndrome, including a distaste for milk, anorexia, weakness, and lethargy.
• If potassium-wasting diuretics or potassium chloride supplements are prescribed, make sure that the patient understands the medication regimen, including the purpose, dosage, and possible adverse effects.

11
Female reproductive disorders

Many interrelated physiologic functions occur in the area of the female reproductive tract. Besides the internal genitalia, the female pelvis contains the organs of the urinary and the gastrointestinal systems. An abnormality in one pelvic organ can readily induce an abnormality in another. Left undetected or untreated, life-threatening conditions, such as hemorrhage or septic shock, can occur as well as fetal demise if the patient is pregnant. Even with prompt treatment, fetal demise may be unavoidable if the mother's life is to be spared.

Life-threatening conditions discussed in this section include ruptured ovarian cyst, ectopic pregnancy, pregnancy-induced hypertension, placenta previa, abruptio placentae, uterine rupture, and postpartal hemorrhage.

Reproductive tract emergencies can arise in any setting—in an obstetrics-gynecology unit, a medical-surgical unit, a walk-in clinic, or the emergency department. Be alert to the possibility of such an emergency in any woman of childbearing age who complains of abdominal pain.

Whatever her age, the woman with a life-threatening reproductive tract disorder needs fast, expert care. Be prepared to conduct a rapid emergency assessment, to institute life-support measures as needed, to assist the doctor with diagnostic and treatment procedures, and to monitor changes in the patient's condition as well as in the fetus, if present.

Initial female reproductive care

Check for:
□ history of reproductive disorders such as polycystic ovarian disease or uterine repair
□ abnormalities in past pregnancies
□ recent amenorrhea or abnormal menses
□ recent abnormal vaginal bleeding, including onset, color, and severity
□ recent onset of abdominal pain, including location and severity
□ signs and symptoms of acute abdomen
□ signs and symptoms of hypovolemic shock
□ hypertension, generalized and pitting edema, or sudden weight gain
□ abnormal neurologic signs such as hyporeflexia, hyperreflexia, seizures, changes in level of consciousness, severe frontal headache, and visual disturbances
□ fever and chills
□ signs and symptoms of pregnancy
□ abnormal fetal presentation, fetal distress, presence and characteristics of uterine contractions.

Intervene by:
□ notifying the doctor of abnormal findings
□ giving patient nothing by mouth
□ inserting a large-bore needle for a peripheral I.V.
□ monitoring vital signs and fetal status
□ initiating external electronic fetal monitoring
□ starting oxygen therapy
□ drawing blood for hemoglobin and hematocrit as well as for typing and crossmatching
□ attempting to keep patient and her family calm.

Prepare for:
□ aggressive fluid resuscitation or fluid restriction
□ administration of emergency medications
□ emergency delivery or surgery.

RUPTURED OVARIAN CYST

An ovarian cyst is a nonneoplastic sac on an ovary, containing fluid or semisolid material. Common cysts result from:
• ovarian endometrial tissue growth that bleeds during menstruation and forms a blood-and-clot-filled cyst
• hemorrhage of a mature corpus luteum into its cavity, creating a blood-filled cyst in the ovarian wall
• an ovarian follicle that fills with serous fluid and becomes distended.

Any ovarian cyst can grow and spontaneously rupture into the peritoneum. When this happens, the ruptured cyst releases fluid that irritates the peritoneum and blood vessels in the ovarian capsule tear, causing hemorrhage. If this life-threatening surgical emergency isn't corrected quickly, shock may rapidly occur.

CAUSES

An ovarian cyst ruptures when the fluid or semisolid material inside the cyst expands until it bursts the outer membranous layer of the cyst. Torsion of the ovary and fallopian tube may also cause a cyst to rupture.

COMPLICATIONS

A ruptured ovarian cyst can cause peritonitis or intraperitoneal hemorrhage, shock, and death.

ASSESSMENT

The patient's history may reveal menstrual irregularities and chronic pelvic pain. She may report sudden onset of sharp or dull pain on one side of her abdomen.

Inspection may reveal the patient to be diaphoretic and pale with signs of an acute abdomen similar to those of appendicitis (abdominal tenderness, distention, and rigidity). She may also have scant to profuse vaginal bleeding. Palpation may reveal guarding of the abdomen or unilateral tenderness during pelvic examination. Auscultation of the heart rate and blood pressure may reveal tachycardia

and mild to severe hypotension, depending on the degree of blood loss.

DIAGNOSTIC TESTS

A ruptured ovarian cyst may be diagnosed by pelvic ultrasonography that shows fluid collection. A pregnancy test may be performed to rule out ectopic pregnancy.

TREATMENT

A ruptured ovarian cyst requires surgical repair at the rupture site to halt bleeding and fluid loss. Fluid replacement with lactated Ringer's solution and transfusions of whole blood, plasma, or plasma components may be necessary if hemorrhage is significant and shock develops.

KEY NURSING DIAGNOSES AND PATIENT OUTCOMES

Fluid volume deficit related to fluid loss and hemorrhage. Based on this nursing diagnosis, you'll establish these patient outcomes. The patient will:
• have her condition identified quickly and treated promptly
• recover and maintain normal fluid and blood volume, as evidenced by stable vital signs and urine output of at least 30 ml/hour.

Pain related to peritoneal irritation. Based on this nursing diagnosis, you'll establish these patient outcomes. The patient will:
• state that she has no further increase in pain before surgery
• express a feeling of comfort and pain relief after surgery.

High risk for infection related to potential for peritonitis. Based on this nursing diagnosis, you'll establish these patient outcomes. The patient will:
• exhibit normal vital signs, especially temperature
• show no signs of severe generalized abdominal pain or abdominal distention
• maintain a normal white blood cell count and differential.

NURSING INTERVENTIONS

• Administer I.V. fluids or blood components, as ordered.
• Insert an indwelling catheter to keep accurate intake and output records.
• Give pain medication, as ordered, and provide supplemental oxygen, as needed.
• Prepare the patient for surgery as you would for any patient undergoing abdominal surgery.

Monitoring

• Assess the patient's vital signs. Report any changes that may signal shock, such as tachycardia, tachypnea, and hypotension.
• Frequently monitor the degree and characteristics of vaginal bleeding.
• Review complete blood count and electrolyte studies, as ordered, comparing values with baseline measurements.
• Monitor the patient's intake and urine output.

Patient teaching

• Explain the patient's condition and treatment to her and her family. Take time to answer their questions and address their concerns.
• Stress the importance of alerting the nurse if symptoms worsen.
• Explain the surgical procedure and expected postoperative care.
• After surgery and before discharge, review the signs and symptoms of infection (fever; increased redness, swelling, or pain at the incision site; pain on urination; voiding only small amounts of urine; and foul-smelling or bright red vaginal discharge). Emphasize the importance of reporting such signs to the doctor.

ECTOPIC PREGNANCY

Implantation of the fertilized ovum outside the uterine cavity, ectopic pregnancy most commonly occurs in the fallopian tube, but other sites are possible. (See *Implantation sites of ectopic pregnancy*, page 270.) In whites, ectopic pregnancy occurs in about 1 in 200 pregnancies; in nonwhites, in about 1 in 120. It's the leading cause of maternal death in the first trimester, accounting for 11% of all maternal deaths in the United States. However, with prompt diagnosis, appropriate surgical intervention, and control of bleeding, the prognosis for the woman is good. Rarely, in cases of abdominal implantation, the fetus may survive to term.

Usually, only one in three women who experience an ectopic pregnancy give birth to a live neonate in a subsequent pregnancy. This is because a woman who has an ectopic pregnancy in one fallopian tube is at increased risk for developing an ectopic pregnancy in the opposite tube.

CAUSES

Conditions that prevent or retard the passage of the fertilized ovum through the fallopian tube and into the uterine cavity include:
• endosalpingitis, an inflammatory reaction that causes folds of the tubal mucosa to agglutinate, narrowing the tube
• diverticula, the formation of blind pouches that cause tubal abnormalities
• tumors pressing against the tube
• previous surgery (tubal ligation or resection, or adhesions from previous abdominal or pelvic surgery)
• transmigration of the ovum (from one ovary to the opposite tube), resulting in delayed implantation.

Ectopic pregnancy may also result from congenital defects in the reproductive tract or ectopic endometrial implants in the tubal mucosa. The increased prevalence of sexually transmitted tubal infection may also be a factor as may the use of an intrauterine device (IUD), which causes irritation of the cellular lining of the uterus and the fallopian tubes.

COMPLICATIONS

Rupture of the tube causes life-threatening complications, including hemorrhage, shock, and peritonitis. Infertility results if the uterus, fallopian tubes, or both ovaries are removed.

Implantation sites of ectopic pregnancy

In roughly 95% of patients with ectopic pregnancy, the ovum implants in the fallopian tube – in the fimbria, ampulla, or isthmus. Other possible abnormal implantation sites include the interstitium, tubo-ovarian ligament, ovary, abdominal viscera, and internal cervical os.

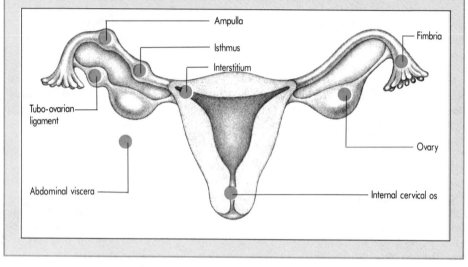

ASSESSMENT

Ectopic pregnancy sometimes produces symptoms of normal pregnancy or no symptoms other than mild abdominal pain (the latter is especially likely in abdominal pregnancy), making diagnosis difficult.

Typically, the patient reports amenorrhea or abnormal menses (after fallopian tube implantation), followed by slight vaginal bleeding and unilateral pelvic pain over the mass. If the tube ruptures, the patient may complain of sharp lower abdominal pain, possibly radiating to the shoulders and neck. She may indicate that this pain is often precipitated by activities that increase abdominal pressure, such as a bowel movement.

During a pelvic examination, the patient may report extreme pain when the cervix is moved and the adnexa are palpated. The uterus feels boggy and is tender.

DIAGNOSTIC TESTS

• *Serum pregnancy test* shows the presence of human chorionic gonadotropin.
• *Real-time ultrasonography* determines intrauterine pregnancy or ovarian cyst (performed if serum pregnancy test results are positive).
• *Culdocentesis* (aspiration of fluid from the vaginal cul-de-sac) detects free blood in the peritoneum (performed if ultrasonography detects the absence of a gestational sac in the uterus).
• *Laparoscopy* may reveal pregnancy outside the uterus (performed if culdocentesis is positive).

TREATMENT

If culdocentesis shows blood in the peritoneum, laparotomy and salpingectomy are indicated, possibly preceded by laparoscopy, to remove the affected fallopian tube (salpingectomy) and control bleeding. Patients who wish to have children can undergo microsurgical repair of the fallopian tube. The ovary is saved, if possible; however, ovarian pregnancy requires oophorectomy.

Interstitial pregnancy may require hysterectomy; abdominal pregnancy requires a laparotomy to remove the fetus, except in rare cases, when the fetus survives to term or calcifies undetected in the abdominal cavity.

Supportive treatment includes transfusion with whole blood or packed red blood cells to replace excessive blood loss, administration of broad-spectrum I.V. antibiotics for sepsis, administration of supplemental iron (given orally or intramuscularly), and institution of a high-protein diet.

KEY NURSING DIAGNOSES AND PATIENT OUTCOMES

Altered cerebral, cardiopulmonary, renal, and peripheral tissue perfusion related to hypovolemia caused by bleeding. Based on this nursing diagnosis, you'll establish these patient outcomes. The patient will:
• have ectopic pregnancy detected quickly and treated promptly
• regain and maintain normal tissue perfusion
• exhibit no residual tissue damage.

Fear related to potential death of self and fetus. Based on this nursing diagnosis, you'll establish these patient outcomes. The patient will:
• express feelings of fear regarding potential death of self and fetus
• use available support systems to cope with fear.

Fluid volume deficit related to hemorrhage caused by ruptured fallopian tube. Based on this nursing diagnosis, you'll establish these patient outcomes. The patient will:
• maintain hemodynamic stability
• regain and maintain adequate fluid volume
• have hemorrhage stop with surgical repair.

NURSING INTERVENTIONS

• Prepare the patient with excessive blood loss for emergency surgery. Administer replacement blood transfusions, as ordered, and provide emotional support.

• Administer analgesics and antibiotics, as ordered.
• If the patient is Rh-negative, administer $Rh_o(D)$ immune globulin (RhoGAM), as ordered. Ask the patient the date of her last menstrual period, and have her describe the character of this period.
• Provide a quiet, relaxing environment, and encourage the patient and her partner to express their feelings of fear, loss, and grief. Help the patient develop effective coping strategies. Refer her to a mental health professional for additional counseling, if necessary.

Monitoring

• Check the amount, color, and odor of vaginal bleeding.
• Monitor vital signs and fluid intake and output for signs of hypovolemia and impending shock. Also monitor cardiopulmonary and neurologic functions for alterations suggesting inadequate cerebral tissue perfusion.
• Monitor and record the location and character of the pain. Also assess the effectiveness of administered analgesics.

Patient teaching

• Teach the patient about the anatomic structures and reproductive processes involved in this disorder. Explain all procedures and treatment options. Prepare her for surgery, and discuss what to expect postoperatively.
• Tell the patient who is vulnerable to ectopic pregnancy not to use an IUD until after she has completed her family.
• To prevent recurrent ectopic pregnancy, advise prompt treatment of pelvic infections to prevent diseases of the fallopian tube. Inform patients who've undergone surgery involving the fallopian tubes or those with confirmed pelvic inflammatory disease that they're at increased risk for another ectopic pregnancy.

PREGNANCY-INDUCED HYPERTENSION

Pregnancy-induced hypertension most commonly develops after the 20th week of preg-

Pathophysiology of pregnancy-induced hypertension

Pregnancy-induced hypertension affects major body systems, including the kidneys, lungs, liver, and uterus. Many changes in these systems—such as tissue ischemia and fibrinogen deposits in the vessel walls—can be identified only through postmortem studies.

Effects on kidneys
Low protein levels cause decreased plasma colloidal pressure and allow fluid to shift from intravascular to interstitial spaces, causing edema. The fluid shift reduces blood flow to the kidneys and diminishes renal perfusion, which in turn triggers the release of renin, leading to the formation of the potent vasopressor angiotensin. As a result, blood pressure increases to offset the effects of diminished renal perfusion. Renal function becomes inefficient and the glomerular filtration rate decreases. Vascular spasms also slow glomerular blood flow and constrict glomerular capillaries. Diminished renal function results in albuminuria and increased blood urea nitrogen levels.

Effects on liver
Vascular spasms result in vessel compression and, in some cases, extravasation (hemorrhage under the liver and in the intra-abdominal cavity). Fibrin clots also may form from elevated plasma fibrinogen levels in gestational hypertension.

Effects on lungs
Pulmonary changes resulting from pregnancy-induced hypertension include pulmonary edema and diffuse intrapulmonary bleeding, which could predispose the patient to bronchopneumonia.

Effects on placenta
Placental changes from pregnancy-induced hypertension affect uteroplacental perfusion. These changes include premature aging, degeneration and calcification of tissues, congested intervillous spaces, and arteriolar thromboses.

nancy. This disorder and its complications are the most common cause of maternal death in developed countries. It most often occurs in nulliparous women and may be nonconvulsive or convulsive.

Preeclampsia, the nonconvulsive form of the disorder, is marked by the onset of hypertension after 20 weeks' gestation. It develops in about 7% of pregnancies and may be mild or severe. The incidence is significantly higher in low socioeconomic groups.

Eclampsia, the convulsive form, occurs between 24 weeks' gestation and the end of the first postpartal week. The incidence increases among women who are pregnant for the first time, have multiple fetuses, and have a history of vascular disease.

About 5% of women with preeclampsia develop eclampsia; of these, about 15% die of eclampsia or its complications. Fetal mortality is high because of the increased incidence of premature delivery.

CAUSES

The cause of pregnancy-induced hypertension is unknown. However, geographic, ethnic, racial, nutritional, immunologic, and familial factors may contribute to vascular disease, which, in turn, may increase the risk of pregnancy-induced hypertension. Age is also a factor. Adolescents and primiparas older than age 35 are at higher risk for preeclampsia.

Other theories postulate a long list of potential toxic sources, such as autolysis of placental infarcts, autointoxication, uremia, maternal sensitization to total proteins, and pyelonephritis. (See *Pathophysiology of pregnancy-induced hypertension.*)

COMPLICATIONS

Generalized arteriolar vasoconstriction is thought to produce decreased blood flow through the placenta and maternal organs. This can result in intrauterine growth retardation, placental infarcts, and abruptio placentae. Severe eclampsia is marked by hemolysis, elevated liver enzyme levels, and a low platelet count (HELLP syndrome). A unique form of coagulopathy is also associated with this disorder.

Other possible complications include stillbirth of the neonate, and seizures, coma, premature labor, renal failure, and hepatic damage in the mother.

ASSESSMENT

A patient with mild preeclampsia typically reports a sudden weight gain of more than 3 lb (1.36 kg) a week in the second trimester or more than 1 lb (0.45 kg) a week during the third trimester.

The patient's history reveals elevated blood pressure readings: 140 mm Hg or more systolic, or a rise of 30 mm Hg or more above the patient's normal systolic pressure, that is measured on two occasions, 6 hours apart; and 90 mm Hg or more diastolic, or a rise of 15 mm Hg or more above the patient's normal diastolic pressure, measured on two occasions, 6 hours apart.

Inspection detects generalized edema, especially of the face. Palpation may reveal pitting edema of the legs and feet. Deep tendon reflexes may indicate hyporeflexia or hyperreflexia.

As preeclampsia worsens, the patient may demonstrate oliguria (urine output of 400 ml/day or less), blurred vision caused by retinal arteriolar spasms, epigastric pain or heartburn, irritability, and emotional tension. She may complain of a severe frontal headache.

A patient whose blood pressure readings during bed rest rise to 160/110 mm Hg or higher on at least two occasions, 6 hours apart, has severe preeclampsia. Also, ophthalmoscopic examination may reveal vascular spasm, papilledema, retinal edema or detachment, and arteriovenous nicking or hemorrhage.

Preeclampsia can suddenly progress to eclampsia with the onset of seizures. The patient with eclampsia may appear to cease breathing, then suddenly take a deep, stertorous breath and resume breathing. She may then lapse into a coma that lasts a few minutes

to several hours. Awakening from the coma, she may have no memory of the seizure. Mild eclampsia may involve more than one seizure; severe eclampsia, up to 20 seizures.

In eclampsia, physical examination findings are similar to those in preeclampsia but more severe. Systolic blood pressure may rise to 200 mm Hg. The patient may have a fever (50% of cases). Inspection may reveal marked edema, but some patients exhibit no visible edema.

DIAGNOSTIC TESTS

Laboratory test findings reveal proteinuria (more than 300 mg/24 hours [1 +] in preeclampsia, and 5 g/24 hours [5 +] or more in severe eclampsia). Test results may suggest the HELLP syndrome.

Ultrasonography, stress and nonstress tests, and biophysical profiles evaluate fetal well-being.

TREATMENT

Therapy for preeclampsia is designed to halt the disorder's progress – specifically, the early effects of eclampsia, such as seizures, residual hypertension, and renal shutdown – and to ensure fetal survival. Some doctors advocate the prompt induction of labor, especially if the patient is near term; others follow a more conservative approach. Therapy may include:

• complete bed rest in the preferred left sidelying position to enhance venous return

• antihypertensive drugs, such as methyldopa and hydralazine

• magnesium sulfate to promote diuresis, reduce blood pressure, and prevent seizures if the patient's blood pressure fails to respond to bed rest and antihypertensives and persistently rises above 160/100 mm Hg, or if central nervous system irritability increases. (See *Identifying drug dosages in PIH*, page 274.)

If these measures fail to improve the patient's condition, or if fetal life is endangered (as determined by stress or nonstress tests and biophysical profiles), cesarean section or induction of labor with oxytocin may be required.

Emergency treatment of eclamptic seizures consists of immediate administration of

DOSAGE FINDER

Identifying drug dosages in PIH

The following two drugs are used for the emergency treatment of pregnancy-induced hypertension (PIH).

Hydralazine
To treat PIH, give an adult 5 mg I.V. or I.M. initially, then 5 to 10 mg every 20 to 30 minutes, as needed.

Magnesium sulfate
To prevent or control seizures in severe preeclampsia or eclampsia, give an adult a loading dose of 4 g I.V. with another 4 g given by deep I.M. injection (using undiluted 50% magnesium sulfate injection) in each buttock. Follow this with 4 to 5 g I.M. q 4 hours, p.r.n. Alternate buttocks with each injection.

Alternatively, give a loading dose of 4 g I.V. in 250 ml dextrose 5% in water followed by 1 to 2 g hourly as a continuous I.V. infusion. The dosage over the next 24 hours depends on the patient's urine and serum magnesium levels. Don't exceed 40 g in 24 hours (30 g in smaller patients); in patients with renal disease, don't exceed 20 g over 48 hours.

When giving magnesium sulfate by I.V. infusion, the concentration should not exceed 20% (200 mg/ml), and the infusion rate should not exceed 150 mg/minute. For I.M. injection, adults usually receive the drug in concentrations of 25% (250 mg/ml) or 50% (500 mg/ml).

magnesium sulfate (I.V. drip), oxygen administration, and electronic fetal monitoring. After the patient's condition stabilizes, cesarean section may be performed.

Adequate nutrition, good prenatal care, and control of preexisting hypertension during pregnancy decrease the incidence and severity of preeclampsia. Early recognition and prompt treatment of preeclampsia can prevent progression to eclampsia.

KEY NURSING DIAGNOSES AND PATIENT OUTCOMES

Altered cerebral tissue perfusion related to hypertensive effects on the brain. Based on this nursing diagnosis, you'll establish these patient outcomes. The patient will:
• have changed condition detected quickly and treated promptly
• regain and maintain normal cerebral tissue perfusion
• exhibit no residual neurologic deficits.

Fluid volume excess related to fluid retention and renal impairment. Based on this nursing diagnosis, you'll establish these patient outcomes. The patient will:
• comply with prescribed treatment measures aimed at keeping blood pressure under control
• exhibit no further signs or symptoms of fluid retention
• maintain a urine output equal to or greater than intake.

High risk for injury related to seizure activity. Based on this nursing diagnosis, you'll establish these patient outcomes. The patient will:
• remain safe and protected during seizure activity
• receive appropriate emergency interventions to halt seizure activity promptly
• experience no injury during seizure activity.

NURSING INTERVENTIONS
• Notify the doctor immediately of any serious change in the patient's condition.
• Establish a peripheral I.V. line and expect to administer parenteral medications, as ordered.
• Keep emergency resuscitative equipment and anticonvulsants available in case of seizures and cardiac or respiratory arrest.
• To protect the patient from injury, maintain seizure precautions. Don't leave an unstable patient unattended. Keep an airway and oxygen available.
• Prepare for emergency cesarean section, if indicated. Alert the anesthesiologist and pediatrician.

• Provide a quiet, darkened room until the patient's condition stabilizes, and enforce absolute bed rest.
• Elevate extremities to promote venous return. Avoid constricting hose, slippers, or bed linens.
• Provide emotional support for the patient and family. Encourage them to verbalize their feelings. If the patient's condition necessitates premature delivery, point out that infants of mothers with pregnancy-induced hypertension are usually small for gestational age but sometimes fare better than other premature babies of the same weight, possibly because they have developed adaptive responses to stress in utero.
• Help the patient and her family to develop effective coping strategies.

Monitoring
• Evaluate the patient regularly for changes in blood pressure, pulse rate, respiratory rate, fetal heart rate, vision, level of consciousness, and deep tendon reflexes and for headache unrelieved by medication. Report changes immediately. Assess these signs before administering medications.
• Monitor the extent and location of edema.
• Assess fluid balance by measuring intake and output and by checking daily weight. Insert an indwelling urinary catheter, if necessary.
• Observe for signs of fetal distress by closely monitoring the results of stress and nonstress tests.
• Carefully monitor the administration of magnesium sulfate, and watch for signs of toxicity: absence of patellar reflexes, flushing, and muscle flaccidity. Keep calcium gluconate at the bedside to counteract any toxic effects.
• Be alert for complications.

Patient teaching
• Teach the pregnant patient and her family to identify and report signs of preeclampsia and eclampsia, such as headache, weight gain, edema, and oliguria.
• Instruct the patient to maintain bed rest, as ordered. Advise her to lie in a left side-lying position to increase venous return, cardiac output, and renal blood flow.

• Stress the importance of adequate nutrition in the prenatal period. Advise the patient to avoid foods high in sodium.
• Emphasize the importance of scheduling and keeping prenatal visits.

PLACENTA PREVIA

In this disorder, the placenta becomes implanted in the lower uterine segment, where it encroaches on the internal cervical os. It may cover all, part, or a fraction of the internal cervical os. (See *Three types of placenta previa*, page 276.) One of the most common causes of bleeding during the second half of pregnancy, placenta previa occurs in about 1 in 200 pregnancies, more commonly in multigravidas.

Among patients who develop placenta previa in the second trimester of pregnancy, less than 15% still have placenta previa at term. This is because the upper and lower uterine segments elongate as the pregnancy progresses, which places the placenta higher on the uterine wall.

Generally, termination of pregnancy is necessary when placenta previa is diagnosed in the presence of heavy maternal bleeding. Although the disorder is potentially life-threatening, maternal prognosis is good if the hemorrhage can be controlled; fetal prognosis depends on gestational age and the amount of blood lost.

CAUSES
Although the specific cause of placenta previa is unknown, factors that may affect the site of the placenta's attachment to the uterine wall include:
• defective vascularization of the decidua
• multiple pregnancy (the placenta requires a larger surface for attachment)
• previous uterine surgery
• multiparity
• advanced maternal age.

COMPLICATIONS
Possible complications of placenta previa include anemia, hemorrhage, disseminated intravascular coagulation, shock, renal dam-

Three types of placenta previa

The degree of placenta previa depends largely on the extent of cervical dilation at the time of examination, because the dilating cervix gradually uncovers the placenta, as shown below.

Marginal placenta previa
If the placenta covers just a fraction of the internal cervical os, the patient has marginal or low-lying placenta previa.

Partial placenta previa
The patient has the partial, or incomplete, form of the disorder if the placenta caps a larger part of the internal os.

Total placenta previa
If the placenta covers all of the internal os, the patient has total, complete, or central placenta previa.

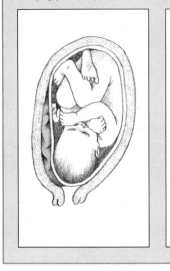
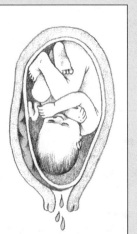
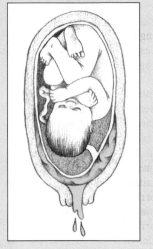

age, cerebral ischemia, and maternal or fetal death.

ASSESSMENT

Typically, a patient with placenta previa reports the onset of painless, bright red vaginal bleeding after the 20th week of pregnancy. Such bleeding, beginning before the onset of labor, tends to be episodic; it starts without warning, stops spontaneously, and resumes later. About 7% of all patients with placenta previa are asymptomatic; in these women, ultrasound examination reveals the disorder incidentally.

Palpation may reveal a soft, nontender uterus. Abdominal examination using Leopold's maneuvers reveals various malpresentations due to interference with the descent of the fetal head caused by the placenta's abnormal location. Minimal descent of the fetal presenting part may indicate placenta previa. The fetus remains active, however, with good heart tones audible on auscultation.

DIAGNOSTIC TESTS

• *Ultrasound examination* determines placental position.

♦ NURSING ALERT. Vaginal and rectal examinations are never performed unless delivery is imminent. If the placenta is located on the posterior wall of the uterus, its lower margin may be obscured. In this case, a vaginal examination is performed with a double setup (preparations for an immediate emergency cesarean section) to confirm the diagnosis. Usually, only the cervix is visualized.

• *Amniocentesis* determines fetal lung maturity before cesarean section.
• *Laboratory studies* may reveal decreased maternal hemoglobin levels (due to blood loss).

TREATMENT

Medical management of placenta previa is designed to assess, control, and restore blood loss; to deliver a viable infant; and to prevent coagulation disorders.

Immediate therapy includes starting an I.V. infusion using a large-bore catheter; drawing blood for hemoglobin and hematocrit levels and for typing and crossmatching; initiating external electronic fetal monitoring; monitoring maternal blood pressure, pulse rate, and respirations; and assessing the amount of vaginal bleeding.

If the fetus is premature (following determination of the degree of placenta previa and necessary fluid and blood replacement), treatment consists of careful observation to allow the fetus more time to mature.

If clinical evaluation confirms complete placenta previa, the patient is usually hospitalized because of the increased risk of hemorrhage. As soon as the fetus is sufficiently mature, or in case of intervening severe hemorrhage, immediate delivery by cesarean section may be necessary. Vaginal delivery is considered only when the bleeding is minimal and the placenta previa is marginal or when the labor is rapid. Because of possible fetal blood loss through the placenta, a pediatric team should be on hand during such delivery to immediately assess and treat neonatal shock, blood loss, and hypoxia.

KEY NURSING DIAGNOSES AND PATIENT OUTCOMES

Altered cerebral tissue perfusion related to cerebral ischemia. Based on this nursing diagnosis, you'll establish these patient outcomes. The patient will:
• have changed condition detected quickly and treated promptly
• regain and maintain normal cerebral function
• exhibit no residual neurologic deficits after the crisis has been resolved.

Fear related to potential fetal death. Based on this nursing diagnosis, you'll establish these patient outcomes. The patient will:
• express feelings of fear regarding the potential death of her unborn child
• use available support systems to cope with her fear
• cooperate with prescribed treatment despite fear.

Fluid volume deficit related to hemorrhage. Based on this nursing diagnosis, you'll establish these patient outcomes. The patient will:
• maintain hemodynamic stability
• regain and maintain adequate fluid volume
• exhibit no further abnormal bleeding.

NURSING INTERVENTIONS

• Notify the doctor immediately if the patient has active bleeding.
• Insert a large-bore catheter to establish a peripheral I.V. line and administer fluids and blood, as ordered.
• Attach an external fetal monitoring device.
• Draw blood for hemoglobin and hematocrit determination as well as for typing and crossmatching.
• If the patient is Rh-negative, administer $Rh_o(D)$ immune globulin (RhoGAM) after every bleeding episode.
• Provide emotional support during labor. Because of the infant's prematurity, the patient may not be given analgesics, so labor pain may be intense. Reassure her of her progress throughout labor, and keep her informed of the fetus's condition.
• Encourage the patient and her family to verbalize their feelings. Help them to develop effective coping strategies, and refer them for counseling, if necessary.

Monitoring

• If the patient with placenta previa shows active bleeding, continuously monitor her blood pressure, pulse rate, respirations, central venous pressure, and intake and output, as well as the amount of vaginal bleeding and the fetal heart rate. Electronic monitoring of fetal heart tones is recommended.

• Assess the patient's response to treatment, and monitor her and the fetus closely for signs of complications.
• During the postpartum period, be alert for signs of hemorrhage and shock caused by the uterus's diminished ability to contract.

Patient teaching

• Teach the asymptomatic patient to identify and report signs of placenta previa (bleeding and cramping) immediately.
• Prepare the patient and her family for the possibility of an emergency cesarean section, the birth of a premature infant, and the physical and emotional changes of the postpartum period.
• Tactfully discuss the possibility of neonatal death. Tell the mother that the infant's survival depends primarily on gestational age, the amount of blood lost, and associated hypertensive disorders. Assure her that frequent monitoring and prompt management greatly reduce the risk of neonatal death.

ABRUPTIO PLACENTAE

Also called placental abruption, abruptio placentae occurs when the placenta separates from the uterine wall prematurely, usually after the 20th week of gestation, producing hemorrhage. This disorder may be classified according to the degree of placental separation and the severity of maternal and fetal symptoms. (See *Degrees of placental separation in abruptio placentae.*)

Abruptio placentae is most common in multigravidas—usually in women over age 35—and is a common cause of bleeding during the second half of pregnancy. Firm diagnosis, in the presence of heavy maternal bleeding, generally necessitates termination of pregnancy. The fetal prognosis depends on gestational age and the amount of blood lost. Although this disorder is potentially life-threatening, maternal prognosis is good if the hemorrhage can be controlled.

CAUSES

The cause of abruptio placentae is unknown. Predisposing factors include traumatic injury (such as a direct blow to the uterus), placental site bleeding from a needle puncture during amniocentesis, chronic or pregnancy-induced hypertension (which raises pressure on the maternal side of the placenta), multiparity, a short umbilical cord, dietary deficiencies, smoking, advanced maternal age, and pressure on the vena cava from an enlarged uterus.

The spontaneous rupture of blood vessels at the placental bed may be due to lack of resiliency or to abnormal changes in the uterine vasculature. The condition may be complicated by hypertension or by an enlarged uterus that can't contract sufficiently to seal off the torn vessels. Consequently, bleeding continues unchecked, possibly shearing off the placenta partially or completely.

COMPLICATIONS

Besides hemorrhage and shock, possible complications of abruptio placentae include renal failure, disseminated intravascular coagulation (DIC), and maternal and fetal death.

ASSESSMENT

Abruptio placentae produces a wide range of clinical effects, depending on the extent of placental separation and the amount of blood lost from maternal circulation.

A patient with *mild abruptio placentae* (marginal separation) may report mild to moderate vaginal bleeding, vague lower abdominal discomfort, and mild to moderate abdominal tenderness. Fetal monitoring may indicate uterine irritability. Auscultation reveals strong and regular fetal heart tones.

A patient with *moderate abruptio placentae* (about 50% placental separation) may report continuous abdominal pain and moderate dark red vaginal bleeding. Onset of symptoms may be gradual or abrupt. Vital signs may indicate impending shock. Palpation reveals a tender uterus that remains firm between contractions. Fetal monitoring may reveal barely audible or irregular and bradycardic fetal

Degrees of placental separation in abruptio placentae

Abruptio placentae is classified by the degree of placental separation from the uterine wall and the extent of hemorrhage.

Mild separation
Internal bleeding between the placenta and uterine wall characterizes mild separation.

Moderate separation
In moderate separation, external hemorrhage occurs through the vagina.

Severe separation
External hemorrhage is also characteristic in severe separation.

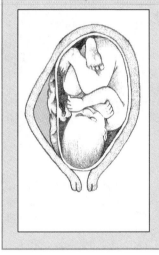

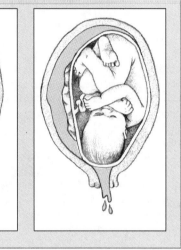

heart tones. Labor usually starts within 2 hours and often proceeds rapidly.

A patient with *severe abruptio placentae* (70% placental separation) will report abrupt onset of agonizing, unremitting uterine pain (described as tearing or knifelike) and moderate vaginal bleeding. Vital signs indicate rapidly progressive shock. Fetal monitoring indicates an absence of fetal heart tones. Palpation reveals a tender uterus with boardlike rigidity. Uterine size may increase in severe concealed abruptions.

DIAGNOSTIC TESTS
Pelvic examination under double setup (preparations for an emergency cesarean) and ultrasonography are performed to rule out placenta previa. Decreased hemoglobin levels and platelet counts support the diagnosis. Periodic assays for fibrin split products aid in monitoring the progression of abruptio placentae and in detecting DIC.

TREATMENT
Medical management of abruptio placentae is designed to assess, control, and restore the amount of blood lost; to deliver a viable infant; and to prevent coagulation disorders.

Immediate measures for abruptio placentae include starting an I.V. infusion (by large-bore catheter) of appropriate fluids (lactated Ringer's solution) to combat hypovolemia; inserting a central venous pressure line and an indwelling urinary catheter to monitor fluid status; drawing blood for hemoglobin and hematocrit determination, coagulation studies, and typing and crossmatching; starting external electronic fetal monitoring; and monitoring maternal vital signs and vaginal bleeding.

After determining the severity of placental abruption and appropriate fluid and blood replacement, prompt delivery by cesarean section is necessary if the fetus is in distress. If the fetus is not in distress, monitoring continues; delivery is usually performed at the first sign of fetal distress. (If placental separation is severe with no signs of fetal life, vaginal delivery may be performed unless uncontrolled hemorrhage or other complications contraindicate it.)

Because of possible fetal blood loss through the placenta, a pediatric team should be ready at delivery to assess and treat the neonate for shock, blood loss, and hypoxia.

Complications of abruptio placentae require appropriate treatment. With a complication such as DIC, for example, the patient will need immediate intervention with heparin, platelets, and whole blood, as ordered, to prevent exsanguination.

KEY NURSING DIAGNOSES AND PATIENT OUTCOMES

Altered cerebral, cardiopulmonary, renal, and peripheral tissue perfusion related to hemorrhage. Based on this nursing diagnosis, you'll establish these patient outcomes. The patient will:
• have changed condition detected quickly and treated promptly
• regain and maintain normal tissue perfusion
• exhibit no residual tissue damage.

Fear related to potential death of fetus. Based on this nursing diagnosis, you'll establish these patient outcomes. The patient will:
• express feelings of fear regarding the potential death of her unborn child
• use available support systems to cope with fear
• cooperate with prescribed treatment despite fear.

Fluid volume deficit related to hemorrhage. Based on this nursing diagnosis, you'll establish these patient outcomes. The patient will:
• maintain hemodynamic stability
• regain and maintain adequate fluid volume
• exhibit no further abnormal bleeding.

NURSING INTERVENTIONS

• Notify the doctor immediately if active bleeding occurs.
• Insert a large-bore catheter to establish a peripheral I.V. line and administer fluids and blood, as ordered.
• Attach an external fetal monitoring device.
• Draw blood for hemoglobin and hematocrit determination as well as for blood typing and crossmatching.
• If vaginal delivery is elected, provide emotional support during labor. Because of the neonate's prematurity, the mother may not receive analgesics during labor and may experience intense pain. Reassure her of her progress through labor, and keep her informed of the fetus's condition.
• Encourage the patient and her family to verbalize their feelings. Help them to develop effective coping strategies. Refer them for counseling, if necessary.

Monitoring

• Assess maternal blood pressure, pulse rate, respirations, central venous pressure, intake and output, and amount of vaginal bleeding every 10 to 15 minutes.
• Monitor the fetal heart rate electronically.
• Evaluate the patient's response to treatment, and monitor her and the fetus closely for signs of complications.

Patient teaching

• Teach the patient to identify and report signs of abruptio placentae, such as bleeding and cramping.
• Explain all procedures and treatments to allay her anxiety.
• Prepare the patient and her family for the possibility of an emergency cesarean section, the delivery of a premature infant, and the changes to expect in the postpartum period. Offer emotional support and an honest assessment of the situation.
• Tactfully discuss the possibility of neonatal death. Tell the mother that the neonate's survival depends primarily on gestational age, the amount of blood lost, and associated hypertensive disorders. Assure her that frequent

monitoring and prompt management greatly reduce the risk of death.

UTERINE RUPTURE

A medical emergency, rupture of the uterus may occur before or during labor. A complete rupture tears all layers of the uterus, establishing direct communication between the uterine and abdominal cavities. In an incomplete rupture, the myometrium tears, but the peritoneal covering of the uterus remains intact. Uterine rupture can be fatal to both the mother and fetus, so make sure that you know what steps to take to help avert grave consequences. (See *Nursing care in uterine rupture*, pages 282 and 283.)

CAUSES

If the uterus undergoes more strain than it's capable of sustaining, uterine rupture occurs. The most common cause is tearing of a scar from a previous cesarean delivery or surgical repair of the uterus. Other factors linked to uterine rupture include prolonged labor, faulty presentation of the fetus, multiple pregnancy, traumatic maneuvers involving forceps or traction, and inappropriate use of oxytocin during labor.

COMPLICATIONS

Uterine rupture may cause such complications as peritonitis, intraperitoneal hemorrhage, shock, and death. Fetal death may also occur.

ASSESSMENT

The patient's history may reveal a previous cesarean delivery or uterine repair as well as the presence of multiple fetuses. The patient will report a sudden, severe pain during a strong labor contraction. If the rupture is incomplete, however, the patient may complain of a localized tenderness and a persistent aching pain over the lower uterine segment.

Inspection reveals that uterine contractions suddenly cease. The contour of the patient's abdomen will change, revealing two distinct swellings (of the retracted uterus and of the extrauterine fetus). As shock develops, the patient quickly becomes pale and diaphoretic with tachypnea and nostril dilation occurring from air hunger. Changes in level of consciousness also occur. Vaginal bleeding may be evident.

Palpation of the abdomen confirms the cessation of uterine contractions. The patient's skin will feel cold and clammy, and her peripheral pulses will be rapid and weak. Auscultation of fetal heart sounds reveals fetal distress or absent heart sounds. Maternal hypotension is evident.

DIAGNOSTIC TESTS

The diagnosis of uterine rupture is based on the patient's clinical presentation.

TREATMENT

Uterine rupture must receive immediate emergency treatment if the mother and, possibly, the fetus are to survive. An emergency laparotomy is performed to remove the fetus, control bleeding, and repair the uterus. A hysterectomy or tubal ligation may be performed at the time of laparotomy to prevent future pregnancies. Supportive measures are instituted to treat shock and blood loss.

Once the fetus is removed from the abdominal cavity, resuscitative measures are implemented to maintain fetal life. The viability of the fetus depends on the extent of uterine rupture and how much time has elapsed between the rupture and abdominal extraction.

KEY NURSING DIAGNOSES AND PATIENT OUTCOMES

Anxiety related to threat of death of self and fetus. Based on this nursing diagnosis, you'll establish these patient outcomes. The patient will:
• verbalize concerns for self and fetus at time of rupture (if conscious) and in recovery period
• use support systems to assist with coping during recovery period
• demonstrate reduced physical symptoms of anxiety in recovery period.

Nursing care in uterine rupture

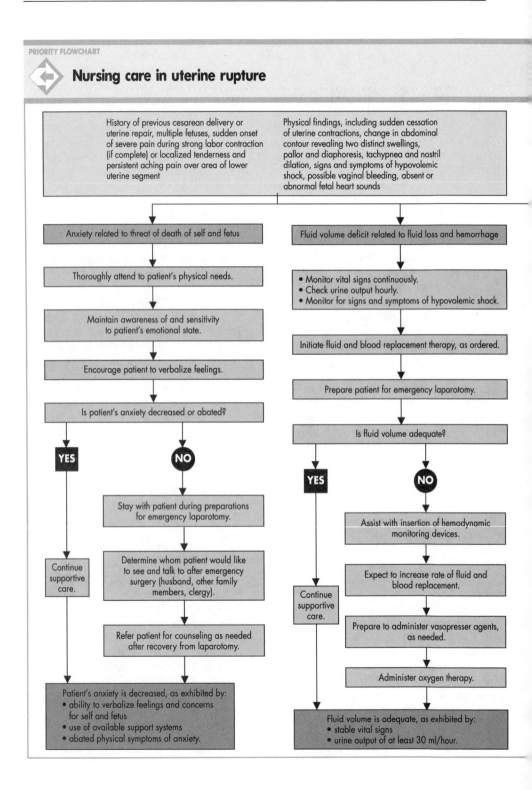

History of previous cesarean delivery or uterine repair, multiple fetuses, sudden onset of severe pain during strong labor contraction (if complete) or localized tenderness and persistent aching pain over area of lower uterine segment

Physical findings, including sudden cessation of uterine contractions, change in abdominal contour revealing two distinct swellings, pallor and diaphoresis, tachypnea and nostril dilation, signs and symptoms of hypovolemic shock, possible vaginal bleeding, absent or abnormal fetal heart sounds

Anxiety related to threat of death of self and fetus

Thoroughly attend to patient's physical needs.

Maintain awareness of and sensitivity to patient's emotional state.

Encourage patient to verbalize feelings.

Is patient's anxiety decreased or abated?

YES / **NO**

Continue supportive care.

Stay with patient during preparations for emergency laparotomy.

Determine whom patient would like to see and talk to after emergency surgery (husband, other family members, clergy).

Refer patient for counseling as needed after recovery from laparotomy.

Patient's anxiety is decreased, as exhibited by:
• ability to verbalize feelings and concerns for self and fetus
• use of available support systems
• abated physical symptoms of anxiety.

Fluid volume deficit related to fluid loss and hemorrhage

• Monitor vital signs continuously.
• Check urine output hourly.
• Monitor for signs and symptoms of hypovolemic shock.

Initiate fluid and blood replacement therapy, as ordered.

Prepare patient for emergency laparotomy.

Is fluid volume adequate?

YES / **NO**

Continue supportive care.

Assist with insertion of hemodynamic monitoring devices.

Expect to increase rate of fluid and blood replacement.

Prepare to administer vasopresser agents, as needed.

Administer oxygen therapy.

Fluid volume is adequate, as exhibited by:
• stable vital signs
• urine output of at least 30 ml/hour.

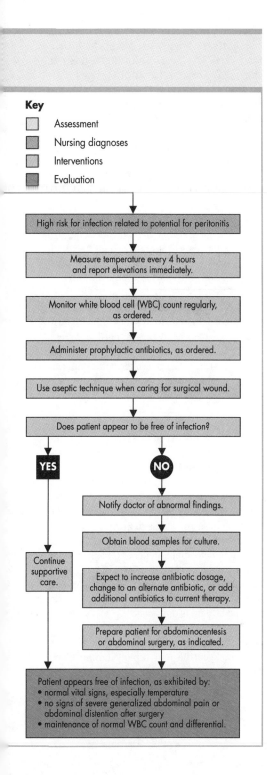

Key

- ☐ Assessment
- ☐ Nursing diagnoses
- ☐ Interventions
- ☐ Evaluation

High risk for infection related to potential for peritonitis

Measure temperature every 4 hours and report elevations immediately.

Monitor white blood cell (WBC) count regularly, as ordered.

Administer prophylactic antibiotics, as ordered.

Use aseptic technique when caring for surgical wound.

Does patient appear to be free of infection?

YES **NO**

Notify doctor of abnormal findings.

Obtain blood samples for culture.

Continue supportive care.

Expect to increase antibiotic dosage, change to an alternate antibiotic, or add additional antibiotics to current therapy.

Prepare patient for abdominocentesis or abdominal surgery, as indicated.

Patient appears free of infection, as exhibited by:
- normal vital signs, especially temperature
- no signs of severe generalized abdominal pain or abdominal distention after surgery
- maintenance of normal WBC count and differential.

Fluid volume deficit related to fluid loss and hemorrhage. Based on this nursing diagnosis, you'll establish these patient outcomes. The patient will:
- have changed condition identified quickly and treated promptly
- regain and maintain a normal fluid and blood volume as evidenced by stable vital signs and a urine output of at least 30 ml/hour.

High risk for infection related to potential for peritonitis. Based on this nursing diagnosis, you'll establish these patient outcomes. The patient will:
- exhibit normal vital signs, especially temperature
- show no signs of severe generalized abdominal pain or abdominal distention after surgery
- maintain a normal white blood cell count and differential.

NURSING INTERVENTIONS
- Notify the doctor immediately if unusual pain and cessation of uterine contractions occur during labor.
- Begin fluid resuscitation measures immediately, and administer oxygen therapy.
- Prepare the patient for emergency laparotomy.

Monitoring
- Continuously monitor the patient's vital signs for evidence of further deterioration.
- Assess fetal condition continuously.
- Check the patient's urine output hourly, and monitor complete blood count, electrolyte, and arterial blood gas levels as ordered.

Patient teaching
- If the patient is conscious, tell her what has happened and what treatment to expect. Reassure her that emergency measures also aim to save the fetus.
- During the recovery period, explain what uterine rupture is and how it occurs.
- Before discharge, teach the patient how to change the incision bandage. Stress the importance of reporting any signs of wound infection or hematoma. Also stress the impor-

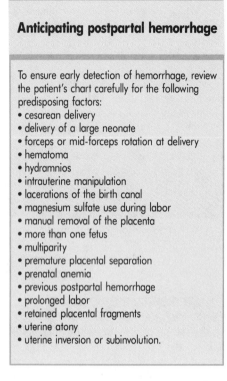

Anticipating postpartal hemorrhage

To ensure early detection of hemorrhage, review the patient's chart carefully for the following predisposing factors:
• cesarean delivery
• delivery of a large neonate
• forceps or mid-forceps rotation at delivery
• hematoma
• hydramnios
• intrauterine manipulation
• lacerations of the birth canal
• magnesium sulfate use during labor
• manual removal of the placenta
• more than one fetus
• multiparity
• premature placental separation
• prenatal anemia
• previous postpartal hemorrhage
• prolonged labor
• retained placental fragments
• uterine atony
• uterine inversion or subinvolution.

tance of reporting bright-red vaginal bleeding.
• Instruct the patient about activity restrictions until healing is complete.
• Inform the patient of the need for follow-up care.
• Provide appropriate referrals, and encourage the patient and her family to seek counseling and supportive therapy if the fetus died.

POSTPARTAL HEMORRHAGE

A life-threatening emergency, postpartal hemorrhage occurs when a patient loses more than 500 ml of blood during or after the third stage of labor. This type of hemorrhage is particularly dangerous because it's hard to measure; for example, actual blood loss at delivery is usually twice that of estimated loss. An added danger is that blood can also collect in the uterus, remaining occult.

Postpartal hemorrhage may occur early or late. Early (or immediate) postpartal hemorrhage occurs within 24 hours after delivery (in about 5% of postpartal patients). Late (or delayed) hemorrhage develops 2 days to 6 weeks postpartum (in about 0.1% of postpartal patients).

CAUSES
Any condition that results in trauma during childbirth can lead to postpartal hemorrhage. The most common causes are uterine atony (poor muscle tone); lacerations of the vagina, cervix, perineum, or labia; and retained placental fragments. Postpartal hemorrhage also may result from various other conditions such as hematomas, episiotomy dehiscence, uterine inversion, and uterine subinvolution.

COMPLICATIONS
This disorder can lead to shock, renal failure from prolonged hypotension, cardiac arrest, and death. A few patients who recover from severe postpartal hemorrhage suffer anterior pituitary gland necrosis, or Sheehan's syndrome.

ASSESSMENT
The patient's history may reveal predisposing conditions such as prolonged labor or prenatal anemia. (See *Anticipating postpartal hemorrhage.*) The patient may report a sudden gush or a slow, steady trickle of blood from the vagina. As shock develops, she may also complain of chills and visual disturbances.

Inspection may reveal the patient quickly becoming pale, diaphoretic, and tachypneic as shock begins. A change in level of consciousness is also likely to occur. Vaginal bleeding may be evident; an estimated blood loss exceeding 500 ml is ominous.

Palpation reveals cold, clammy skin and a rapid, weak peripheral pulse. Auscultation reveals tachycardia and rapidly falling blood pressure.

DIAGNOSTIC TESTS

Diagnosis of postpartal hemorrhage is based on the patient's clinical presentation. However, pelvic ultrasonography may detect retained placental fragments.

TREATMENT

Postpartal hemorrhage warrants immediate emergency treatment to prevent life-threatening complications. Emergency measures to control bleeding include I.V. oxytocin, methylergonovine, ergonovine maleate, or prostaglandin. (See *Identifying drug dosages in postpartal hemorrhage.*) Volume expanders, blood products, or both are used if a large amount of blood is lost or if the patient is in shock.

Although currently controversial, curettage (formerly a standard treatment) may be performed to control bleeding. Other surgical procedures, such as incision and drainage of a hematoma or episiotomy dehiscence, may be required, depending on the underlying cause. Antibiotics are prescribed to prevent infection.

KEY NURSING DIAGNOSES AND PATIENT OUTCOMES

Altered cardiopulmonary, cerebral, and renal tissue perfusion related to hypovolemia. Based on this nursing diagnosis, you'll establish these patient outcomes. The patient will:
• regain and maintain adequate cardiac output exhibited by normal vital signs; being alert and oriented to time, person, and place; and urine output of at least 30 ml/hour
• demonstrate no permanent residual damage when tissue perfusion returns to normal.

Fluid volume deficit related to active postpartal hemorrhage. Based on this nursing diagnosis, you'll establish these patient outcomes. The patient will:
• have her changed condition identified quickly and treated promptly
• recover and maintain a normal fluid and blood volume as evidenced by stable vital signs and a urine output of at least 30 ml/hour.

High risk for infection related to the underlying cause of postpartal hemorrhage, such

---

DOSAGE FINDER

Identifying drug dosages in postpartal hemorrhage

These two drugs are used to control bleeding in postpartal hemorrhage.

Ergonovine
For emergency treatment of postpartal or postabortion hemorrhage caused by uterine atony or subinvolution, give an adult 0.2 mg I.V. or I.M. in a single dose. Repeat the dose every 2 to 4 hours, as necessary, up to a total of five doses.

Methylergonovine
For emergency treatment of severe postpartal and postabortion hemorrhage caused by uterine atony or subinvolution, give an adult 0.2 mg I.V. or I.M. over at least 60 seconds. If necessary, repeat the dose every 2 to 4 hours up to a total of five doses.

---

as lacerations or retained placental fragments or membranes. Based on this nursing diagnosis, you'll establish these patient outcomes. The patient will:
• exhibit normal temperature and white blood cell count and differential
• show no signs of infection, such as foul-smelling, purulent vaginal discharge.

NURSING INTERVENTIONS

• Estimate blood loss and notify the doctor immediately.
• Insert a peripheral I.V. line and initiate fluid replacement therapy as prescribed. If large amounts of blood have been lost, expect to administer volume expanders, blood products, or both.
• Give supplemental oxygen therapy at 6 liters/minute, as prescribed.
• Administer an I.V. oxytocic agent (such as oxytocin or methylergonovine), as prescribed.
• Assist with insertion of a central venous pressure line (if one hasn't been previously inserted).
• Insert an indwelling urinary catheter, as prescribed.

• Lower the head of the bed, and help the patient into a supine position.
• Massage the fundus gently but firmly, as needed. Support the uterus with one hand at the symphysis pubis to prevent inversion.
• Prepare the patient for surgery, as indicated.

Monitoring

• Assess the patient's vital signs every 5 to 15 minutes until her condition has stabilized.
• Monitor the fundal status of the uterus. Document the amount and frequency of uterine massage and the size and amount of any blood clots expressed.
• Check the number of perineal pads used, the percentage of pad saturation, and the time required to saturate the pad (weigh pads to assess blood loss).
• Frequently review complete blood count for the effects of blood loss.
• Monitor the amount, color, consistency, and odor of lochia.
• Monitor fluid intake and urine output.
• Evaluate the patient's mental status closely, and report any changes to the doctor.

Patient teaching

• If the patient is alert, explain why postpartal hemorrhage is occurring and how it's treated.
• Stress the importance of notifying the nurse if bleeding increases or other symptoms worsen.
• Tell the patient to save all used pads for assessment purposes.
• Teach the patient how to perform perineal hygiene, and explain its importance in decreasing the risk of infection.
• If appropriate, teach the patient about the surgical procedure and what to expect postoperatively.
• Stress the importance of close follow-up care.

Appendices and Index

Appendix I

CODE MANAGEMENT

The goals of any code are to restore the patient's spontaneous heartbeat and respirations and to prevent hypoxic damage to the brain and other vital organs. Fulfilling these goals requires a team approach. Ideally, the team should consist of health care workers trained in advanced cardiac life support (ACLS), although nurses trained in basic life support (BLS) may also be a part of the team. Sponsored by the American Heart Association, the ACLS course incorporates BLS skills with advanced resuscitation techniques.

In most hospitals, ACLS-trained nurses provide the first resuscitative efforts to cardiac arrest patients, often administering cardiac medications and performing defibrillation before the doctor's arrival. Because ventricular fibrillation commonly precedes sudden cardiac arrest, initial resuscitative efforts focus on rapid recognition of arrhythmias and, when indicated, defibrillation. If monitoring equipment isn't available, you should simply perform BLS measures. Of course, the scope of your responsibilities in any situation depends on your hospital's policies and procedures and your state's nurse practice act.

Indications for instituting a code include absent pulse, apnea, ventricular fibrillation, ventricular tachycardia, and asystole. Contraindications include a no-code order written by the patient's doctor or an advance directive from the patient or his family requesting that the patient not be resuscitated.

EQUIPMENT

Oral, nasal, and endotracheal (ET) airways ▪ one-way valve mask (if available before the emergency equipment arrives) ▪ mask ▪ oxygen source ▪ oxygen flowmeter ▪ intubation supplies ▪ hand-held resuscitation bag ▪ suction supplies ▪ nasogastric (NG) tube ▪ goggles, masks, and gloves ▪ cardiac arrest board ▪ peripheral I.V. supplies, including 14G and 18G peripheral I.V. catheters ▪ central I.V. supplies, including an 18G thin-wall catheter, a 6-cm needle catheter, and a 16G 15- to 20-cm catheter ▪ I.V. administration sets (including microdrip and minidrip) ▪ I.V. fluids, including dextrose 5% in water (D_5W), 0.9% sodium chloride solution, and lactated Ringer's solution ▪ electrocardiogram (ECG) monitor ▪ cardioverter or defibrillator ▪ conductive medium ▪ ECG leads ▪ cardiac medications, including epinephrine, lidocaine, procainamide, bretylium, atropine, isoproterenol, dopamine, calcium chloride, and dobutamine ▪ optional: external pacemaker, percutaneous transvenous pacer, cricothyrotomy kit, end-tidal carbon dioxide detector.

PREPARATION

Because effective emergency care depends on reliable and accessible equipment, the equipment as well as the personnel must be ready for a code at any time. You also should be familiar with the cardiac drugs you may have to administer. (See *Reviewing code drugs*, pages 291 to 293.)

Always be aware of your patient's code status as defined by the doctor's orders, the patient's advance directives, and the family's wishes. If the doctor has ordered a "no code," make sure he has written and signed the order. If possible, have the patient or a responsible family member cosign the order.

For some patients, you may need to consider whether the family wishes to be present during a code. If the family wants to be present, and if a nurse or clergyman can remain with the family, consider allowing them to remain during the code.

IMPLEMENTATION

• If you're the first to arrive at the site of a code, assess the patient's level of consciousness (LOC), airway, breathing, and circulation, and then begin cardiopulmonary resuscitation (CPR). Use a one-way valve mask, if available, to ventilate the patient.

• Call for help. When a second BLS provider arrives, have that person call a code and retrieve the emergency equipment.

• Once the emergency equipment arrives, have the second BLS provider place the cardiac arrest board under the patient and then assist with two-rescuer CPR. Meanwhile, have the nurse assigned to the patient relate the patient's medical history and describe the events leading to the arrest.

• A third person, either a nurse certified in BLS or a respiratory therapist, will then attach the hand-held resuscitation bag to the oxygen source and begin to ventilate the patient with 100% oxygen.

• When the ACLS-trained nurse arrives, she'll expose the patient's chest and apply defibrillator pads. She'll then apply the paddles to the patient's chest to obtain a "quick look" at the patient's cardiac rhythm. If the patient is in ventricular fibrillation, ACLS protocol calls for defibrillation as soon as possible with 200 joules. The ACLS-trained nurse will act as code leader until the doctor arrives.

• If not already in place, apply ECG electrodes and attach the patient to the defibrillator's cardiac monitor. Avoid placing electrodes on bony prominences or hairy areas. Also avoid the areas where the defibrillator pads will be placed and where chest compressions will be given.

• As CPR continues, you or an ACLS-trained nurse will then start two peripheral I.V. lines with large-bore I.V. catheters. Be sure to use only a large vein, such as the antecubital vein, to allow for rapid fluid administration and to prevent drug extravasation.

• As soon as the I.V. catheter is in place, begin an infusion of 0.9% sodium chloride solution or lactated Ringer's solution to help prevent circulatory collapse. D_5W continues to be acceptable but the recent ACLS guidelines encourage the use of 0.9% sodium chloride solution or lactated Ringer's solution because D_5W can produce hyperglycemic effects during a cardiac arrest.

• While one nurse starts the I.V. lines, the other nurse will set up portable or wall suction equipment and suction the patient's oral secretions as necessary to maintain an open airway.

• The ACLS-trained nurse will then prepare and administer emergency cardiac drugs as needed. Keep in mind that drugs administered through a central line reach the myocardium more quickly than those administered through a peripheral line.

• If the patient doesn't have an accessible I.V. line, you may administer medications such as epinephrine, lidocaine, and atropine through an ET tube. To do so, dilute the drugs in 10 ml of 0.9% sodium chloride solution or sterile water and then instill them into the patient's ET tube. Afterward, manually ventilate the patient to distribute the drug throughout the bronchial tree, which aids in absorption.

• The ACLS-trained nurse will also prepare for and assist with ET intubation. During intubation attempts, take care not to interrupt CPR for longer than 30 seconds.

• Suction the patient as needed. After the patient has been intubated, assess the patient's breath sounds to ensure proper tube placement. If the patient has diminished or absent breath sounds over the left lung field, the doctor will pull back the ET tube slightly and reassess. When the tube is correctly positioned, tape it securely. To serve as a reference, mark the point on the tube that's level with the patient's lips.

• Throughout the code, check the patient's carotid or femoral pulses before and after each defibrillation. Also check the pulses frequently during the code to evaluate the effectiveness of cardiac compressions.

• Meanwhile, other members of the code team should keep a written record of the events. Other duties include prompting participants about when to perform certain activities (such as when to check a pulse or take vital signs), overseeing the effectiveness of CPR, and keeping track of the time between therapies. Each team member should know what each participant's role is to prevent duplicating effort. Finally, someone from the team should make sure that the primary nurse's other patients are reassigned to another nurse.

• If the family is at the hospital during the code, have someone, such as a clergy member or social worker, remain with them. Keep the family informed of the patient's status.

• If the family isn't in the hospital, contact them as soon as possible. Encourage them not to drive to the hospital, but offer to call someone who can give them a ride.

• When the patient's condition has stabilized, assess his LOC, breath sounds, heart sounds, peripheral perfusion, bowel sounds, and urine output. Take the patient's vital signs every 15 minutes and continuously monitor his cardiac rhythm.

• Make sure the patient receives an adequate supply of oxygen, whether through a mask or a ventilator.

• Check the infusion rates of all I.V. fluids, and use infusion pumps to deliver vasoactive drugs. So that you can evaluate the effectiveness of fluid therapy, insert an indwelling urinary catheter if the patient doesn't already have one. Also insert an NG tube to relieve or prevent gastric distention.

• If appropriate, reassure the patient and explain what is happening. Allow the patient's family to visit as soon as possible. If the patient dies, notify the family and allow them to see the patient as soon as possible.

COMPLICATIONS

Even when CPR is performed correctly, complications may include fractured ribs, a lacerated liver, a punctured lung, and gastric distention.

DOCUMENTATION

• During the code, document the events in as much detail as possible. Note whether the arrest was witnessed or unwitnessed, the time of the arrest, the time CPR was begun, the time the ACLS-trained nurse arrived, and the total resuscitation time. Also document the number of defibrillations, the times they were performed, the joule levels, the patient's cardiac rhythm before and after the defibrillation, and whether or not the patient had a pulse.

• Document all drugs administered, including dosages, routes of administration, and patient response. You'll also want to record all procedures, such as peripheral and central line insertion, pacemaker insertion, and ET tube insertion, with the time performed and the patient's tolerance of the procedure. Also keep track of all arterial blood gas results.

• Finally, record any complications and the measures taken to correct them. Have the doctor and ACLS nurse review and then sign the document.

• Be sure to document all of your findings. Record whether the patient is transferred to another unit or facility, the patient's condition at the time of transfer, and whether the family was notified.

• To make sure your code team performs optimally, schedule a time to review the code.

Reviewing code drugs

Use this chart to review drugs typically stocked in the emergency cart and administered during a code. Note the drug indications and dosages as well as the special considerations for code team members administering each medication.

DRUG USES AND DOSAGES	SPECIAL CONSIDERATIONS
Adenosine • *For paroxysmal supraventricular tachycardia (PSVT):* initial dose of 6 mg by rapid I.V. push over 1 to 3 seconds, followed by 20-ml saline flush; if no response within 1 to 2 minutes, administer 12-mg dose by rapid I.V. push	• Keep in mind that this drug depresses atrioventricular (AV) node and sinus node activity. It's used for PSVT because most common forms of this arrhythmia involve a reentry pathway. If the arrhythmia isn't from reentry involving the AV node or sinus node, adenosine won't stop the arrhythmia but may clarify the diagnosis. • Watch for transient sinus bradycardia and ventricular ectopy. • Be aware that PSVT may recur after drug delivery because of adenosine's short half-life (under 5 seconds). Consider giving additional doses or a calcium channel blocker to treat recurrences. • Recognize that this drug produces few, if any, hemodynamic effects because of its short half-life, but facial flushing is common.
Atropine • *For sinus bradycardia with hemodynamic compromise or frequent ventricular ectopic beats:* 0.5 to 1 mg by I.V. push, repeated every 3 to 5 minutes to a maximum dose of 0.04 mg/kg • *For ventricular asystole:* 1 mg repeated in 3 to 5 minutes if asystole persists; a total dose of 3 mg (0.04 mg/kg) results in full vagal blockade	• Don't use a full vagal blocking dose (except for asystole): This can trigger tachyarrhythmias and increase myocardial oxygen demand. • Give the drug endotracheally if quick peripheral I.V. access is unavailable. Increase dose to 2 to 2½ times the I.V. dose, diluted in 10 ml of 0.9% sodium chloride solution or distilled water. Administer using a syringe with a catheter tip that protrudes beyond the end of the endotracheal tube; administer quickly and follow with several insufflations to ensure adequate drug dispersal. • Keep in mind that this drug slows the heart rate at doses below 0.5 mg but may induce tachycardia at regular doses.
Bretylium • *For resistant ventricular fibrillation:* 5 mg/kg by I.V. push followed by defibrillation; if fibrillation persists, increase to 10 mg/kg and repeat at 5-minute intervals (maximum: 30 mg/kg) • *For resistant ventricular tachycardia:* 5 to 10 mg/kg diluted to 50 ml with dextrose 5% in water (D₅W) and injected I.V. over 8 to 10 minutes; infuse continuously at 2 mg/minute if tachycardia persists	• Because bretylium isn't a first-line drug, use it only as follows: if ventricular fibrillation doesn't respond to drug therapy and defibrillation, if ventricular fibrillation recurs despite epinephrine and lidocaine therapy, if lidocaine and procainamide fail to control ventricular tachycardia associated with palpable pulse, or if lidocaine and adenosine fail to control wide-complex tachycardias.
Calcium salts • *For hypocalcemia, hyperkalemia, or calcium channel blocker toxicity:* calcium chloride 10%—1.4 to 2.8 ml I.V.; calcium gluceptate 22%—5 to 7 ml I.V.; calcium gluconate 10%—5 to 8 ml I.V.	• Avoid routine use of calcium salts in resuscitation efforts; they may be detrimental.
Dobutamine • *For low cardiac output, hypotension, or pulmonary congestion:* 2 to 20 mcg/kg/minute by I.V. infusion; use smallest effective dose, as indicated by hemodynamic parameters	• Be aware that the drug may induce reflex peripheral vasodilation. • Monitor the heart rate closely; a rise of 10% or more may increase myocardial ischemia.

(continued)

Reviewing code drugs *(continued)*

DRUG USES AND DOSAGES	SPECIAL CONSIDERATIONS
Dopamine • *For hypotension with bradycardia:* initial dose of 2.5 to 5 mcg/kg/minute by I.V. infusion, titrated until desired response occurs	• Expect drug effects to vary with dosage. At 1 to 2 mcg/kg/minute, the drug dilates renal and mesenteric vessels without increasing heart rate or blood pressure. At 2 to 10 mcg/kg/minute, the drug increases cardiac output without peripheral vasoconstriction; at over 10 mcg/kg/minute, the drug causes peripheral vasoconstriction and a marked increase in pulmonary artery wedge pressure.
Epinephrine • *For cardiac arrest:* 1 mg I.V. (10 ml of 1:10,000 solution); repeat every 3 to 5 minutes during resuscitation if necessary	• Expect some clinicians to use a 1-mg dose initially, then raise subsequent doses to 5 mg. • Give the drug endotracheally if quick peripheral I.V. access is unavailable. Increase dose to 2 to 2½ times the I.V. dose, and dilute in 10 ml of 0.9% sodium chloride solution or distilled water. Administer using a syringe with a catheter tip that protrudes beyond the end of the endotracheal tube; administer quickly and follow with several insufflations to ensure adequate drug dispersal. • Give the drug by intracardiac injection only if venous and endotracheal routes are unavailable.
Isoproterenol hydrochloride • *For torsades de pointes or temporary control of bradycardia:* 2 mcg/ml I.V. (obtained by diluting 1 mg [5 ml] in 500 ml of D₅W and infusing 2 to 10 mcg/minute), titrated according to heart rate and rhythm	• Use for immediate temporary control of hemodynamically significant bradycardia in heart transplant recipients, but not for cardiac arrest. • Be aware that this drug increases the cardiac workload and worsens ischemia and arrhythmias in patients with ischemic heart disease. • Use only until pacemaker therapy begins.
Lidocaine • *For ventricular tachycardia, ventricular fibrillation, premature ventricular contractions (PVCs), or cardiac arrest:* loading dose of 1 to 1.5 mg/kg by I.V. bolus, followed by 0.5 to 1.5 mg/kg by I.V. bolus every 5 to 10 minutes to a maximum of 3 mg/kg (300 mg over 1 hour) • *For persistent ventricular fibrillation if defibrillation and epinephrine fail:* 1.5 mg/kg by I.V. bolus initially, followed by a continuous infusion at 2 to 4 mg/minute (dilute 1 g of lidocaine in 250 ml of D₅W for a 0.4% solution, or 4 mg/ml)	• Avoid giving the drug prophylactically to prevent ventricular ectopy when myocardial infarction is suspected but unconfirmed, unless the electrocardiogram (ECG) shows PVCs. • Keep in mind that this drug improves response to defibrillation if the patient has ventricular fibrillations. • Give the drug endotracheally if quick peripheral I.V. access is unavailable. Increase dose to 2 to 2½ times the I.V. dose, and dilute in 10 ml of 0.9% sodium chloride solution or distilled water. Administer using a syringe with a catheter tip that protrudes beyond the end of the endotracheal tube; administer quickly and follow with several insufflations to ensure adequate drug dispersal.
Magnesium sulfate • *For ventricular fibrillation or ventricular tachycardia:* 1 to 2 g in 100 ml of D₅W administered over 1 to 2 minutes • *For magnesium deficiency:* loading dose of 1 to 2 g mixed in 50 to 100 ml of D₅W over 5 to 60 minutes	• Use for torsades de pointes and to decrease the incidence of postinfarction arrhythmias. • Monitor the patient closely for significant hypotension and asystole.

Reviewing code drugs (continued)

DRUG USES AND DOSAGES	SPECIAL CONSIDERATIONS
Nitroglycerin • *For congestive heart failure or unstable angina:* continuous I.V. infusion (50 or 100 mg in 250 ml of D₅W or 0.9% sodium chloride solution) at 10 to 20 mcg/minute, increased by 5 to 10 mcg/minute every 5 to 10 minutes until desired hemodynamic or clinical response occurs	• Monitor for hypotension, which could worsen myocardial ischemia. • Provide a mean dosage range of 50 to 500 mcg/minute. Most patients respond to 200 mcg/minute or less. • Special I.V. administration sets from the manufacturer may elicit an increased drug effect. With regular I.V. tubing, expect a decreased drug effect from increased binding to tubing. • Prolonged continuous administration (over 12 hours) may produce tolerance.
Nitroprusside • *For heart failure or hypertensive crisis:* add 50 to 100 mg to 250 ml of D₅W or 0.9% sodium chloride solution; dosage range is 0.1 to 0.5 mcg/kg/minute up to 10 mcg/kg/minute	• Wrap the drug container in opaque material to prevent drug deterioration. • Monitor blood pressure with an intra-arterial line.
Norepinephrine • *For severe hypotension with low total peripheral resistance:* add 4 mg of norepinephrine or 8 mg of norepinephrine bitartrate to 250 ml of D₅W with or without 0.9% sodium chloride solution to yield a concentration of 16 mcg/ml of norepinephrine or 32 mcg/ml of norepinephrine bitartrate; initial dosage is 0.5 to 1 mcg/minute titrated to effect; refractory shock may require 8 to 30 mcg/minute	• Avoid giving this drug if the patient has hypovolemia. • Monitor blood pressure with an intra-arterial line; a false-low blood pressure reading may occur with a standard cuff. • Be aware that cardiac output may increase or decrease, depending on vascular resistance, left ventricular function, and reflex response. • Avoid prolonged use, which may cause ischemia of vital organs. • Don't administer in the same I.V. line as alkaline solutions, which may inactivate the drug.
Procainamide • *For ventricular arrhythmias:* 20 mg/minute by I.V. infusion until arrhythmia is suppressed, hypotension ensues, QRS complex widens by 50% of original width, or a total of 17 mg/kg infuses; maintenance infusion rate is 1 to 4 mg/minute	• Use for ventricular arrhythmias, such as PVCs or tachycardia, when lidocaine is contraindicated or ineffective. • Lower the maintenance dosage for patients with renal failure. • Too-rapid infusion causes acute hypotension. • Monitor the ECG carefully; if the QRS complex widens more than 50% or if the PR interval appears prolonged, notify the doctor and discontinue the infusion as ordered. Don't administer to patients with a preexisting prolonged QT interval or torsades de pointes.
Sodium bicarbonate • *For metabolic acidosis:* 1 mEq/kg initially, followed by half of the dose every 10 minutes thereafter	• If arterial blood gas analysis is available, guide therapy by the calculated base deficit or bicarbonate concentration. • Avoid giving this drug for initial resuscitation unless the patient clearly has preexisting acidosis (hyperventilation should be the primary therapy to control acid-base balance).
Verapamil • *For atrial arrhythmias:* initial dose of 2.5 to 5 mg I.V. over 2 minutes; if no therapeutic response, repeat doses of 5 to 10 mg may be administered every 15 to 30 minutes to a maximum dose of 20 mg	• Use for atrial arrhythmias, especially PSVT with AV node conduction. • Don't use to treat atrial arrhythmias in patients with Wolff-Parkinson-White syndrome. • Use cautiously and in lower doses for patients receiving beta blockers. • Monitor the patient for hypotension, severe bradycardia, and congestive heart failure.

Appendix II

CARDIOPULMONARY RESUSCITATION

Cardiopulmonary resuscitation (CPR) seeks to restore and maintain the patient's respiration and circulation after his heartbeat and breathing have stopped. CPR is a basic life support (BLS) procedure performed on victims of cardiac arrest. Clearing an obstructed airway is another BLS procedure.

Most adults in sudden cardiac arrest develop ventricular fibrillation and require defibrillation; CPR alone does not improve their chances of survival. Therefore, you must assess the victim and then contact emergency medical services (EMS) or call a code *before* starting CPR. Timing is critical. Early access to EMS, early CPR, and early defibrillation greatly improve chances of survival.

In most instances, you perform CPR to keep the patient alive until advanced cardiac life support (ACLS) can begin. Basic CPR consists of assessing the victim, calling for help, and then following the ABC scheme: opening the **a**irway, restoring **b**reathing, and then restoring **c**irculation. After the airway has been opened and breathing and circulation have been restored, drug therapy, diagnosis by electrocardiogram (ECG), or defibrillation may follow. CPR is contraindicated in "no code" patients.

EQUIPMENT

CPR requires no special equipment except a hard surface on which to place the patient.

IMPLEMENTATION

• The following illustrated instructions provide a step-by-step guide for CPR as currently recommended by the American Heart Association.

One-person rescue

• If you're the sole rescuer, expect to call for help; then open the patient's airway, check for breathing, and assess for circulation before beginning compressions.

• Assess the victim to determine if he's unconscious. Gently shake his shoulders and shout, "Are you okay?" This helps ensure that you don't start CPR on a person who's conscious. Check whether he has an injury, particularly to the head or neck. If you suspect a head or neck injury, move him as little as possible to reduce the risk of paralysis.

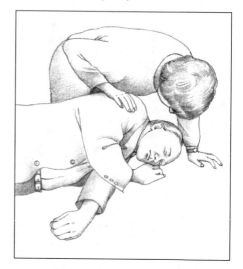

• Call out for help. Send someone to contact the EMS or call a code, if appropriate. Place the victim in a supine position on a hard, flat surface. When moving him, roll his head and torso as a unit. Avoid twisting or pulling his neck, shoulders, or hips.

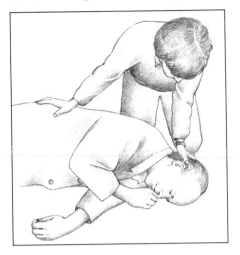

Open the airway
• Kneel near his shoulders. This position will give you easy access to his head and chest.

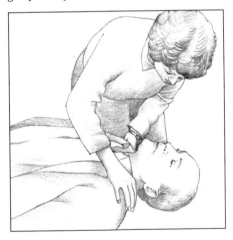

• In many cases, the muscles controlling the victim's tongue will be relaxed, causing the tongue to obstruct the airway. If the victim doesn't appear to have a neck injury, use the *head-tilt/chin-lift maneuver* to open his airway. To accomplish this, first place your hand that's closer to the victim's head on his forehead. Then apply firm pressure. The pressure

should be firm enough to tilt the victim's head back. Next place the fingertips of your other hand under the bony part of his lower jaw near the chin. Now lift the victim's chin. At the same time, keep his mouth partially open.

Avoid placing your fingertips on the soft tissue under the victim's chin because doing so may inadvertently obstruct the airway you're trying to open.

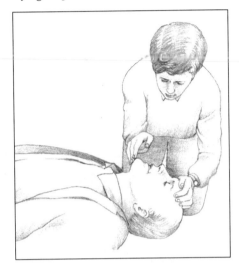

• If you suspect a neck injury, use the *jaw-thrust maneuver* instead of the *head-tilt/chin-lift maneuver*. Kneel at the victim's head with your elbows on the ground. Rest your thumbs on his lower jaw near the corners of the mouth, pointing your thumbs toward his feet. Then place your fingertips around the lower jaw. To open the airway, lift the lower jaw with your fingertips.

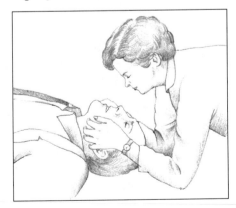

Check for breathing

• While maintaining the open airway, place your ear over the victim's mouth and nose. Now, listen for the sound of air moving, and note whether his chest rises and falls. You may also feel airflow on your cheek. If he starts to breathe, keep the airway open and continue checking his breathing until help arrives.

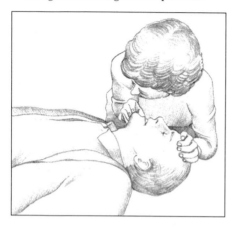

• If the victim doesn't start breathing after you open his airway, check for a foreign body obstructing the airway and follow the procedure for clearing an airway obstruction if necessary. Then begin rescue breathing. Pinch his nostrils shut with the thumb and index finger of the hand you've had on his forehead.

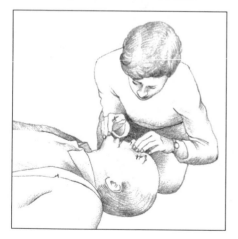

• Take a deep breath and place your mouth over the victim's mouth, creating a tight seal. Give two full ventilations, taking a deep breath after each to allow enough time for his chest to expand and relax and to prevent gastric distention. Each ventilation should last 1½ to 2 seconds.

• If the first ventilation isn't successful, reposition the victim's head and try again. If you're still not successful, he may still have a foreign body obstructing the airway. Perform five quick abdominal thrusts followed by breathing assessment in sequence until you clear the airway.

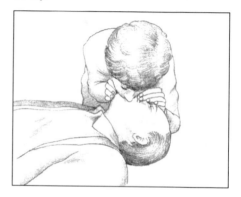

Assess circulation

• Keep one hand on the victim's forehead so his airway remains open. With your other hand, palpate the carotid artery that's closer to you. To do this, place your index and middle fingers in the groove between the trachea and the sternocleidomastoid muscle. Palpate for 5 to 10 seconds.

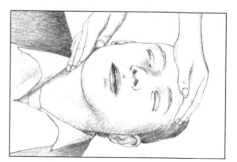

• If you detect a pulse, don't begin chest compressions. Instead, perform rescue breathing by giving the victim 12 ventilations per minute (or one every 5 seconds). After every 12 ventilations, recheck his pulse.

• If there's no pulse, start giving chest compressions. Make sure your knees are apart for a wide base of support. Using the hand closer to his feet, locate the lower margin of the rib cage next to you. Then move your fingertips along the margin to the notch where the ribs meet the sternum.

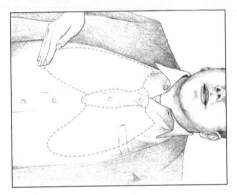

• Place your middle finger on the notch and your index finger next to your middle finger. Your index finger will now be on the bottom of the sternum.

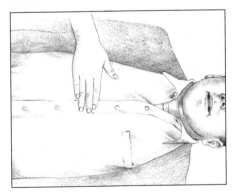

• Put the heel of your other hand on the sternum, next to the index finger. The long axis of the heel of your hand will be aligned with the long axis of the sternum.

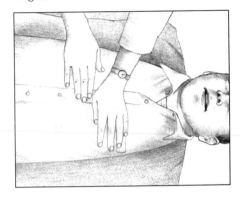

• Take the first hand off the notch and put it on top of the hand on the sternum. Make sure you have one hand directly on top of the other and your fingers aren't on his chest. This position will keep the force of the compression on the sternum and reduce the risk of a rib fracture, lung puncture, or liver laceration.

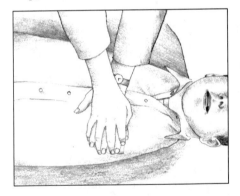

• With your elbows locked, arms straight, and your shoulders directly over your hands, you're ready to give chest compressions. Using the weight of your upper body, compress the victim's sternum 1½″ to 2″ (3.8 to 5 cm), delivering the pressure through the heels of your hands. After each compression, release the pressure and allow the chest to return to its normal position so that the heart can fill with blood. Don't change your hand position during compressions—you might injure the victim.

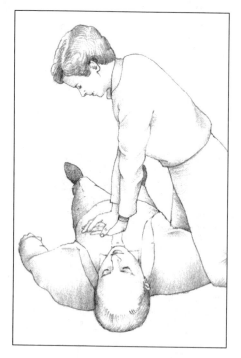

• Give 15 chest compressions at a rate of 80 to 100 per minute. Count "One and two and three and" up to 15. Open the airway and give 2 ventilations. Then find the proper hand position again and deliver 15 more compressions. Do four complete cycles of 15 compressions and 2 ventilations.

• Palpate the carotid pulse again. If there's still no pulse, continue performing CPR in cycles of 15 compressions and 2 ventilations. Every few minutes, check for breathing and a pulse at the end of a complete cycle of compressions and ventilations. If you detect a pulse but the victim isn't breathing, give 12 ventilations per minute and monitor his pulse. If he has a pulse and is breathing, monitor his respirations and pulse closely. You should stop performing CPR only when his respirations and pulse return, he's turned over to the EMS, or you're exhausted.

Two-person rescue

If another rescuer arrives while you're giving CPR, follow these steps:

• If the EMS team hasn't arrived, tell the second rescuer to repeat the call for help. If he's not a health care professional, ask him to stand by. Then, if you become fatigued, he can take over one-person CPR.

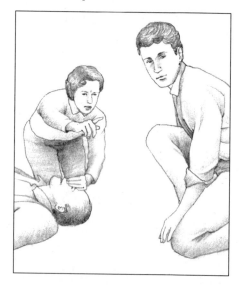

• Have him begin by checking the victim's pulse for 5 seconds after you've given two ventilations. If he doesn't feel a pulse, he should give two ventilations and begin chest compressions.

• If the rescuer is another health care professional, the two of you can perform two-person CPR. He should start assisting after you've finished a cycle of 15 compressions, two ventilations, and a pulse check.

• As shown at the top of the opposite page, the second rescuer should get into place opposite you. While you're checking for a pulse, he should be finding the proper hand placement for delivering chest compressions.

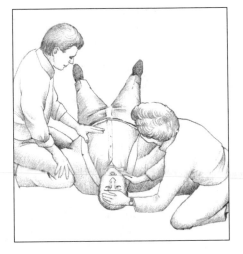

• If you don't detect a pulse, say, "No pulse, continue CPR," and give one ventilation. Then the second rescuer should begin delivering compressions at a rate of 80 to 100 per minute. Compressions and ventilations should be administered at a ratio of 5 compressions to 1 ventilation. The compressor (at this point, the second rescuer) should count out loud so the ventilator can anticipate when to give ventilations. To ensure that the ventilations are effective, the rescuer performing the chest compressions should stop briefly or at least long enough to observe the victim's chest rise with the air supplied by the rescuer giving ventilations.

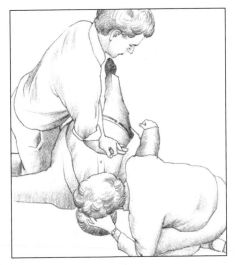

• As the ventilator, you must check for breathing and a pulse. Signal the compressor to stop giving compressions for 5 seconds so you can make these assessments.

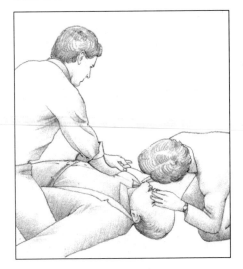

• After a minimum of 10 cycles, the compressor (second rescuer) may call for a switch. This should be done clearly to allow for a smooth transition. The compressor can substitute the word "switch" for the word "one" as he counts compressions. In other words, he'd say, "Switch and two and three and four and five." You'd then give a ventilation and become the compressor by moving down to the victim's chest and placing your hands in the proper position.

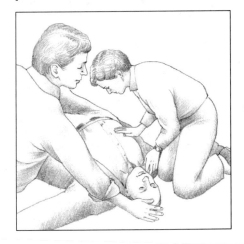

• The second rescuer would become the ventilator and move to the victim's head. He'd check the pulse for 5 seconds. If he found no pulse, he'd say, "No pulse," and give a ventilation. You'd then give compressions at a rate of 80 to 100 per minute – or five compressions for each ventilation. Both of you should continue giving CPR in this manner until the victim's respirations and pulse return, he's turned over to the EMS, or both of you are exhausted.

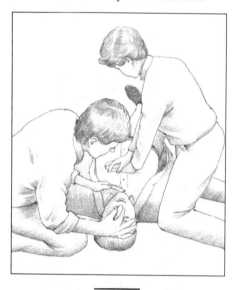

SPECIAL CONSIDERATIONS

Although acquired immunodeficiency syndrome (AIDS) isn't known to be transmitted in saliva, some health care professionals may hesitate to give rescue breaths – especially if the victim has AIDS. For this reason, the American Heart Association recommends that all health care professionals learn how to use disposable airway equipment.

A second rescuer may instinctively take the victim's pulse without waiting for the end of a cycle. This is *not* part of the American Heart Association recommendations and may confuse some rescuers. The recommendations aim to have all rescuers act in the same way so that time isn't wasted and all efforts help restore the victim's respirations and heartbeat.

COMPLICATIONS

CPR can cause certain complications – especially if the compressor doesn't place her hands properly on the sternum. These complications include fractured ribs, a lacerated liver, and punctured lungs. Gastric distention, a common complication, results from giving too much air during ventilation.

DOCUMENTATION

Whenever you perform CPR, document why you initiated it, whether the victim suffered from cardiac or respiratory arrest, when you found the victim and started CPR, and how long the victim received CPR. Note his response and any complications. Also include any interventions taken to correct complications.

If the victim also received advanced cardiac life support, document which interventions were performed, who performed them, when they were performed, and what equipment was used.

Appendix III

MANUAL VENTILATION

In this procedure, oxygen or room air is manually delivered to the lungs of a patient who can't breathe by himself. The procedure uses a hand-held resuscitation bag—an inflatable device that can be attached to a face mask or directly to an endotracheal or tracheostomy tube.

Usually performed in an emergency, manual ventilation is also used while a patient is temporarily disconnected from a mechanical ventilator—for example, during a tubing change, during transport, or before suctioning. Using the hand-held resuscitation bag maintains ventilation. Oxygen administration with a resuscitation bag improves oxygenation.

EQUIPMENT

Hand-held resuscitation bag ▪ mask ▪ oxygen source (wall unit or tank) ▪ oxygen tubing ▪ nipple adapter attached to oxygen flowmeter ▪ optional: positive end-expiratory pressure valve, oxygen accumulator, suction equipment.

IMPLEMENTATION

• Select a mask that fits snugly over the mouth and nose unless the patient is intubated or has had a tracheotomy. Attach the mask to the resuscitation bag.
• If oxygen is readily available, connect the hand-held resuscitation bag to the oxygen. Attach one end of the tubing to the bottom of the bag and the other end to the nipple adapter on the flowmeter of the oxygen source.
• Turn on the oxygen and adjust the flow rate according to the patient's condition. For example, if the patient has a low partial pressure of oxygen in arterial blood, he'll need a higher fraction of inspired oxygen (FIO_2). To increase the concentration of inspired oxygen, you can add an oxygen accumulator (also called an oxygen reservoir). This device, which attaches to an adapter on the bottom of the bag, permits an FIO_2 of up to 100%. Then, if time allows, set up the suction equipment.
• Before using the hand-held resuscitation bag, check the patient's upper airway for foreign objects. If you find any, remove them because this alone may restore spontaneous respirations in some instances. Also, foreign matter or secretions can obstruct the airway and impede resuscitation efforts. Suction the patient to remove any secretions that may obstruct the airway. If necessary, insert an oropharyngeal or nasopharyngeal airway to maintain airway patency. If the patient has a tracheostomy or endotracheal tube in place, suction the tube.
• If appropriate, remove the bed's headboard and stand at the head of the bed to help keep the patient's neck extended and to free space at the side of the bed for other activities, such as cardiac compressions.
• Tilt the patient's head backward, if not contraindicated, and pull his jaw forward to move the tongue away from the base of the pharynx and prevent potential airway obstruction. (See *Applying a hand-held resuscitation bag and mask,* page 302.)
• Keeping your nondominant hand on the patient's mask, exert downward pressure to seal the mask against his face. Use your dominant hand to compress the bag every 5 seconds to deliver about 1 liter of air.
• Deliver breaths with the patient's own inspiratory effort, if present. Don't attempt to deliver a breath as the patient exhales.
• Observe the patient's chest to ensure that it rises and falls with each compression. If ventilation fails to occur, check the fit of the mask and the patency of the patient's airway. If necessary, reposition the patient's head and ensure patency with an oral airway.

Applying a hand-held resuscitation bag and mask

Place the mask over the patient's face so that the apex of the triangle covers the bridge of his nose and the base lies between his lower lip and chin.

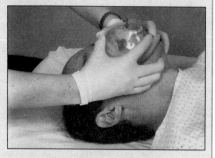

Make sure that the patient's mouth remains open underneath the mask. Attach the bag to the mask and to the tubing leading to the oxygen source.

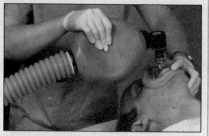

Or, if the patient has a tracheostomy or endotracheal tube in place, remove the mask from the bag and attach the hand-held resuscitation bag directly to the tube.

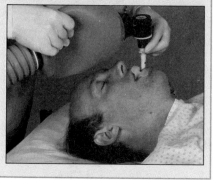

SPECIAL CONSIDERATIONS

Avoid neck hyperextension if the patient might have a cervical injury; instead, use the jaw-thrust technique to open the airway. If you need both hands to keep the patient's mask in place and maintain hyperextension, have another person compress the bag or, if necessary, use the lower part of your arm to compress the bag against your side.

Observe for vomiting through the clear part of the mask. If vomiting occurs, stop the procedure immediately, lift the mask, wipe and suction the vomitus, and resume resuscitation.

Underventilation commonly occurs because the hand-held resuscitation bag is difficult to keep positioned tightly on the patient's face while ensuring an open airway. What's more, the volume of air delivered to the patient varies with the type of bag used and the hand size of the person compressing the bag. An adult with a small or medium-sized hand may not consistently deliver 1 liter of air. For these reasons, have someone assist with the procedure, if possible.

COMPLICATIONS

Gastric distention may result from air forced into the patient's stomach; this distention can cause vomiting, aspiration, and pneumonia.

DOCUMENTATION

Document the use of manual ventilation. Be sure to note how long it was given, if room air or oxygen therapy was used (including liters/minute of oxygen and FIO_2), complications (if any), and the outcome.

Selected references

American Joint Committee on Cancer. *Manual for Staging of Cancer,* 4th ed. Philadelphia: J.B. Lippincott Co., 1992.

Braunwald, E. *Heart Disease: A Textbook of Cardiovascular Medicine,* 4th ed. Philadelphia: W.B. Saunders Co., 1992.

Clinical Laboratory Tests: Values and Implications. Springhouse, Pa.: Springhouse Corp., 1991.

Cohen, S.M., et al. *Maternal, Neonatal, and Women's Health Nursing.* Springhouse, Pa.: Springhouse Corp., 1991.

Farzan, S., et al. *A Concise Handbook of Respiratory Diseases,* 3rd ed. East Norwalk, Conn.: Appleton & Lange, 1992.

Gulanick, M., et al. *Nursing Care Plans: Diagnosis and Interventions,* 2nd ed. St. Louis: Mosby–Year Book, Inc., 1990.

Horne, M., and Swearingen, P.L. *Pocket Guide to Fluids, Electrolytes, and Acid-Base Balance,* 2nd ed. St. Louis: Mosby–Year Book, Inc., 1992.

Ignatavicius, D., and Bayne, M.V. *Medical-Surgical Nursing: A Nursing Process Approach.* Philadelphia: W.B. Saunders Co., 1991.

Illustrated Guide to Diagnostic Tests. Springhouse, Pa.: Springhouse Corp., 1994.

Illustrated Manual of Nursing Practice, 2nd ed. Springhouse, Pa.: Springhouse Corp., 1994.

Long, B.C., et al. *Medical-Surgical Nursing: A Nursing Process Approach,* 3rd ed. St. Louis: Mosby–Year Book, Inc., 1992.

Luckmann, J., and Sorensen, K. *Medical-Surgical Nursing: A Psychophysiologic Approach,* 4th ed. Philadelphia: W.B. Saunders Co., 1993.

Mandell, G.L., et al. *Principles and Practices of Infectious Diseases,* 3rd ed. New York: Churchill Livingstone, 1990.

Nurse's PhotoLibrary. Springhouse, Pa.: Springhouse Corp., 1994.

Patrick, M.L., et al. *Medical-Surgical Nursing: Pathophysiological Concepts,* 2nd ed. Philadelphia: J.B. Lippincott Co., 1991.

Phipps, W.J., et al. *Medical-Surgical Nursing: Concepts and Clinical Practice,* 4th ed. St. Louis: Mosby–Year Book, Inc., 1991.

Rakel, R.E., ed. *Conn's Current Therapy 1993.* Philadelphia: W.B. Saunders Co., 1993.

Sexton, D.L. *Nursing Care of the Respiratory Patient.* East Norwalk, Conn.: Appleton & Lange, 1990.

Smeltzer, S.C., and Bare, B.G. *Brunner and Suddarth's Textbook of Medical-Surgical Nursing,* 7th ed. Philadelphia: J.B. Lippincott Co., 1992.

Sparks, S.M., and Taylor, C.M. *Nursing Diagnosis Reference Manual,* 2nd ed. Springhouse, Pa.: Springhouse Corp., 1993.

Swearingen, P. *Manual of Nursing Therapeutics: Applying Nursing Diagnoses to Medical Disorders,* 2nd ed. St. Louis: Mosby–Year Book, Inc., 1990.

Ulrich, B.T., ed. *Nephrology Nursing: Concepts and Strategies.* East Norwalk, Conn.: Appleton & Lange, 1989.

Whaley, L.F., and Wong, D.L. *Nursing Care of Infants and Children,* 4th ed. St. Louis: Mosby–Year Book, Inc., 1991.

Wilson, J.D., et al., eds. *Harrison's Principles of Internal Medicine,* 12th ed. New York: McGraw-Hill Book Co., 1992.

Index

i refers to an illustration; t, to a table

i refers to an illustration; t, to a table

i refers to an illustration; t, to a table